Human Flourishing in
an Age of Gene Editing

T0177736

Human Flourishing in an Age of Gene Editing

Edited by
ERIK PARENS
JOSEPHINE JOHNSTON

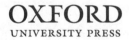

OXFORD
UNIVERSITY PRESS

OXFORD
UNIVERSITY PRESS

Oxford University Press is a department of the University of Oxford. It furthers
the University's objective of excellence in research, scholarship, and education
by publishing worldwide. Oxford is a registered trade mark of Oxford University
Press in the UK and certain other countries.

Published in the United States of America by Oxford University Press
198 Madison Avenue, New York, NY 10016, United States of America.

CIP data is on file at the Library of Congress
ISBN 978-0-19-094036-2

This material is not intended to be, and should not be considered, a substitute for medical or other
professional advice. Treatment for the conditions described in this material is highly dependent on the
individual circumstances. And, while this material is designed to offer accurate information with respect
to the subject matter covered and to be current as of the time it was written, research and knowledge about
medical and health issues is constantly evolving and dose schedules for medications are being revised
continually, with new side effects recognized and accounted for regularly. Readers must therefore always
check the product information and clinical procedures with the most up-to-date published product
information and data sheets provided by the manufacturers and the most recent codes of conduct and
safety regulation. The publisher and the authors make no representations or warranties to readers, express
or implied, as to the accuracy or completeness of this material. Without limiting the foregoing, the
publisher and the authors make no representations or warranties as to the accuracy or efficacy of the drug
dosages mentioned in the material. The authors and the publisher do not accept, and expressly disclaim,
any responsibility for any liability, loss or risk that may be claimed or incurred as a consequence of the use
and/or application of any of the contents of this material.

3 5 7 9 8 6 4

Printed by Marquis, Canada

Contents

Acknowledgments

This volume is one outcome of The Hastings Center's project "Gene Editing and Human Flourishing," led by Erik Parens, Josephine Johnston, and Mildred Z. Solomon. That project was made possible through the support of a grant from the John Templeton Foundation. The opinions expressed in this publication are those of the editors and authors and do not necessarily reflect the views of the John Templeton Foundation. Kevin Arnold, Senior Program Officer for Life Sciences & Genetics, supported and guided the project. Invaluable editorial and research assistance was provided by Elizabeth Dietz and Ben C. Wills. Lucy Randall and Hannah Doyle at Oxford University Press welcomed and expertly shepherded this volume and two anonymous reviewers offered edits that strengthened its contents. The editors thank the volume's authors for their insightful chapters and their engagement with both the issues and each other's work.

Contributors

Gaymon Bennett, Arizona State University, Associate Professor of Religion, Science, and Technology, is the author of *Technicians of Human Dignity: Bodies, Souls and the Making of Intrinsic Worth* (Fordham University Press, 2015) and coauthor of *Designing Human Practices: An Experiment with Synthetic Biology* (University of Chicago Press, 2012).

Michael Burdett, University of Nottingham, Assistant Professor in Christian Theology, is the author of *Beyond Genetic Engineering: Technology and the Rise of Transhumanism* (Grove Books, 2014) and *Eschatology and the Technological Future* (Routledge, 2015).

Celia Deane-Drummond, University of Notre Dame, Professor of Theology and Director of the Center for Theology, Science, and Human Flourishing, is trained as both a scientist and a theologian. She is the author, most recently, of *The Wisdom of the Liminal: Evolution and Other Animals in Human Becoming* (Eerdmans, 2014) and editor, with Rebecca Artinian Kaiser, of *Theology and Ecology across the Disciplines: On Care for Our Common Home* (Bloomsbury, 2018).

John H. Evans, University of California, San Diego, Tata Chancellor's Chair in Social Sciences, Associate Dean of Social Sciences, and Codirector of UCSD's Institute for Practical Ethics. His most recent book is *Morals Not Knowledge: Recasting the Contemporary US Conflict between Religion and Science* (University of California Press, 2018).

Rosemarie Garland-Thomson, Emory University, a bioethicist and Professor of English, is a disability justice and culture thought leader and humanities scholar. She is the author of several books, including *Staring: How We Look* (Oxford University Press, 2009), and co-editor of *About Us: Essays from the* New York Times *about Disability by People with Disabilities* (Liveright, 2019).

Michael Hauskeller, University of Liverpool, Professor of Philosophy, writes about transhumanism and the philosophy of human enhancement and, more recently, on death and meaning. His most recent book is *Mythologies of Transhumanism* (Palgrave Macmillan, 2016).

Daniel M. Haybron, Saint Louis University, Theodore R. Vitali C. P. Professor of Philosophy, is interested in the connection between human nature and the good life. He is the author of *The Pursuit of Unhappiness: The Elusive Psychology of Well-Being* (Oxford University Press, 2008) and *Happiness: A Very Short Introduction* (Oxford University Press, 2013).

Sheena Iyengar, Columbia University, S. T. Lee Professor of Business, is author of *The Art of Choosing* (Twelve, 2010). Her research challenges the basic assumption that choice is always preferred and unilaterally beneficial.

Emma A. Jane, University of New South Wales, Senior Lecturer in the School of the Arts and Media, researches the social and ethical implications of emerging technologies. Her most recent book is *Misogyny Online: A Short (and Brutish) History* (Sage, 2017).

Bruce Jennings, Vanderbilt University School of Medicine, Adjunct Associate Professor, Department of Health Policy and Center for Biomedical Ethics and Society, is also Senior Fellow at the Center for Humans and Nature and Senior Advisor and Fellow at The Hastings Center. His most recent book is *Ecological Governance: Toward a New Social Contract with the Earth* (West Virginia University Press, 2016).

Josephine Johnston, The Hastings Center, Research Scholar and Director of Research, works on the ethical, legal, and social implications of emerging technologies, with a focus on genetics and human reproduction.

Gregory E. Kaebnick, The Hastings Center, Research Scholar and the Editor-in-Chief of *Hastings Center Report*, is the author of *Humans in Nature: The World as We Find It and the World as We Create It* (Oxford University Press, 2013).

Richard Kim, Loyola University Chicago, Assistant Professor of Philosophy, works on ethics, moral psychology, and East Asian philosophy with a view to deepening our understanding of the nature of well-being and relevant concepts, including emotion, virtue, and friendship.

Tucker Kuman, University of Virginia, is pursuing his PhD in English. He received his BA from Columbia University in 2013 and subsequently worked as a research associate in the lab of Dr. Iyengar at Columbia Business School.

Erik Parens, The Hastings Center, Senior Research Scholar and Director of the Initiative in Bioethics and the Humanities, is the author of *Shaping Our Selves: On Technology, Flourishing, and a Habit of Thinking* (Oxford University Press, 2015).

Dorothy Roberts, University of Pennsylvania, George A. Weiss University Professor of Law and Sociology and Raymond Pace and Sadie Tanner Mossell Alexander Professor of Civil Rights, is founding director of the Penn Program on Race, Science and Society in the Center for Africana Studies. Her most recent book is *Fatal Invention: How Science, Politics, and Big Business Re-create Race in the Twenty-first Century* (New Press, 2011).

Maartje Schermer, Erasmus MC Rotterdam, Professor of the Philosophy of Medicine, has degrees in medicine and philosophy. She has published widely on philosophical, ethical, and social implications of new technologies, especially human enhancement, neurotechnologies, early diagnosis and screening, concepts of health and disease, and patient autonomy and informed decision-making. She is chair of the standing committee on ethics and law of the Dutch Health Council.

Jackie Leach Scully, Newcastle University, Professor of Social Ethics and Bioethics and Executive Director of the Policy, Ethics, and Life Sciences (PEALS) Research Center, is the author of *Disability Bioethics: Moral Bodies, Moral Difference* (Rowman & Littlefield, 2008).

Robert Sparrow, Monash University, Professor in the Department of Philosophy, works on bioethics, political philosophy, and applied ethics.

Nicole A Vincent, University of Technology Sydney, Senior Lecturer in the Faculty of Transdisciplinary Innovation, and Honorary Fellow in the Department of Philosophy at Macquarie University, conducts research on a range of social, legal, and ethical issues raised by emerging technologies like smart drugs, blockchain, and autonomous vehicles, with a special focus on the notion of responsibility and futures.

Human Flourishing in an Age of Gene Editing

Introduction to *Human Flourishing in an Age of Gene Editing*

Erik Parens and Josephine Johnston

In 2015, in the journal *Science*, a highly regarded group of scientists, science policy experts, and ethicists called for a public conversation about the ethical questions raised by a new technology that could be used to alter the genomes of human beings.[1] Among these ethical questions were ones regarding safety. Most simply, could the new technology be deployed without posing an unreasonable risk of causing physical harms? The authors of the commentary in *Science* also alluded to broader ethical questions that have been raised ever since the 1970s, when it first seemed it would be possible to use gene transfer technologies to alter human genomes.[2] These broader questions have nothing to do with medically detectable harms to people's bodies: Might such technologies push us toward thinking of human beings in increasingly mechanistic terms? Might they push us toward ever-narrower conceptions of acceptable ways to be human? Might they undermine healthy relationships between parents and children? Might they exacerbate the obscene gap between the haves and have-nots? These harms are "nonphysical" in the sense that they wouldn't immediately diminish the functioning of any bodily system. Rather, if they occurred, they would be harms to what we can call people's psyches. They would do harm to people's experience of being persons. They would threaten relationships and strain communities. The broadest form of the question concerning nonphysical harms is: might this technology be used in ways that would inadvertently thwart human flourishing? That is the question motivating this book.

But saying what we mean when we say we're worried about nonphysical harms in general and about flourishing in particular is much harder than saying what we mean when we say we're worried about physical harms. And it is that harder task we have set for ourselves in this volume. We aim for this collection to serve as a resource for people, including those who are not familiar with the formal study of bioethics, to engage in the sort of public conversation called for by the authors of the commentary in *Science*. It is through this public conversation that citizens can influence laws and the distribution of funding for science and medicine; that professional leaders can shape understanding and use of gene editing and related technologies by scientists, patients, and practitioners; and that individuals can make decisions about their own lives and the lives of their families.

What We Mean by *An Age of Gene Editing*

The specific technology that precipitated the *Science* commentary is called CRISPR-Cas9, and in 2012 it was unveiled as the first in a series of so-called gene editing technologies.[3] These gene editing technologies marked a huge leap forward in researchers' ability to engage in what, since at least the 1970s, has been called "genetic engineering." Whereas the older technologies only allowed researchers to transfer copies of whole genes to targeted genomes, the newer gene editing technologies allow them to make changes to as large or as small a part of a gene as they desire. The newer gene editing technologies also enable researchers to make such changes far more easily, cheaply, and reliably than was possible with the old-fashioned "gene transfer" technology.

The technical details regarding CRISPR-Cas9 and related gene editing technologies are complicated, but the basic idea is simple. These technologies can be programmed to target and then cut one or more specific stretches of DNA. The targeted gene can be shut off (deleted) or new DNA can be pasted in. Although CRISPR gene editing technologies are far more accurate than previously available tools, they can accidently cause unintended or "off-target" changes or fail to make all hoped-for changes, resulting in a mixture of edited and unedited cells within an organism (otherwise known as mosaicism). For an excellent written introduction to the technical details, you might consult Chapter 3 of the 2017 National Academy of Science report on gene editing.[4] Numerous video introductions to the scientific details of CRISPR technologies can be found on the Internet.[5]

The ethical conversation about gene-altering technologies, whether of the old-fashioned gene transfer variety or the newer gene editing variety, has traditionally employed some basic distinctions. One of those regards the difference between efforts to alter genomes in somatic cells and efforts to alter genomes in germ cells. If the DNA in germ cells (including sperm, eggs, and early embryos) is altered, those alterations appear not only in the DNA of the people who are created from those cells, but also in those people's children. In contrast, if the DNA in somatic cells (all the cells in the body that aren't germ cells) is altered, those alterations are not passed on to future generations.

Another of those basic distinctions seeks to draw a line between treatment and enhancement uses of gene editing technologies. In the case of treatment, a disease-causing bit of the genome is deleted or silenced, with possibly a healthy bit pasted in. In contrast, we can imagine efforts to use the same technology to enhance some human trait, where a healthy bit of the genome is cut out and a "better-than-healthy" bit pasted in. In principle, gene editing could be used to alter the somatic cells of living persons to enhance their traits, and it could also be used to alter germ cells to enhance the traits of future persons. Efforts of the latter sort are referred to as germline genetic enhancement and, if attempted, would be the most ethically controversial application of gene editing technology.

Those observers, however, who think it would be an ethical mistake to attempt germline genetic enhancement can find some comfort in knowing that, for the foreseeable future, it will likely be very difficult to achieve such interventions with respect to the traits that human beings in our society seem to care about most. The more we know about the staggeringly complex ways in which genes interact with each other and the environment to produce the sorts of enhancements that people might want most for themselves or their children—say, more intelligence, more musical ability, or more resilience—the less likely it seems that it will be possible to produce such traits by editing genes. That is, in practice, CRISPR technologies may not provide the level of control over the shape of our children and ourselves that critics dread and enthusiasts desire.

But this volume is not about any one technology, and it does not assume that it will be technically feasible to achieve the fabulous level of control that would be required to produce children who were more intelligent, musical, or resilient. Rather, it is about a large set of technologies that coexist with gene editing and are sometimes called "reprogenetic," and it is about the increased level of control over the genetic makeup of our children that these technologies are already beginning to provide. The phrase *in an age of gene editing* in our title is meant to indicate that, while gene editing may be an emblematic technology for the time we live in, it is but one of many related technologies, all of which raise the same set of ethical issues.

Among the other technologies pertinent to our reflections here are preimplantation genetic diagnosis and prenatal genetic testing. Preimplantation genetic diagnosis allows a person who wants to become pregnant to choose which of several embryos with different genomic profiles she wants to have transferred to her uterus. Prenatal genetic testing enables people who are already pregnant to choose whether to bring a fetus with a given genomic profile to term. Neither preimplantation genetic diagnosis nor prenatal genetic testing provides the level of control over the genetic makeup of the child-to-be that is dreamt of by some would-be gene editors, but all of these techniques share the aspiration to increase control over the shape of future generations. It is that aspiration to control, and what it means for the prospects of human flourishing, that we reflect on in this volume.

What We Mean by *Flourishing*

When we use the English word *flourishing* in the title of this volume, we are thinking of it as a translation of the ancient Greek word *eudaimonia*, which Aristotle used to name what he said all human beings want.[6] Other common translations of eudaimonia are "well-being" and "happiness." According to Aristotle, human beings don't want to flourish because they think that flourishing will get them something else like, say, power or money. Flourishing (or happiness or well-being) is what humans want for the sake of itself. It isn't a means for achieving some other end that humans desire; it is the desired end that they desire. People want to flourish because they want to flourish.

So, what more can we say about the meaning of flourishing that is a bit less abstract? It can help to start by distinguishing flourishing from health. Everyone wants to be healthy. But people don't want health for the sake of itself. They want to be healthy so that they can engage in activities that they find meaningful. They want to be at work in, engaged with, the world. For many human beings, those meaningful activities include engaging in various forms of loving relationships and in various forms of work.

As we try to get a bead on what we mean by flourishing or well-being or happiness, it's important to notice that we are not talking about a psychological state, say of the sort people would expect to enjoy if they won the lottery or got a job promotion or received a rave review. We're talking about an experience of being engaged in activities in the world that people find meaningful, which can actually entail temporarily painful psychological states. Being in loving relationships entails negotiating inevitable and sometimes-painful conflicts and, too often, entails the excruciating pain of losing to death the people we love. To be engaged in meaningful work can require sacrificing time that might be spent in other activities that would entail temporarily pleasurable psychological states. Yet both are paradigmatic instances of flourishing.

Flourishing is the experience of being fully alive, exercising whatever particular set of capacities we were thrown into the world with. And, as several contributors to this volume will remind you, flourishing depends less on the particular capacities that one has than on one's opportunities for exercising them. A corollary of that view is that using genetic technologies in attempts to shape our children's capacities is less urgent than the even more difficult (if less costly) business of creating environments in which people can exercise whatever capacities they have. The idea that achieving more control over the nature of children might not always promote their flourishing or that of their parents might sound strange at first, but that is one of the central claims we are exploring in this volume.

Acceptance Can Conduce to Flourishing

In the first section of our book, three authors open up the discussion from very different levels and perspectives, previewing themes and questions taken up in subsequent chapters. English Professor and bioethicist Rosemarie Garland-Thomson, writing from her and others' experience of disability, argues that for a greater openness to the fact that people with all sorts of bodies can flourish magnificently. She argues that to promote flourishing, instead of changing bodies or genes, individuals and societies should invest in changing environments in ways that make them more welcoming of different kinds of bodies. Philosopher Daniel Haybron introduces a very brief history of the idea of flourishing in the West before exploring the significance for human well-being of authenticity, a value that is arguably at stake when considering altering genomes to enhance human capacities. Sociologist John Evans offers a history of the way in which some prominent thinkers about public policy have, lamentably, discounted concerns about human flourishing.

In the next section of the book, three contributors pick up an argument introduced by Garland-Thompson: that one way to promote human flourishing is to honor the stance of, or attitude of, what might be called acceptance. We say "might be called acceptance" for at least two reasons. First, the word *acceptance* can have a connotation of passivity, which is not what our authors intend; accepting what is requires attention and energy. Second, acceptance might not perfectly capture the resonance of being grateful for or affirming what is, which some, if not all, of our authors do intend. Those caveats aside, acceptance is not a bad term to name the attitude or stance toward our children and ourselves that the authors in this volume are converging on. We should add that while they are converging on a defense of the attitude or stance of acceptance, they are surely not absolutist in that defense. They are doing no more or less than offering what they take to be a critique of the status quo—where the status quo assumes that more control, or more shaping, is better.[7] They are making the claim that if human beings could became less preoccupied with transforming the bodies of themselves and their children, they might flourish more.

Philosopher Michael Hauskeller makes an argument that expands the notion of acceptance to the notion of cherishing. If people can learn to cherish children and the world as they are (as opposed to how people might think they should be) everyone would flourish more. Whereas Hauskeller draws on the insights of Western philosophy, Richard Kim draws on the insights of Eastern philosophy to make the case for learning to let things be. And philosopher Gregory Kaebnick explains that, while the case for accepting nature as we find it is under constant challenge today, that case can be made with intellectual integrity, and it warrants respect.

Choice and Control Can Be Overrated

To endorse the value of acceptance is of course to run up against one of Western culture's fundamental articles of belief: that more choice is good. From three different angles, our contributors challenge that belief. Psychologist Sheena Iyengar and her collaborator Tucker Kuman, a former member of her Columbia research lab, write on the large empirical psychological literature regarding choice, arguing that it simply is not true that more choice leads to more flourishing. They offer the figure of the inverted U-shaped curve to describe the relationship between choice and sense of well-being: sense of well-being does increase with more choice, but only up to a point, where more choice is associated with a decreased sense of well-being. Bioethicist and lawyer (and co-editor of this volume) Josephine Johnston explores the possibility that good parents will, with a view to promoting their own flourishing, sometimes choose against availing themselves of the panoply of technological options on offer. Along very similar lines, philosophers Nicole A Vincent and Emma A. Jane argue that choosing to use reprogenetic technologies to shape one's children should be an option, but in no way a requirement, for people who aspire to be good parents.

Seeking Balance between Competing Values

If we lived in a culture where there was too much emphasis on the ethical value of acceptance, this volume would have emphasized the need to remember the ethical value of shaping. But the contributors to this volume agree that in this cultural moment there is a bias toward the goodness of intervention and the value of controlling the shape of oneself and one's progeny. And for that reason they are making the case for the goodness of eschewing intervention and for accepting our children and ourselves as we've been thrown into the world.

It is essential to notice, however, that no one in this volume is arguing that acceptance is an absolute or ultimate value. Indeed, their point isn't that there is a single ethical value to be embraced, but a balance to be achieved between important ethical values that push in different directions. They are arguing for a better balance between control and acceptance—a point one of us (Erik Parens) has sought to elaborate previously.[8]

Four of our contributors, from very different angles, make the case for balance. Sociologist Jackie Leach Scully, drawing on interviews with laypeople in the United Kingdom, suggests that they, often much better than many professional bioethicists, recognize the profound importance of balancing commitments to control and acceptance when thinking about reprogenetic technologies. Philosopher Rob Sparrow is deeply impressed by the argument from the disability rights community that accepting the fact of genetic diversity is important, and he also cautions against taking that argument too far: not all genomic diversity deserves to be conserved. Michael Burdett, who does research in religion, science, and technology, explains that mainline Christianity holds the ethical commitments to acceptance and to shaping in a fruitful tension. Burdett invites readers to see that they needn't choose between, but ought rather balance, those commitments. (One of us [Parens] would argue that Judaism also seeks such a balance and would guess that any religious or cultural tradition that endures has to honor both commitments.) Theologian Celia Deane-Drummond offers an extended explication of the virtue of practical wisdom as a tool for finding the sort of balance that is required to deploy a technology like gene editing.

Seeing the Bigger Picture

The contributors to this volume acknowledge that gene editing, in working at the level of DNA, can do much good to advance human health. But they also want to say that, to promote human flourishing, human beings need to get much better at working at the level of the social. To promote more flourishing, societies need to get exceedingly better at building environments that support people with whatever genome they happen to have. And, our contributors are suggesting, building such environments will sometimes have to be accompanied by the articulation of some limits on the uses to which technologies like gene editing are put.

In her essay, lawyer, bioethicist, and race studies scholar Dorothy Roberts argues that a real commitment to the flourishing of the most disadvantaged members in society wouldn't look first to genomics, but to building social environments that are more supportive of more people. Philosopher Maartje Schermer explains how the Dutch, in balancing the value of self-determination (held so dear in the United States) and the value of solidarity (held far less dearly), accept limits on some reprogenetic services that are made available. That is, the Dutch make peace with the fact that if to make basic reprogenetic testing available to everyone, they are not going to make nonbasic forms of testing available to anyone, regardless of ability to pay. Anthropologist and scholar of science studies Gaymon Bennett describes the development of the idea of human dignity and argues for deploying a rich conception of it to recognize and redress the powerful forces promoting the uses of technologies like gene editing. Finally, political theorist and bioethicist Bruce Jennings argues that to create just and sustainable environments that can support human flourishing requires a better understanding of the philosophical underpinnings of the view that gives technologies like gene editing such a prominent place in society. He argues that doing so can help people cultivate the values of humility and restraint, which can seem to be in short supply in our age of gene editing.

Public Oversight and Public Conversation

The contributors to this volume all think that public conversation about flourishing is deeply important for making good public policy. And we are aware that citizens of democracies can resist engaging in such conversation for good reasons and for bad ones. A good reason is the desire to honor individual liberty. Public conversation about what human flourishing consists in for human beings in general can lead to constraining the liberty of individuals who have minority conceptions of what that concept means. A bad reason is the notion that conceptions of human flourishing are too "speculative"[9] or "nebulous"[10] to inform public policy.

In fact, the question isn't whether conceptions of human flourishing can inform public policy. They frequently do. Though hardly the only, one of the reasons that policymakers make the policies they do is to promote the flourishing of their constituents as they understand it. So, the real question is whether policymakers—and others—are willing to be explicit about what their conception is or would prefer to leave it implicit. Plainly, the contributors to this volume want more explicit talk.

But how might more explicit public conversation about human flourishing and nonphysical harms inform public policy? Is there, for example, a way to directly plug such concerns into a public oversight mechanism responsible for a new technology like gene editing? To briefly respond to that question, it helps to consider some historical context.

The summit in Napa, California, out of which came the 2015 commentary in *Science* mentioned in the beginning of this introduction, was a sort of sequel to a summit that occurred in Pacific Grove, California, in 1975. The 1975 summit, referred to as "the Asilomar conference" (because it was held at the Asilomar conference center in Pacific Grove), occurred in the wake of the discovery that recombinant DNA could, at least in principle, be used to "engineer" somatic and germ cells.

Five years after the Asilomar conference, three religious leaders wrote a letter to then-President Jimmy Carter.[11] Albeit in traditionally religious language about the dangers of "playing God," those leaders were worried about what we here are calling nonphysical harms in particular and human flourishing concerns more generally. More to the point, those leaders suggested that, to manage potential harms, this new genetic technology needed "oversight."

Two years later, in 1982, a presidential bioethics commission (which was created during President Carter's tenure) responded to the letter from the religious leaders with the first national report on genetic engineering, *Splicing Life*. The authors of *Splicing Life* rejected the idea that it was possible to integrate concerns about what we are calling nonphysical harms into oversight mechanisms. In fact, the tone of that 1982 report was rather dismissive of such concerns.

Whereas the Asilomar conference was followed by the presidential bioethics commission's 1982 report on genetic engineering, the Napa summit was followed by an international summit, as well as a 2017 report on genome editing from the National Academy of Sciences (NAS).[12] When the authors of the NAS report on human genome editing looked back and described *Splicing Life*, they observed that their predecessors had taken the concerns of the three religious leaders and had "*reformulated* the ethical debate so that [their report] would be 'meaningful to public policy consideration'" (italics added).[13] This "reformulation" of the ethical debate meant essentially removing from the public policy table any questions concerning what we're calling nonphysical harms—and what the NAS authors called "cultural harms." The NAS authors wrote:

> To make ethical claims legally actionable meant [that the authors of *Splicing Life* moved] away from arguments about future cultural harms or claims that it is not the role of humanity to modify itself. Consequences needed to be *more concrete and near-term, not speculative.* (italics added)[14]

Yet the NAS authors distanced themselves from this view. Instead, they concluded that the prospect of germline genetic enhancement raises "broader and longer-term social effects"[15] that warrant careful consideration. In contrast to their predecessors, the NAS authors didn't require that concerns be "concrete and near-term." They didn't dismiss such concerns as merely "speculative," and they didn't insinuate that the only people who might hold them are Luddites or religious kooks or people with what some more recent commentators have begun to suggest are hyperactive amygdalae. Instead, they called for sustained public reflection on these concerns.

The NAS report did not, however, begin to say how an "oversight mechanism" might actually integrate concerns about nonphysical harms into the creation of public policy. Instead, the NAS report called for public conversation, which might sound, at best, like a punt. This call for public conversation—or public engagement—echoes similar calls in other recent national and international reports, including the statement from the organizing committee of the first and second international gene editing summits. Because detail is seldom given about how to hold such conversation or how to feed it into policy, calling for public conversation can begin to sound more like a mantra than policy-relevant advice. But it also might be the most reasonable thing that a NAS committee can say. It may be that systems as complex as modern societies just don't admit of the sorts of "mechanistic" interventions into public policy imagined by the three religious leaders who wrote to President Carter back in 1980. After all, even the authors of the 2003 report on enhancement by the US President's Council on Bioethics, who took concerns about nonphysical harms with the utmost seriousness, declined to suggest how such concerns might be integrated into oversight mechanisms. In the end, their primary policy recommendation was that the public move forward "with its eyes wide open."[16]

The contributors to this volume are making the case for opening one's eyes wide to the simple fact that, to promote human flourishing, one ought not first look to increase control over the DNA of children by means of reprogenetic technologies like gene editing. This is not to deny the value of using a technology like gene editing to cure disease. Nor is it to deny the value in some cases of the ability to alter the DNA of children. It is to affirm the value of acceptance and to suggest that if a society really cares about human flourishing, it will first create environments that welcome people with all sorts of genomes. Creating such environments requires social policies that invest in public goods like housing and public health and education. Alas, those efforts won't usually require technologies that are as sexy or potentially profitable as gene editing, but they might deliver more flourishing bang-for-buck.

To create such policies, communities and societies need to talk together about what human flourishing consists in, which policies and practices and technologies can promote human flourishing and which can jeopardize it. Creating such policies should involve remembering what health is for, as well as what enhancement might—and might not—help individuals and societies achieve. Along with the contributors to this volume, we hope that this book will serve as a useful resource for all those who want to engage in that conversation.

Notes

1. David Baltimore, Paul Berg, Michael Botchan, Dana Carroll, R. Alta Charo, George Church, Jacob E. Corn, et al., "A Prudent Path Forward for Genomic Engineering and Germline Gene Modification," *Science* 348, no. 6230 (2015): 36–38.
2. Michael Hamilton, ed., *The New Genetics and the Future of Man* (Grand Rapids, MI: Eerdmans, 1972).
3. Martin Jinek, Krzysztof Chylinski, Ines Fonfara, Michael Hauer, Jennifer A. Doudna, and Emmanuelle Charpentier. "A Programmable Dual-RNA–Guided DNA Endonuclease in Adaptive Bacterial Immunity," *Science* 337, no. 6096

(2012): 816–821; Le Cong, F. Ann Ran, David Cox, Shuailiang Lin, Robert Barretto, Naomi Habib, Patrick D. Hsu, et al. "Multiplex Genome Engineering Using CRISPR/Cas Systems," *Science* 339, no. 6121 (2013): 819–823; Prashant Mali, Luhan Yang, Kevin M. Esvelt, John Aach, Marc Guell, James E. DiCarlo, Julie E. Norville, and George M. Church. "RNA-Guided Human Genome Engineering via Cas9," *Science* 339, no. 6121 (2013): 823–826.

4. National Academies of Sciences, Engineering, and Medicine. *Human Genome Editing: Science, Ethics, and Governance*. (Washington, DC: The National Academies Press, 2017). https://doi.org/10.17226/24623, see especially Chapter 3.

5. For example, consult https://www.youtube.com/watch?v=2pp17E4E-O8 or https://www.ted.com/talks/jennifer_doudna_we_can_now_edit_our_dna_but_let_s_do_it_wisely#t-61154.

6. Aristotle, *Nicomachean Ethics*, trans. H. Rackham (Cambridge, MA: Harvard University Press, 1926).

7. Cf. Nick Bostrom and Toby Ord, "The Reversal Test: Eliminating Status Quo Bias in Applied Ethics," *Ethics* Vol. 116, No. 4 (July 2006): 656–679.

8. Erik Parens, *Shaping Our Selves: On Technology, Flourishing, and a Habit of Thinking* (Oxford: Oxford University Press, 2014).

9. President's Commission for the Study of Ethical Problems in Medicine and Biomedical and Behavioral Research, *Splicing Life: A Report on the Social and Ethical Issues of Genetic Engineering with Human Beings* (Washington, DC: President's Commission, 1982).

10. Steven Pinker, "The Moral Imperative for Bioethics" *The Boston Globe*, August 1, 2015. https://www.bostonglobe.com/opinion/2015/07/31/the-moral-imperative-for-bioethics/JmEkoyzlTAu9oQV76JrK9N/story.html.

11. Claire Randall, Bernard Mandelbaum, and Thomas Kelly, "Letter from Three General Secretaries." In President's Commission, *Splicing Life*, 95–96.

12. National Academies of Sciences, Engineering, Medicine, *Human Genome Editing: Science, Ethics, and Governance* (Washington, DC: National Academies Press, 2017).

13. National Academies, *Human Genome Editing*, 120.

14. National Academies, *Human Genome Editing*, 120.

15. National Academies, *Human Genome Editing*, 156.

16. President's Council on Bioethics, *Beyond Therapy: Biotechnology and the Pursuit of Happiness* (Washington, DC: President's Council, 2003).

PART I
WHAT IS HUMAN FLOURISHING?

1

Welcoming the Unexpected

Rosemarie Garland-Thomson

We four women gather together for dinner whenever we can, often at academic conferences, for research trips, or when we find ourselves in the same city for professional obligations. We favor California-style farm-to-table restaurants these days, most always with good French wines. We are modern career women, each credentialed with a PhD, supported by a reliable income with good benefits, accommodated by advanced technology, and sustained by a network of colleagues and family. We are writers, educators, managers, institutional leaders, and recognized experts in our chosen fields. While some of us have husbands, none of us depends on them primarily for our social status or economic security. Although we have followed different paths to converge in these moments of professional fellowship, one aspect of our lives that draws us together is our access to unprecedented opportunities available to people like us in the last four decades.

We are part of the first generation of women who entered into places in America where we could accumulate the social and economic capital that undergirds a life of flourishing in liberal capitalist societies. Structural barriers in the form of males-only policies, laws, and practices kept women out of jobs, schools, military, government, clubs, sports, and public spaces of power and prestige and limited most American women to low-status jobs and domestic confinement. In short, gender restrictions before the policy and practice changes that began in the 1970s in the United States kept women from direct access to economic resources and consigned us to derivative status through husbands and fathers. Until the 1860s, married women could not own any property or have money of their own; until 1920, women could not vote; until the 1970s, women could not serve in the military, attend most prestigious universities, or participate in mainstream sports. We could be excluded from anything simply because we were women. In the first decades of the twenty-first century in the United States, however, the condition of being female can even be an advantage now that most structural barriers that disadvantaged women and benefited men are removed. Indeed, some men have not adjusted to the current social and economic landscape that my friends and I enjoy. Living out our shared gender identity in an era of unprecedented opportunity and attendant obligations bonds us together in both the celebrations and the struggles of womanhood. We four women understand our femaleness as an advantage in our current moment.

But we share another bond besides the common condition of being women that draws us together. We each live with a rare genetic condition that shapes us and the way we live our lives.[1] One of us developed hereditary blindness early in life. Another is congenitally deaf, like her grandmother. The other of us has a genetic muscular condition. I was born with asymmetrical unusual hands and forearms, a genetic anomaly that occurs in fewer than one of ninety thousand people. Each of us has an "orphan disease"—that odd, almost-poetic, faintly Dickensian, phrase for rare genetic conditions that captures the unexpected outsiderness of our being and bespeaks the sundered connection between people like us and the human family of ordinary people. And yet, we are anything but "orphans." Indeed, we are inextricably linked to ancestors and descendants who vanish into horizons lost to us whether we look back or forward. The genetic etiology of our being binds us to our progenitors through an ancestral inheritance hidden deep in the elegant whirls of that double helix, steadfastly awaiting manifestation in unwitting descendants like us.

Before the human genome map appeared in 2003 to give us genetic origin stories for all manner of unexpected human variation, our blindness, deafness, crippledness, and weakness were understood as defects, for sure, often with diagnostic disease labels. But usually the origin of our rarity was inexplicable. When we were children, the cause and development of congenital disabilities was often unrecognized and unrecognizable. Modern versions of the ancient stories of "maternal impression" crowded around the fundamental question of our being: What went wrong? In the world before modern medicine, the narrative of maternal impression—the idea that a pregnant woman's emotional state might cause congenital or other disorders in the fetus—might have found the etiology of my unusual arms in my mother having scrutinized too closely, for some baffling reason, the fins of fish or the flippers of seals while she carried me. Committing, or even witnessing, a moral transgression was thought to imprint an unborn child with some singular sign, either mysterious or revelatory. Modern versions of this fear haunt the mothers of today's congenitally disabled children with a corrosive guilt about unwitting or, worse yet, intentional exposure to toxins ranging from face cream and nail polish, alcohol and cigarettes, to thalidomide and the BPA (bisphenol A) in our plastic bottles. We were then and are now prophecies: cautions or warnings of bad things past or future, canaries in the coal mine of human existence. The unexpected or unusual arrival of anything into human life demands explanation because it threatens the stability, the coherence, of predictable mundane existence so crucial to simply getting through our days.

We four women emerged into the world, then, as strangers to our parents, interruptions in the continuity of sameness that forges familial solidarity. To use Andrew Solomon's invocation of the folk expression, we landed "far from the tree," somehow the wrong child, a changeling for the nondisabled child our parents had expected.[2] Not that we were unloved; indeed, our outsiderness in the world was to our parents a vulnerability they by turns protected, indulged, or betrayed. My Deaf friend's family pretended she was hearing and just not paying attention. As my other friend's blindness developed, she hugged the front row at school and paid careful attention to everything her fully sighted classmates and teachers said, making her an excellent, parent-pleasing student. I was simply not permitted to retreat from barriers I encountered, either physical or social ones. We all learned endurance and resourcefulness from managing in a world not made for us. Our parents were responsible for us in both senses of the word. The source of our differences from our parents, our siblings, and other children may have been understood as some unintentional or inadvertent act on the part of our parents, but not as a harm for which we held them responsible.

But the mystery and unsettling lore of congenital disability has now given way to the certainty of genetic narratives. The geneticist who recently identified the genetic condition that yielded my arms scoffed when I explained that doctors in the past had considered my disability a random occurrence. The genetic origin stories that now account for our unusual ways of being establish a fundamental new network of relationships stamped in every cell of our kin, starting first with our parents and extending far from that tree into the distant, unknowable past and future. This vast, previously unknowable kinship network is newly legible through the technologies of genetic testing and recorded for us in the disease pedigree trees by which our doctors and genetic counselors represent for us our extended genetic tribe. Each of my women friends now belongs to a distinctive genetic diagnostic category that replaces the vague derivation stories of intrusive substances, external violation, maternal inadequacy, divine intervention, or just random occurrence. Now, the geneticist assured me, I "have" *complicated ectrodactyly*.

In this post–human genome world in which we find ourselves, medical science has identified approximately 7,000 different types of rare diseases, with more being discovered each day.[3] Determining which variations count as disease and which as mere difference is complicated. Human biology tolerates abundant variation within the basic form that will sustain life. We humans have a surprisingly distinctive array of structure, arrangement, and function that maintains vitality. Our distinctive variation is disorder reined in only by the order viability requires. A live birth is the threshold for what range of human variation is tolerable. The classical tradition of the ideal—expressed so aptly in Leonardo's famous *Vitruvian Man*—exalts human regularity, symmetry, and order. That tradition has given us a low tolerance for human variation both aesthetically and medically. In contrast, aesthetic traditions such as the grotesque or the baroque honor the wide swath of human variation that embodies the unpredictable, anomalous, asymmetrical, illogical, or gratuitously ornate. The very fact of rarity's vitality—its persistence in human form—flies in the face of *Vitruvian Man*'s lofty display of normalcy. Those of us born with congenital disabilities, now even more those of us with genetic congenital disabilities, crossed over the viability threshold with admirable endurance, only to be unwelcome surprises on our arrival.

People like the four of us have long been the "bad news" of lying-in hospitals, delivery rooms, neonatal units, and prenatal imaging and testing—unexpected arrivals delivered by the Black Stork.[4] In the swiftly developing world of genetic engineering, however, people like us are identifiable, legible in our distinctiveness and rarity, much earlier in the trajectory of medicalized human procreation than in the past. Detecting disability through selective testing is carried out now at all developmental stages of human reproduction, from the gametic to the embryonic to the fetal to the neonatal. Germline interventions would seek to prevent people with rare diseases and congenital disabilities from coming into being. This pruning of human variation at the genetic level proceeds with little consideration of our perspectives as people who live out these genetic narratives. Enthusiasts about genetic engineering cite facts against us such as those described by the Global Burden of Disease Project, which calculates our supposed collective costs without accounting for our contributions.[5] We are a vanishing tribe, those of us now detectable earlier and earlier in the process of human procreation. We are now often culled out before the traits that embryonic and fetal testing reveal are brought into being in a lived life.

Certainly not all people with rare genetic diseases or congenital disabilities affiliate with their conditions in the way that we four women do. Pain, dysfunction, frailty, and other so-called comorbidities inflect our attachments to our individuality and our group alignments in different ways. In his Chapter 11 in this volume, Robert Sparrow argues that elimination of some genetic conditions might advance the welfare of future persons. My friend Alice Wexler, Board of Directors member and secretary of the Hereditary Disease Foundation, a nonprofit organization devoted to research on Huntington's disease, a condition present in Alice's family, tells me that everyone in the Huntington's community would like to see that disease obliterated from the human genetic line. Whether that aspiration is achievable through genetic engineering without unacceptable unintended consequences is another thing, she is quick to add. Yet the increasing expansion of what counts as genetic disease and thus the pathologizing of human anomaly and variation concerns people like us who understand our way of being as essential to our human individuality and flourishing.

The story of our ways of being in the world as people with rare genetic diseases emerged gradually for the four of us. My Deaf and my blind friends were recognized as such only in mid-childhood because each had enough hearing and sight to manage what life asked of them in the first few years. My friend with muscular weakness and I were, in contrast, floridly disabled from the get-go. My accommodation needs were less clear than hers, but we both in time got access to what we needed to flourish. The gradual expression of genetic blindness and deafness or late-onset disabilities can create its own disadvantage by sandwiching a person between the categories of fully able-bodied and disabled. It can be a boon to get an early start on disability, to be recognized for who we are, to get on with learning how to most effectively use the world we live in, and to be comfortable as ourselves. These are in truth the life tasks for any person; having disabilities simply requires resourcefulness in mustering such skills and supports for flourishing in a world built for other kinds of people.

Our genetic imprints have shaped our bodies, our senses of self, our relations with others, and the ways we use the world. The distinctive form and function of our bodies bequeathed to us by our rare genetic conditions are the ground from which the lives we live have arisen. As with all human beings, our bodies carry out our lives in idiosyncratic ways; we become who we are through the bodies we have. Human enfleshment both restricts and enables undertaking the scope of aspirations that comprise a life. The manifestations of embodiment we consider disability, disease, and anomaly are aspects of our being that intertwine with an array of characteristics we think of as normal in the shifting patterning of particularity that comprises a human person. Our lived life emerges from the encounter between animated flesh and vibrant world. The human person is dynamic, constantly re-formed by this call and response between body and environment.

The contours of the world into which each of us was born have determined our life quality much more than have our genetic profiles and the distinctive ways of being those genes produced. That we were born into adequately economically stable families, had good enough mothering, learned at appropriate public schools, built sustaining social networks, acquired economic resources through employment, obtained access to the technology and skills we needed to accomplish the tasks of everyday life, and benefited from general good fortune in our life events gave us the good lives we live. In short, we flourished as the genetically distinctive human beings we were because we were embedded in environments that sustained our emotional, psychological, social, physical, and material needs.

We have flourished, not in spite of our disabilities, but rather with our disabilities. This counterintuitive claim sits uneasily with modern medicine's framing of disease, disability, and anomaly.[6] Nonetheless, the way we understand our lives is that the limitations to our life projects due to blindness, deafness, weakness, and deformity are not inherent in the conditions themselves but exist largely because the world that we live in was built by and for hearing, sighted, walking, strong, and fully handed people. That we do not experience our way of being in the world as disadvantage, diminishment, or distress can be difficult to grasp for people who understand themselves as nondisabled, as Jackie Leach Scully also observes in Chapter 10 in this volume. The experience of minorities is always challenging for those in the majority to imagine. While disability can occasion suffering, living with disabilities is not necessarily a limitation, a reduction of future opportunities, or a predictor of distress or suffering. And the state of being we think of as perfect health or able-bodiedness is no guarantee of flourishing. Indeed, sometimes a too easeful fit into one's social and material world can breed complacency and stunt the development of resourcefulness, adaptability, and strong life management skills. As the geneticist and Nobel laureate Mario R. Capecchi recently recognized in a conversation about CRISPR, "There is benefit to adversity."

Certainly, we four suffer in our particular ways, as do all human beings, but we are not likely to suffer any more than the nondisabled suffer. The sources of human suffering are complex, ineluctable, and deeply embedded in all of us. Any bright boundary in the likely apportionment of human suffering is a comforting folly to those who hope to find themselves on the protected side of such a border.

Our genetic conditions gave us a head start in accessing multiple opportunities for expression, creativity, resourcefulness, and relationships—for human flourishing. Living in a world not built for us and in a community where the majority of members understand themselves and are understood by others as being more fortunate, advantaged, better, more able, or healthier than we are has been an opportunity. From that place where we have lived our lives, many of us have developed a vibrant resourcefulness, interdependence, an alternative knowledge base, and a consciousness sometimes perceptible only in the recesses of our being, all of which have served us well. Our genetic conditions have offered us the occasion to ripen early the life skills we will all need as enfleshed beings for navigating the unwelcoming attitudes and structuring of our environment. We flourished as we were supported by adequate resources, benefits, and goods that sustain anyone's well-being. Ours is not the cliché of overcoming disability; indeed, is the fresh story of coming fully into disability and flourishing just as we are.

We came of age as people with disabilities in the newly equitable and accessible world of the late twentieth century. This world opened doors and paths that had been closed to us and our fellow disabled citizens before the civil rights movements and the social and material changes it introduced literally changed the landscape for us and other people with disabilities. Starting early with our congenital and early-onset disabilities and supported by adequate economic, familial, and educational resources, we had a sustaining environment in which we could flourish. The human and civil rights movements reconceptualized all of us as full and equal citizens rather than genetic errors. Over our lifetimes, it became possible for us to move from isolation to community, from ignorance to knowledge about who we are, from shame to pride, and from exclusion to access. The disabled poet Sheila Black affirmed our experience when she wrote, "To be human often entails finding ways to make what appears a disadvantage a point of strength or pride."[7]

One way to think about how we four women with rare genetic conditions have flourished is to consider the grammatical meaning making of the word *flourish*. We shape language, and language shapes us. Flourish is a verb, and as such expresses action. To flourish is to *do* something. In English, there are two kinds of verbs. One kind is a transitive verb, used when the action of the verb is a transaction in which an actor (the subject) does an action (the verb) to a thing (the direct object). As the word *transitive* suggests, the transitive verb establishes a connecting action between two things, a subject and an object, that can never be the same. Something always does something to something else, as in "I hit the ball." A transitive verb can even separate out parts of the same entity, as in "I broke my leg." There is an inherent differentiation, even alienation, at work with transitive verbs. As an intransitive verb, flourish expresses a different kind of action, one complete in the relationship between the actor and action so that the work of *flourishing* that the subject enacts loops back onto the subject itself rather than being passed on to another object. *She flourishes*—period. This snug syntactic dyad of subject and verb form a reflexive story in which actor and action, cause and effect, time and place tangle tightly. The *Oxford Living Dictionary* tells us that to flourish is to "grow or develop . . . in a vigorous way" within "a particularly congenial environment."[8] To flourish, then, is a story in which an actor emerges as itself through time and across space in a good way. This is exactly what we four women have done.

The philosopher Jürgen Habermas offered a story similar to ours in his 2004 Kyoto Prize lecture, "Public Space and Political Public Sphere—The Biographical Roots of Two Motives in My Thought."[9] This lecture, we learn, answers the request to "tell us something instructive about the path of your life." What Habermas told is that the experiences that came to him from being born with a congenital disability shaped his development in positive ways, even when the experiences themselves were negative. He explained this seeming contradiction. Born with a cleft palate in 1929 Germany, just as the Nazi regime marched toward totalitarianism, Habermas's experiences of disability led him to become the philosopher he is today. Being "exposed to the traumatic experience of surgery" several times in childhood, he developed an early "awareness of how one person always depends on others," which is a crucial element in his philosophy of the ethical dimensions of the public sphere as the space of mutual recognition and deliberation among equal citizens. In addition, because he spoke, and indeed still speaks, in an unu-sual way due to his congenital disability, "other people did not understand [him] very well and they responded with annoyance or rejection." He recognized now that such "rejection" was manifest in "those more or less harmless acts of dis-crimination which many children suffer in the schoolyard or street if they appear somehow different from the others." Habermas forged a direct and strong link between the "difficulties [he] encountered when trying to make [himself] un-derstood" and the struggles and fragility of direct communication in liberal self-governing social orders. This disability gain—if you will—also made it possible for him to comprehend the terrible consequences of the failures of communica-tion among equals and the acts of discrimination against people who appeared somehow different that characterized the Nazi regime.

What this story makes clear is that determining what life experience counts as bad or good, beneficial or detrimental, positive or negative is far more compli-cated than what the accepted scripts of disease, disability, and deformity would have us believe about quality of life or human flourishing.[10] Even more uncertain is genetic engineering's premise that we can conclude in advance how the trajec-tory of development we call human life will unfold according to a legible, stable, and tractable code.

Jürgen Habermas, like we four women, flourishes not in spite of but in part because of the lived experience of disability. The experiences Habermas's cleft palate generated made a significant contribution to his flourishing. And those particular experiences would not have come to him without that congenital characteristic. Like us, he did not overcome his congenital disability, but rather the unusual feature we call a cleft palate intertwined with the cumulative char-acteristics that comprise his human individuality to grow, to come into being dynamically as itself, through time and space and relations into a human life of flourishing. This is not to deny that his "congenital abnormality," like ours, occasioned negative experiences or disadvantage. Rather it was at the same time an occasion for flourishing. Like us, he benefited from an early start at being disa-bled, at being "different." His life perspective and projects, then, arose organically from his personhood as he lived out his distinctive life through his particular body. Simply put, as our differences were for us, his cleft palate was integral to his being, shaping his experience and development in unpredictable, unexpected, and marvelous ways.[11] Perhaps more important than contributing to Habermas's own individual flourishing, his experience of living with congenital disability in-formed a theory of collective human flourishing laid out in his premises about mutual communication in public space as the essence of the liberal democratic promise.

In his 2003 book, *The Future of Human Nature*, Habermas-as-philosopher proposed a useful moral theory for thinking about human flourishing in the

age of genetic engineering.[12] Here Habermas put forward what I would call—
following my grammatical analysis of the word *flourishing*—a model of human
development that recognizes the open future inherent in human embodied variation and distinctiveness. Persons, according to Habermas, should *grow* rather
than be *made*. Grow can be an intransitive verb, expressing an action complete in
itself, whereas *made* is usually transitive, expressing an action done by a subject
to an object. A *grown* person develops, then, out of the way he or she was thrown
into the world by forces that no person made, not by the preferences of another
person. A made person is fabricated according to the will of another. What's
wrong with *making* people through genetic engineering is that someone else's
priorities, even if intended to be in their own best interests, govern the selections
either for or against the traits that make up our unique personhood.

To flourish, then, is to grow over a lifetime into a particular rather than generic individual human person. Habermas's concept of the grown conflicts
with modern medicine's identification of much human variation and anomaly
as pathology that can be excised from an otherwise-generic, or *normal*, human
person. Many of the genetic and congenital traits that medicine considers disease
or pathology would in Habermas's account be essential parts of who we are—
perhaps like his cleft palate—out of which our particular form of flourishing
grows. Liberty, then, is to grow from our distinctive individuality, not according
to conceptions of health, normalcy, advantage, or future quality of life imposed
through parental will or medical authority and justified as the best interests of
the child.

Determining which elements of our being are essential and which are sepa-
rable from our being through vaccination, medical treatment, surgical shaping,
or even genetic engineering is the challenge of Habermas's concept of the organically grown human person. But if we fail to meet that challenge, and continue
uncritically to medically form individuals rather than recognize their potential
to grow into unique beings with their own distinctive ways of emerging into personhood, we fail the promise of the freedom to become ourselves that is fundamental to liberal modern orders. Once we begin medically making individuals
rather than imagining them as either creations of an inexplicable divine will or
an existential contingency that throws into the world singular beings with their
own inherent logic and distinctive essence that will emerge as they grow over a
lifetime, we are engaging in what Habermas calls "a liberal eugenics regulated by
supply and demand."[13]

The proper relation between living and future persons is one of stewardship,
rather than instrumental shaping. Such stewardship requires protecting the
interests of future persons by creating a communal shared environment that
supports our unique being and protects us from interventions by individuals,
the collective, or institutions that hinder our emergence as distinctive persons.

Flourishing depends not so much on what our individual human variations might be but rather on whether the collection of characteristics that make up our distinctive being develops in harmonious relation with the environment. Hostile environments thwart flourishing; congenial environments promote it. Such a notion of personhood sustained by networks of social and material relationships departs from the classical image of the human represented in da Vinci's iconic *Vitruvian Man*, the at once generic and normative Aristotelian unmoved mover suspended in a sealed circle of enforced static symmetry. Flourishing, then, is emerging as our distinctive selves in reciprocity with a shared environment that recognizes and supports our distinct particularity.

In modern liberal societies, government or civic culture carries out this communal obligation to support the distinctiveness of its members according to the egalitarian principals of justice, equality, and liberty.[14] To maintain such commitments, liberal orders should build environments that anticipate, recognize, and support the widest spectrum of embodiments, building a kind of moral ecosystem, in which human embodied existence can successfully thrive as it is.[15] Bruce Jennings's Chapter 17 in this collection expands on this idea. Such a congenial environment is a just environment, one that supports what Valerie Fletcher, director of the Institute for Human Centered Design, calls "social sustainability." Such sustainable environments promote human flourishing by providing a material context of received and built resources ranging from accessibly designed built public spaces, welcoming natural surroundings, communication devices, tools, and implements, as well as other people.

To support some of the human variations we think of as genetic disorder, disease, anomaly, or disability does not preclude appropriate interventions—sometimes medical, sometimes social—that ameliorate pain and suffering or promote human functioning and flourishing. Supporting disability in this way also includes using technology as a bridge between flesh and world. A call for such a moral ecosystem is not status quo bias, passive acceptance, moral timidity, or resistance to imagining something better than the present circumstances. Instead, it is a caution against an aggressive normalization imperative that eliminates rather than accommodates (or as Michael Hauskeller puts it in Chapter 4, "respects" and "cherishes"). It is an outlook of humility about the human capacity to control future circumstances through present actions and works against the arrogance of what the writer Chimamanda Ngozi Adichie called "the danger of a single story."[16] This morality of human flourishing has at its core the concept of active accommodation that is fundamental to the disability rights movement: change the environment, not the person; protect rather than regularize; abide rather than improve; accommodate rather than eliminate.

What the lived experience of we four women with genetic conditions offers is a provocation to contemplate how we all understand ourselves as enfleshed beings and how we can build a shared world that honors the wide variation of human embodiment. Recognizing the lived experience of disability as an informing principal of full moral personhood is essential to understanding what is required for human flourishing.

Such an attitude of humility and welcome toward the human experience of disability can serve to guide practice, policy, world building, and technology making in the world we inhabit together. Technologies devoted to making rather than growing human beings based on values and preferences of others should not be used to shape human communities or individuals. It is challenging to make distinctions between medical treatments that allow us to grow into ourselves flourishing in our full distinctiveness and interventions that standardize us according to narrow and current versions of traits thought to be advantageous. The enterprise of shaping human communities should be shared across our communities broadly and go beyond the perspectives and entangled interests of science, medicine, and commerce. CRISPR is only one example of this kind of technology. In setting practice and policy about such technologies, we should recognize relationships to the larger cultural and commercial project of making rather than growing individuals and communities that is being carried out largely today within the procreative economy. In the larger enterprise of considering human futurity—of intentional deliberations about how our actions now shape a future then—this provocation to conserve and welcome a wider range of human variations within our communities allows us to reconsider the logic and practice of a velvet eugenics that would standardize human variation in the interest of individual, market-driven liberty and at the expense of social justice and the common good.[17]

We need a bioethics for intentionally and ethically shaping society instead of shaping bodies. The late Nancy Mairs, who lived with multiple sclerosis for decades, expressed this idea in two ways: First, she told us that if a cure were developed for multiple sclerosis she would take it, but that to flourish she did not need such a cure. Second, Mairs explained that her task in writing about living with multiple sclerosis was "to conceptualize not merely a habitable body but a habitable world: a world that wants me in it."[18] The shape of the material world we build and occupy together governs who inhabits human communities. We are shaping communities with medical technologies, carried out most fully in our human enterprise of procreation, that limit the diversity of our human communities by targeting and selecting against a broad range of human variations identified as illness and disability. Rather than aim to reduce human variations in the interest of making this the same as an advantage, I invite us to use the technologies of disability culture, disability justice, and inclusive technologies—from medicine to laws, tools, and stories—to make a shared world inhabitable by the widest range of human users. Such an enterprise would shift our attention and resources to conserving the human variations we think of as disabilities rather than eliminating them. This world will strengthen the cultural, political, institutional, and material climate in which people with and without disabilities can most effectively flourish.

Notes

1. Some of the material in this chapter appeared in an earlier form in opinion pieces published in the *New York Times* as part of the series on disability written by people with disabilities. See Rosemarie Garland-Thomson, "Becoming Disabled," *New York Times*, August 19, 2012, https://www.nytimes.com/2016/08/21/opinion/sunday/becoming-disabled.html; Rosemarie Garland-Thomson, "My Orphan Disease Has Given Me a New Family" [disability series], *New York Times*, October 26, 2017, https://www.nytimes.com/2017/10/26/opinion/my-orphan-disease-has-given-me-a-new-family.html.
2. Andrew Solomon, *Far from the Tree: Parents, Children and the Search for Identity* (New York: Scribner, 2012).
3. "Facts and Statistics about Rare Disease," Global Genes, last modified 2015, https://globalgenes.org/wp-content/uploads/2015/12/2016-WRDD-Fact-Sheet.pdf. Other significant rare disease facts are as follows: Of rare diseases, 80% are genetic in origin and thus are present throughout a person's life, even if symptoms do not immediately appear; approximately 50% of the people affected by rare diseases are children; 30% of children with rare disease die before age five; rare diseases are responsible for 35% of deaths in the first year of life; 80% of all patients with a rare disease are affected by approximately 350 rare diseases. Also see Marilyn J. Field and Thomas F. Boat, eds., *Rare Diseases and Orphan Products: Accelerating Research and Development* (Washington, DC: National Academies Press, 2010).
4. Martin S. Pernick, *The Black Stork* (New York: Oxford University Press, 1996); Luke Camery, "The Black Stork; Eugenic Infanticide in Twentieth Century America," (unpublished manuscript, June 14, 2012), https://docs.google.com/file/d/0B9BESb-X9dvza00wRmFzZjRkUTA/edit
5. Steven Pinker, "The Moral Imperative for Bioethics" *The Boston Globe*, August 1, 2015, https://www.bostonglobe.com/opinion/2015/07/31/the-moral-imperative-for-bioethics/JmEkoyzlTAu9oQV76JrK9N/story.html.
6. See: Ron Amundson and Shari Tresky, "Bioethics and Disability Rights: Conflicting Values and Perspectives," *Journal of Bioethical Inquiry* 5, no. 2 (May 2008): 111–123; Tom Shakespeare, "Disability: Suffering, Social Oppression, or Complex Predicament?" In *The Contingent Nature of Life: Bioethics and Limits of Human Existence*, ed. Marcus Düwell, Christoph Rehmann-Sutter, and Dietmar Mieth (Dordrecht: Springer Netherlands, 2008), 235–246; Gary L. Albrecht and Patrick J.

Devlieger, "The Disability Paradox: High Quality of Life against All Odds," *Social Science & Medicine* 48, no. 8 (April 1999): 977–988.

7. Sheila Black, "Trying to Embrace a 'Cure,'" *The New York Times*, June 4, 2017, https://www.nytimes.com/2017/05/31/opinion/trying-to-embrace-the-cure.html.

8. *Oxford Living Dictionary*, s.v. "Flourish, v," 2017, accessed April 11, 2019, https://en.oxforddictionaries.com/definition/flourish.

9. Jürgen Habermas, "Public Space and Political Public Sphere–The Biographical Roots of Two Motifs in My Thought" (commemorative lecture, Kyoto, Japan, November 11, 2004), 5.

10. A 2005 case in the United Kingdom in which several late-term abortions were approved due to the presence of cleft palate, which was judged by a National Health Service board to be serious enough to merit termination, illustrates the complexity of determining which human traits are benefits and which are liabilities in future quality of life and well-being. See "No Charges in Late Abortion Case," *BBC News*, March 16, 2005, http://news.bbc.co.uk/2/hi/uk_news/england/hereford/worcs/4354469.stm

11. Habermas intriguingly added, "You find, by the way, an experience of illness or physical handicap in the biographies of many philosophers," Habermas, Public Space, 2.

12. Jürgen Habermas, *The Future of Human Nature* (Malden, MA: Polity Press, 2003). Habermas argued here against enhancement and reproductive selection, calling such medical practices "a liberal eugenics regulated by supply and demand." See Habermas, *The Future*, i.

13. Habermas, *The Future*, 14.

14. Rosemarie Garland-Thomson, "Human Biodiversity Conservation: A Consensual Ethical Principle," *The American Journal of Bioethics* 15, no. 6 (June 2015): 13–15.

15. For an account of the relationship between human embodied existence and a sustaining environment, see Rosemarie Garland-Thomson, "Misfits: A Feminist Materialist Disability Concept," *Hypatia* 26, no. 3 (2011): 591–609; for an explication of human rights in relation to human embodied existence, see Brian S. Turner, *Vulnerability and Human Rights* (University Park: Penn State University Press, 2006).

16. Chimamanda Ngozi Adichie, "The Danger of a Single Story." Filmed July 2009 in Oxford, UK. TEDGlobal video, 18:49. http://www.ted.com/talks/chimamanda_adichie_the_danger_of_a_single_story?language=en.

17. For an explanation of disability conservation, see Rosemarie Garland-Thomson, "Human Biodiversity Conservation: A Consensual Ethical Principle," *The American Journal of Bioethics*, 15, issue no. 6 (2011): 13–15, http://dx.doi.org/10.1080/15265161.2015.1028663. Disability conservation may not preclude editing out specific human conditions such as Huntington's disease or Tay Sachs on the same logic that through vaccination, polio or smallpox has been largely eliminated. Disability conservation may also include preserving genetic traits considered to be disabilities, such as deafness or dwarfism. The morality of selecting for disability—with deafness as our case study—has been vigorously debated and generally rejected by

nondisabled bioethicists. My intention here is to promote conserving the lived experience of disability rather than arguing for and against specific human traits understood as genetic that might be eliminated from the human condition.

18. Nancy Mairs, *Waist High in the World: A Life among the Nondisabled* (Boston: Beacon Press, 1996), 63.

2

Flourishing and the Value of Authenticity

Daniel M. Haybron

Notoriously, biotechnologies like gene editing raise deep philosophical questions, not least of which is what it means for humans to flourish—that is, to achieve well-being, as philosophers today usually put it. Some of those questions have to do with the notion of *authenticity*: whether such technologies might threaten authenticity and thereby, perhaps, personal well-being. While the notion of authenticity has received considerable attention in the bioethics literature,[1] it remains poorly understood and has been far less present in philosophical writings on well-being.[2] In what follows I argue that there are good reasons to view authenticity as an aspect of well-being, and I discuss some implications of this view for gene editing technologies. As some readers may not be conversant in the philosophical literature on well-being, I also briefly survey the relevant landscape. But my chief goal here is to make the case that authenticity merits serious consideration as an aspect of well-being. Even if one concludes that it has no role in the best theory of well-being, the notion of authenticity is deeply embedded in ordinary thinking about the good life, and merits attention from policymakers and others for that reason alone.

I do not take a stand on the advisability of gene editing, or whether the benefits to individuals are likely to outweigh the harms. Nor do I discuss the social dimensions of authenticity—whether authenticity concerns emerge at collective levels or how far notions of authenticity should inform social norms and deliberation. Focusing just on the individual case, I suggest that, though some applications of gene editing likely have no bearing on authenticity, others may enhance authenticity, diminish it, or both. While I argue that authenticity is important for well-being, I assume that well-being depends as well on other factors. Indeed, most views that accord fundamental value to authenticity count it only as one among other aspects of well-being. It is not, in my view, a suitable foundation for an entire ethic.[3]

In what follows I draw on exotic science fiction scenarios, such as "soulscramblers." This a standard philosopher's tactic, famously employed in the "experience machine" example. Reflecting on such cases can be useful, not because we shall ever encounter them, but because doing so can help us to isolate important variables. For instance, gene editing will never allow us straightforwardly to manufacture very many of an individual's characteristics, but it does promise to give us *some* degree of control over people's traits—that's the point. Is that in any way problematic? In ordinary life it can be hard to tell: A variety of potentially relevant factors will be in play, with a mix of pros and cons, and effects may be subtle. Exotic cases of extreme control let us screen out possible sources of noise to see what matters in such interventions. If a factor seems important in the extreme case, then it may also be significant in ordinary cases. Such thought experiments aren't foolproof and require caution as our intuitions may not always be reliable in unusual situations. But "unusual" doesn't entail "baffling": Darth Vader strangling folks with the Force may be exotic, but I suspect one needn't puzzle for long to figure out that it isn't a nice thing to do.

Philosophical Theories of Flourishing or Well-Being

What is a theory of well-being? In philosophy, it is a theory that tells us what, ultimately, is good or bad for people; what benefits or harms them; or what makes their lives go better or worse for them. We are talking about a kind of value here, and *well-being* is the most common term now used by philosophers for this value. Other terms include *flourishing, welfare, thriving,* and, for the ancient Greeks, *eudaimonia.* In one older sense of the word, *happiness* also belongs on this list, for instance in translations of Aristotle's eudaimonia.

For the most part, philosophical accounts of human flourishing or well-being fall into one of four approaches[4]:

1. Hedonism
2. Desire theories
3. List theories
4. Nature-fulfillment ("eudaimonistic") theories

Hedonism

According to hedonism, most famously championed by Jeremy Bentham and John Stuart Mill, well-being consists of pleasure: how pleasant or unpleasant our experience of life is—whether we enjoy life, are suffering, and so on. There's no uncontroversial way of defining the view, but the general idea is easy enough to grasp. Despite the connotations of the name, hedonists needn't claim that we should focus on sensory pleasures, or that we should aim at pleasure at all. Perhaps the most pleasant life, as the Greek hedonist Epicurus maintained, is a simple life of virtue, leaving us free from pains of the body and troubles of the mind.

Desire Theories

Desire theories—or "desire-fulfillment" theories—identify well-being roughly with getting what you want. A version of this approach is standard among economists and accordingly is pretty much the default approach in public policy.[5] Desire theories can take many forms, with a popular variant focusing on the satisfaction of informed desires: the desires we *would* have if fully informed about all our options. Desire theories can seem very similar to hedonism, and both approaches are commonly deemed "subjectivist": what's good for you depends entirely on how things stand from your perspective. One major difference is that desire theories focus on things *actually* going the way you want; hedonism only concerns how you feel. In the famous example of an experience machine, you might be perfectly happy plugged forever into a virtual reality machine, blissfully unaware that your mother, your friends, your job, are illusory, nothing more than routines in the program.[6] Hedonism can say nothing against such a life: what you don't know can't hurt you. Desire theories, by contrast, can say that such a life is sad, a failure, because you're not *actually* getting what you want: You're not really doing anything, your "mother" doesn't actually love you, and so on. Whereas hedonism identifies well-being with a state of mind, desire theories identify it with a state of the world: things actually going as you want them to go.

A further difference is that desire theories are able to ground your well-being in what you care about, and chances are good that you care about things other than pleasure; in fact, many people would gladly sacrifice some pleasure to lead a life of achievement. Philosophers, athletes, soldiers, and many others often seem to have such priorities and think they are better off in such a life. According to hedonism, however, they are wrong: they would be better off in more pleasant lives with less struggle and frustration.

For convenience, I will follow the common practice of referring to both hedonistic and desire-fulfillment theories as "subjectivist" accounts of well-being. There are good questions about whether hedonism is really a subjectivist view given the point made in the last paragraph, but we need not enter that debate here.

List Theories

List theories, also called objective list theories, are "objectivist" in an uncontroversial sense: They hold that what's good for you is to possess the items on some standard list; your well-being doesn't depend entirely on what you want, like, or enjoy. Common list items include knowledge, achievement, friendship, and pleasure, but just about every list theorist posits a distinct list. While list theorists do not make well-being entirely dependent on the person's wants or tastes, neither do they generally make it entirely independent: An objectively worthwhile life will presumably also have some compensations from the subjective point of view. Few have claimed that you could thrive in a life of agony that you detest. And friendship presupposes that you care about your friends. But whereas a desire theorist or a hedonist must allow that there would be nothing missing in a person's life if he or she were fundamentally asocial and happy to live without friends, a list theorist can claim, plausibly, that there's something lacking in such a life.

Nature-Fulfillment Theories

The fourth family of philosophical accounts of flourishing or well-being is concerned with the fulfillment of our natures. These views claim that what's good for a person is a function of what he or she is like: his or her nature. The claim is stronger than it may appear: The idea is that certain goals are "written into" a person's constitution, and that one flourishes insofar as one reaches those goals (realizing one's potential, for example). Such theories make their account of well-being dependent on some prior account of persons' natures.[7] For Aristotle, the most influential of nature-fulfillment theorists, the relevant nature is one's nature as a member of the human species: we flourish by leading characteristically human lives, which is to say—given that we are rational animals by nature—lives of rational, virtuous activity. Some other theorists, notably in the modern era, adopt a less species-based and more individualized conception of a person's nature: what matters for your flourishing is what *you* are like as a person, *who* you are: the self. On such views, well-being is a matter more specifically of *self*-fulfillment and accordingly depends on how the self is constituted.[8] If, as many people think, the self is defined by what one values or cares about, then self-fulfillment might consist of fulfilling one's values[9]; if instead the self is defined more by matters of temperament and emotional propensities, then self-fulfillment might involve being happy, in the familiar (non-Aristotelian) sense of being in a particular psychological state.[10] Or perhaps the self has multiple aspects, in which case well-being likewise will have multiple facets.

This may all seem very airy and theoretical, but it is important for our purposes to see the attractions of nature-fulfillment theories. One advantage, as I just suggested, is that they offer an elegant theoretical structure that can accommodate a lot of complexity. We don't need to make up a list, with accompanying mysteries about how we ended up with that list and not some other; the list of human goods can flow naturally from the varied dimensions of human nature. Moreover, such theories naturally extend to a wide range of life forms and indeed can help illuminate why flourishing varies across species: each has a different nature, given, for instance, by its characteristic makeup or form of life. So for acorns, flourishing involves growing into full-bodied, healthy oaks; for wolves, flourishing includes hunting in packs—wolves are social hunters by nature, and so fulfill their natures by leading characteristically lupine lives. Human beings are rational, emotional, and social and thus (perhaps) flourish through the rational exercise of their agency in social lives that suit their emotional natures.

The acorn-oak example is apt; it nicely illustrates one of the chief themes of nature-fulfillment theorizing about well-being: the idea of realizing one's potential. "Be all you can be." Don't be a couch potato; make something of yourself; live life to the fullest; don't let your talents go to waste. Such sentiments probably explain why the term *flourishing* is so often associated with nature-fulfillment views: it strongly connotes the realization of potential. These sentiments are also very widespread, and not just in Western societies. Ideals of nature-fulfillment can be found in a variety of cultures, including classical Indian and Chinese thought, and may indeed prove to be somewhat universal.[11] (Even if you refuse to judge the slacker out of a wish to be tolerant, you may not aspire to be one yourself; perhaps your refusal to judge isn't that you don't view well-being as involving nature-fulfillment or realizing one's potential, but that you don't see it as your place to pass judgment on other people's personal ideals.) There are probably few cultures where people would see nothing lacking in a life passed in some variant of an opium den, even if it were equipped with amazing drugs from the future that guaranteed everlasting ecstasy. The den dweller might be leading an eminently pleasant life and getting all he or she wants. Yet it still will strike many as a sad, impoverished life.

In relation to many biotechnologies such as gene editing, nature-fulfillment views have some interesting features. Such theories tend to accord an individual's "given" nature special status, as something to be honored or respected. It would not be quite accurate to say that the person's nature serves as a fixed point, as it may well evolve significantly over time; becoming a philosopher or musician, for instance, can change who you are, altering your identity, commitments, what makes you happy, and so forth. But most—or at least many—nature-fulfillment accounts arguably hold that such transformations must somehow be "true" to who or what one most fundamentally is, representing a natural development of one's capacities or goals and not rank manipulation.

A common worry about biotechnologies like gene editing is that they can appear to violate this constraint by being manipulative in ways that may diminish the individual's flourishing. To express the concern in an exaggerated form, how could it be so important to be yourself, or be all you can be, if "you" are just what someone else decided you should be? Say, if "being yourself" means being the great swimmer your parents engineered you to be? What could being yourself even amount to in that case?

Many philosophers have been skeptical about the very idea of nature-fulfillment and see no reason to worry about such questions at all. As I suggest in the next section, however, one reason for concern has to do with *authenticity*, which appears to be the value at issue. This value has a long, distinguished history and is neither as obscure nor as mysterious as many believe. Indeed, even hedonists, desire theorists, and other subjectivists seem to have taken authenticity seriously as a value.[12] Whether the worry points to any incompatibility between gene editing and flourishing, however, is another question.

Before proceeding I want briefly to set aside one common source of objections to notions like authenticity, nature-fulfillment, or the self, namely that they rely on metaphysically dubious assumptions that sit ill with a scientific worldview. I have rebutted this concern elsewhere, as have others, but simply note that my own perspective is strongly naturalistic. If we have reason to value authenticity or nature-fulfillment, it is because those notions are deeply embedded in our sensibilities—in the way we see and think about human life.[13]

The Value of Authenticity

Independent Reasons for Caring about Authenticity

> You're beautiful, but you're empty. . . . One couldn't die for you. Of course, an ordinary passerby would think my rose looked just like you. But my rose, all on her own, is more important than all of you together, since she's the one I've watered. . . . Since she's my rose.
> Antoine de Saint-Exupéry, *The Little Prince*

Crudely speaking, authenticity has to do with being "the genuine article." Somewhat less crudely, a person is authentic insofar as how she (or he) is, or presents herself, reflects who she truly is (to which some would add: and she is truly her own person). A person's desires, emotions, thoughts, or actions might also be authentic or otherwise, depending on whether they reflect who the person really is. There is no need to tender a precise definition of authenticity here as it may reasonably be understood in a variety of ways, and my purpose in this chapter is just to make plausible that *some* notion of authenticity is relevant to the question of gene editing. The notion of authenticity can draw a fair amount of hostility as it is so often associated with highly individualistic, if not narcissistic, ideals of living. But authenticity does not need to be understood as a self-indulgent "I gotta be me" ideal or any kind of ideal that one strives toward. It can also be understood simply as a fairly minimal requirement or constraint, which precludes certain (inauthentic) ways of living.[14] Such a requirement could be just as well at home in "collectivist" as in individualistic cultures, and indeed it is plausible that authenticity in human lives is prized in some form in just about all cultures.[15]

Most people seem pretty clearly to care about authenticity in various guises. We value original works of art more than copies, for instance. Likewise for many natural objects, landmarks, and other places: We'd rather see the real thing, and we tend not to care very much about preserving, say, Las Vegas Venice. We feel similarly about treasured heirlooms, pets, friends, and family. Think of the Little Prince, in the epigraph to this section, and his beloved rose: his attachment is to *her*. One cannot simply grow another, as she is unique and irreplaceable by virtue of her relationship to him. The authenticity of his rose—that it is really *her*— is not just significant; it is crucial. And we, too, find authenticity to be crucial in certain matters. (Here I'd be willing to wager a modest sum: it really is "we," as in just about all normally constituted human beings except for the wise guy sitting in the back of Philosophy 101. Take the most nonindividualistic culture you can think of: Would they really find it hard to relate to the Little Prince's attachment to his flower? Would they not mind if we were to replace Granny with RepliGranny?)

Why should we care about authenticity? This is a good question, which I'll not try fully to settle here. But a plausible conjecture is that, perhaps among other things, a concern for authenticity is crucial for healthy relationships. It is good for us, and our relationships, to form strong attachments to particular individuals. In turn, such attachments require a concern that it actually be *those* individuals to whom we devote our attentions. It is hard to imagine what human life would be like if we really saw our parents as replaceable. In turn, it may be that concerns for authenticity help underwrite—or at least are inextricably linked with—important parts of ordinary moral cognition, such as the idea that persons should be treated with respect, as ends in themselves and not as mere means: what grounds this idea, at least in part, may be a view of people as irreplaceable. If it didn't matter to us whether we were dealing with the authentic Granny, why should we not be content to replace her (painlessly, and maybe with a few improvements) with RepliGranny? And could we still be said to regard her as an end rather than a mere means—to be treating her with respect?

More generally, authenticity may be significant in any context where personhood matters—or at least, where it matters *which* person, or *who*, is involved. In assigning moral responsibility, for instance, it matters whether your actions issue from *you* and reflect what manner of person you are. If they are merely the product of compulsion, drugging, manipulation—of processes that don't reflect the character of your self—then your responsibility for them seems diminished, or eliminated altogether. Moral responsibility seems to require that your actions be genuinely—authentically—yours.[16]

Authenticity and Well-Being

It should not be surprising that the notion of authenticity plays a signifi-cant role in ordinary thinking about well-being. From brainwashing victims to drugged lotus eaters, opium den dwellers, and Brave New Worlders and from repressed conformists to oppressed LGBT (lesbian, gay, bisexual, trans-gender) persons to the inappropriately lobotomized McMurphy in *One Flew Over the Cuckoo's Nest*, commonsense thinking is replete with various forms of the thought that we are worse off insofar as our lives or states of mind are not authentic—if they are not genuinely or fully our own. McMurphy's case is particularly striking: his friend Chief, seeing that he is no longer himself, euthanizes him. We are given no evidence that McMurphy faces a life of suf-fering or frustrated desires; the act is incomprehensible on, for example, a hedonistic account of well-being. Yet probably few viewers of the film have trouble relating to Chief's choice, and it is plausible that the preoperation McMurphy would have wanted it.

To distill the insight at work in these kinds of examples, we might imagine a device that can arbitrarily change a person's brain to yield whatever psychological characteristics one might wish. I shall call this imaginary device a *soulscrambler* since I wish to focus on its ability to manipulate the sorts of characteristics that have traditionally been associated with the soul, but which I will assume are merely the aspects of ordinary psychology that we deem especially important. Let's assume we have the device set on "full scramble," so that no recognizable features of the individual's personality remain.[17] With this device one could change Mother Teresa into someone with the personality of Imelda Marcos or vice-versa. Dour Wittgenstein could be transformed into a bubbly extrovert like Richard Simmons. Violent offenders could, with shades of *A Clockwork Orange*, be turned into upstanding citizens, and so forth. Whatever worries arise in the fa-miliar examples noted previously, they are presumably at least as pronounced in the case of soulscrambling. Were such a device possible, I suspect the market for it would be small indeed, perhaps confined to buyers with less-than-benevolent intentions.

Perhaps some will be tempted to dismiss the whole family of intuitions suggesting that authenticity is an important element of well-being. One could, for example, embrace a skeptical or deflationary view of the self, thus leaving little work for any notion of being true to one's self. This possibility needs to be taken seriously, and I do not try to rebut it here. But I hope it is clear how deeply revisionary such a move would be: to expunge concerns about authenticity would, at least arguably, entail a radical departure from commonsense thinking about who we are and how we ought to live.

If we want the concept of authenticity to have teeth, we shall need (a) some notion of a person's "true nature" that they can authentically realize and (b) a real possibility that a person's "manifest nature" (or life) can diverge significantly from their "true nature," yielding some diminution of authenticity. Hedonistic and desire theories rarely offer any such specification.[18] List theories generally do not even try to make room for authenticity since they simply posit a list of goods, unmoored in any account of the characteristics of those for whom the list is supposed to be good.[19]

The notion of authenticity is most clearly at home—and indeed may be unavoidable—within the fourth sort of account of well-being that we began with: a nature-fulfillment framework. Plausibly, one cannot flourish, fulfilling one's nature, if one is not even really oneself or if one's true character is being suppressed. This is not to say that the notion of authenticity is always or even usually made explicit in this sort of theorizing about well-being or flourishing. One will not encounter the term in a translation of Aristotle's *Nichomachean Ethics*, for instance. Yet Aristotelian responses to cases of brainwashing, lobotomy, drugging, and so forth would arguably reveal an implicit commitment to authenticity:

> It may even be held that [the intellect] is the true self of each, inasmuch as it is the dominant and better part; and therefore it would be a strange thing if a man should choose to live not his own life but the life of some other than himself. Moreover ... that which is best and most pleasant for each creature is that which is proper to the nature of each; accordingly the life of the intellect is the best and the pleasantest life for man, inasmuch as the intellect more than anything else is man.[20]

In short, the most distinctive philosophical concerns about well-being raised by human enhancement technologies, including applications of gene editing toward that end, have to do with the notion of authenticity. And the notion of authenticity, in turn, is most clearly at home within the framework of nature-fulfillment theories of well-being and their associated ideals of flourishing. Note that this leaves open how exactly authenticity figures in well-being; perhaps it is a weak requirement that only becomes salient in fairly unusual cases and only makes a modest impact on well-being. Or perhaps it is a much more important practical concern—maybe so important that being authentic suffices for well-being. This last possibility seems implausible—it seems one can perfectly well be authentically unhappy, say, and even that authenticity sometimes demands being unhappy, as when a family member dies. But we can leave those questions aside here.

Gene Editing, Authenticity, and Flourishing

Suppose authenticity does play some fundamental role in well-being. How does this bear on the potential benefits or harms of gene editing technologies? Compared to most other implements for human modification, gene editing presents a special puzzle: Standard examples of inauthenticity take existing persons as starting points and then transform them, raising questions about whether the result is true to the original. Yet germline gene editing, at least as it concerns us here, intervenes at or before the point of an individual's creation, or perhaps soon enough after conception as effectively to amount to the same thing. There is no original to whom the resulting individual might be more or less faithful: the edited version, it seems, *is* the original. For this reason, gene editing might be thought to raise no questions of authenticity and in turn to have no special impact on the individual's flourishing.

Yet popular concerns about such technologies having to do with "designer babies" and the like *do* seem very much to be worries about authenticity, with much the same form as concerns about other enhancement technologies that might be applied further along in a person's development. And it is not clear why anyone should care very much about authenticity if it made no difference whether the person's basic makeup was another person's creation—if, in a sense, the "original" wasn't really an original. Again putting the matter in stark terms, imagine a companion device to the soulscrambler, the *soulmaker*, differing only in that it does not need an existing person to work with: it can build a person from scratch, with whatever psychological characteristics are desired.[21] It seems odd to posit diminished flourishing as the product of soulscrambling, but not soulmaking: In both cases the person is substantially someone else's creation, and any meaningful notion of authenticity seems at best compromised. "Be true to the laboratory staff's designs" is not very inspiring, whether the designing was done at age zero or thirty.

It appears to matter, not only that one's state of mind, actions, and life reflect one's true self, but also that the self be truly one's own and not the product of another's will. That is, part of authenticity is what we might call *nonheteronomy*: that one's character and life not be determined by others.[22] We might thus say that soulmaking undermines authenticity by making individuals heteronomous in a certain way.[23]

Does gene editing diminish flourishing in any way by threatening authenticity? I do not take a stand on this question here, as the issues are complex and my chief purpose is to show that authenticity concerns need to be taken seriously when thinking about human modification technologies. Depending on the application, at least one of two philosophical issues needs to be addressed in settling whether a given form of gene editing diminishes flourishing:

1. Where an individual undergoes change (as with somatic cell gene editing): What counts as an *authenticity-preserving transformation*? Rational persuasion is presumably authenticity preserving, whereas brainwashing seems not to be. Some cases are not so clear, especially in the context of human enhancement.
2. Where there isn't a transformation of an existing person but an intervention that occurs at or before the individual's creation (as with germline gene editing): Does the intervention compromise authenticity, or its value,[24] in the resulting person?

Deciding these questions is not a trivial undertaking, but even without a systematic framework we can make some preliminary suggestions about the well-being implications of gene editing.

Gene editing may compromise authenticity in some cases, especially where person-level characteristics are targeted—intelligence, empathy, cheerfulness, and so on.[25] Were a young man with artistic talent to learn that this owes to his parents having selected the "Picasso Special" at his conception, he might reasonably find his reasons to take up painting to be less compelling: the talent ultimately owes not to some brute fact about him, but to his parents' choice to have a certain kind of child. Concerns of this sort are open to challenge, however: such enhancements will usually do no more than bias development in certain ways, leaving ample room for environmental influences and individual decisions to yield different outcomes. What we are talking about may in practice be fairly distant from soulscramblers and soulmakers.

In very many cases, at least, gene editing probably poses no threat to authenticity. Most applications presently under consideration, or likely to be pursued in the near future, are therapeutic, not "enhancements" (I set aside the difficulty of drawing a sharp line here). Modifying a genome to prevent cystic fibrosis does not approximate soulmaking even to a tiny degree: the resulting healthy teenager has no reasons—or no more reasons than usual—for an existential crisis.[26] "Am I really my own person?" is not a question that arises in this scenario.

In fact, gene editing might sometimes *enhance* authenticity.[27] Depression, for instance, can suppress much of one's personality. Editing out a predisposition toward this condition, even if it bears some costs in authenticity—maybe having a depressive personality is part of who you are—may enhance authenticity sufficiently in other respects by allowing a fuller expression of one's character to yield, on the whole, an increase in authenticity. It is also possible that one's depressive tendencies are simply disordered and form no part of one's true self. For similar reasons, many patients experience antidepressants as enhancing the authenticity of their responses to their lives, though others see them as diminishing authenticity if, for example, the enhanced mood doesn't reflect their personality.[28]

Even if authenticity is somewhat compromised by an intervention, such costs might sometimes be partly or wholly offset by gains of other sorts: It may be good, for instance, that someone's life is made more pleasant, with less suffering, whether it is fully authentic or not. Similarly, one might regard the use of antidepressants to treat ordinary, healthy grieving as reducing the authenticity of one's emotional responses somewhat, but still think it beneficial on the whole: the loss of authenticity is perhaps quite small and the hedonic gains well worth it. Similarly, one might engage in minor acts of self-deception, say about one's children or parents, for peace of mind. Such cases are a far cry from the *Cuckoo's Nest* scenario.

Importantly, authenticity need not be understood in the "thick" manner I've been assuming here (for more on "thick" vs. "thin" thinking, see John Evans' Chapter 3 in this volume). For some, authenticity is a matter of self-creation, and to attempt to conform one's life to some substantial notion of a given nature, or essence, is to be inauthentic.[29] With this sort of approach, gene editing of just about any sort is no cause for concern: so long as one's capacity for free choice remains intact, one can perfectly well be authentic. Indeed, if they enhance the individual's powers of self-creation, even quite extreme interventions, including soulmaking or self-imposed soulscrambling, might promote authenticity.

The thin conception of authenticity may be coherent, but it cannot make sense of some of the worries that, we saw, motivate ordinary concern for authenticity: Cases of drug-induced happiness and brain procedures, for instance, tend to evoke the relevant intuitions regardless of whether the individual chose it for himself. Had McMurphy arranged the lobotomy himself, the standard reaction would, if anything, have been to find his vacant condition even more lamentable than it was. For the most part, the arguments for valuing authenticity caution against the thin conception. To adopt a thin notion of authenticity is effectively to take the highly revisionary skeptical position described previously: perhaps the right move, for all I have argued, but a very costly one.

As well, defenses of thin approaches sometimes assume that the alternative to authenticity as self-creation is authenticity as "self-discovery," where the goal is to conform our lives to some given, and apparently fixed, nature.[30] But any sane view of authenticity will recognize that human beings are dynamic and constantly evolving. A thick conception of authenticity could also allow ample room for projects of self-creation to promote flourishing: A given individual might just as authentically choose to be an accountant as an artist if both pursuits suit his personality. Similarly, an artist might, authentically in any reasonable sense, leave behind an unhappy childhood, adopt a new identity, and lead a radically unorthodox lifestyle. Perhaps with the right technology he (or she) even engages in manipulations of personality, temperament, or memory; these might compromise authenticity in some respects but enhance it in others, liberating him from the burdens of an oppressive past. Even if authenticity is somewhat compromised, bringing some cost in well-being, perhaps he gains enough in other respects, like relieving considerable suffering, to make it beneficial on balance. Finally, there are plausibly other values in life besides well-being, and even if he is worse off for the manipulations he might realize enough in terms of other values, such as artistic accomplishment, to make it worthwhile. (Good art is, notoriously, not always in the artist's own best interests.)

I have suggested that a plausible account of well-being will include a fairly robust conception of authenticity, regarding many manipulations—including perhaps some applications of gene editing—as exacting significant costs on the individual's well-being. But this leaves open that there may also be significant benefits, or other reasons not having to do with well-being, to engaging in them. And it leaves open the possibility that each of us might authentically flourish in any of a radically diverse array of futures, some of them quite transformative. Self-discovery, if that's the right word for it, need not preclude, and might sometimes demand, self-creation.

Conclusion

A central goal in this chapter has been to show that the notion of authenticity and attendant concerns about the use of certain technologies aimed at enhancement are deeply embedded in ordinary thinking about the good life, are not as obscure or mysterious as commentators sometimes suggest, and deserve to be taken seriously: we have good reason to care about authenticity in matters of human well-being. One might wonder why authenticity isn't more widely discussed in the well-being literature and why the concept is so often associated with modern individualism. The answer may be that, for most of human history, authenticity was not generally a major practical concern: Most people have not chosen to be lotus eaters or otherwise in obvious ways to suppress or tamper with their personalities. For the most part, people tend to be themselves and to manifest who they are in how they live. What modernity may instead have brought about was, first, a more or less new way of thinking about authenticity: as an ideal of living that many of us are too conventional, unreflective, or hidebound to satisfy. Whatever its merits, this is indeed an ideal that many people reject. A second likely factor is the proliferation of technologies capable of influencing our psychologies in ways that raise questions of authenticity even on more traditional conceptions. We are learning how to shape the soul, far more than human beings ever could, and this makes matters of authenticity a live practical concern, far more than they ever were. What was largely implicit in thinking about the good life must now be made explicit and thought through more clearly.

There will of course be many, including many hedonists, desire theorists, and list theorists, who remain unconvinced that authenticity has any deep role in human well-being.[31] For those readers I want to close with a parting observation: Very many of our fellow citizens, perhaps most, see things otherwise and, like the Little Prince, are deeply committed to the value of authenticity. They are not unreasonable in this conviction. Indeed, the eccentric view may be puzzlement about why McMurphy's lobotomy should be such a big deal that his friend would see euthanasia as the only fitting response. When setting policy regarding emerging biotechnologies, including gene editing, we need to take those values seriously, whether we agree with them or not.[32]

Notes

1. See, for example, Erik Parens, *Shaping Ourselves: On Technology, Flourishing, and a Habit of Thinking* (Oxford: Oxford University Press, 2015); Neil Levy, "Enhancing Authenticity," *Journal of Applied Philosophy* 28, no. 3 (2011): 308–318; David Degrazia, "Enhancement Technologies and Human Identity," *The Journal of Medicine and Philosophy* 31 no. 3 (2005): 261–283; Carl Elliott, *Better Than Well: American Medicine Meets the American Dream* (New York: Norton, 2003).

2. A seminal recent discussion, which heavily influenced the present discussion, is L. Wayne Sumner, *Welfare, Happiness, and Ethics* (Oxford: Oxford University Press, 1996). I discuss authenticity in relation to well-being at length in Daniel M. Haybron, *The Pursuit of Unhappiness: The Elusive Psychology of Well-Being* (New York: Cambridge University Press, 2008).

3. Cf. Charles Taylor, *The Ethics of Authenticity* (Cambridge, MA: Harvard University Press, 1991).

4. Other philosophers divide up the field differently. For a review of the literature, see Haybron, *Pursuit of Unhappiness*, ch. 2. An excellent recent collection is Guy Fletcher, ed., *The Routledge Handbook of Philosophy of Well-Being* (New York: Routledge, 2015).

5. Danial Hausman, *Preferences, Value, Choice, and Welfare* (New York: Cambridge University Press, 2011).

6. Robert Nozick, *Anarchy, State, and Utopia* (New York: Basic Books, 1974).

7. For a related discussion, see Michael Burdett's Chapter 12 in this volume; also, Celia Deane-Drummond's Chapter 13.

8. My reading of Mill is based on his discussion of individuality in *On Liberty*, which is arguably a classic statement of an ideal of self-fulfillment. John Stuart Mill, *On Liberty*, ed. John Gray (New York: Oxford, 1991).

9. For example, Benjamin Yelle, "Alienation, Deprivation, and the Well-Being of Persons," *Utilitas* 26, no. 4 (2014): 367–384.

10. For example, Daniel M. Haybron, "Happiness, the Self and Human Flourishing," *Utilitas* 20, no. 1 (2008): 21–49.

11. The idea of self-realization plays a major role in Hindu thought; for nature-fulfillment ideals in the Confucian tradition, see Richard Kim, "Well-Being and Confucianism," in *The Routledge Handbook of Philosophy of Well-Being*, ed. Guy Fletcher (New York: Routledge, 2015), 40–55.

12. For example, arguably, Sumner, *Welfare*; Mill, *On Liberty*; John Harsanyi, "Morality and the Theory of Rational Behaviour," in *Utilitarianism and Beyond*, eds. Amartya Sen and Bernard Williams (Cambridge: Cambridge University Press, 2011), 39–62.

13. See Haybron, *Pursuit of Unhappiness*; Daniel M. Haybron, "The Philosophical Basis of Eudaimonic Psychology," in *Handbook of Eudaimonic Well-Being*, ed. Joar Vitterso (New York: Springer, 2016), 27–53. If we have reason to value authenticity or nature-fulfillment, it is because those notions are deeply embedded in our sensibilities—in the way we see and think about human life. It bears remarking that ideas resembling nature-fulfillment seem to inform a good deal of practice in the healthcare professions. For instance, the notions of health and disorder are commonly defined in Aristotelian-sounding terms, via conformity to species norms, even in ostensibly "value-free" theories (see Christopher Boorse, "Health as a Theoretical Concept," *Philosophy of Science* 44, no. 4 (1977): 542–573). If functioning in species-typical ways partly defines health, it may not be so odd to think it also plays a role in defining flourishing. In fact it might be odd to hold one view and not the other.

14. On authenticity as an ethical ideal, and not merely an aspect of well-being, see, for example, Taylor, *Ethics of Authenticity*; Charles Guignon, *On Being Authentic* (London: Routledge, 2004). Note that these authors were also keen to distance the notion of authenticity from popular associations with self-indulgence.

15. See, for example, L. Slabu, A. P. Lenton, C. Sedikides, and M. Bruder, "Trait and State Authenticity Across Cultures," *Journal of Cross-Cultural Psychology* 45, no. 9 (2014): 1347–1373. The Daoist tradition discussed in Richard Kim's Chapter 5 in this volume may also endorse something akin to authenticity.

16. See the previous references to "deep self" views of responsibility.

17. Those concerned that this would amount to replacing a person with a numerically different one may imagine dialing down the machine so that it merely makes a radical change.

18. In general, subjectivist theories struggle to accommodate these demands, though an important exception is Sumner's account of well-being as "authentic happiness" (see Sumner, *Welfare*). On this view, to be authentically happy, hence doing well, is for one's happiness to be informed and autonomous—reflecting one's life as it truly

is and constituting a response to that life that is truly one's own. But there is some question about whether the authenticity constraint is really compatible with his subjectivism (see Mark Lebar, "Good for You," *Pacific Philosophical Quarterly* 85, no. 2 (2004): 195–217; Habron, "Happiness" and *Pursuit of Unhappiness*).

19. In this respect subjectivist and nature-fulfillment theories resemble each other more than either do most objective list theories; both make your good dependent on the sort of creature you are. For list theories, things like knowledge or friendship are just good to have, period. If you're a rock or a lizard, so much the worse for you. And so much the worse for us humans, compared to ET, who can rack up even more of the list items than we can—and presumably knows of list items we can't even imagine.

20. Aristotle, *Nicomachean Ethics*, trans H. Rackham (Cambridge, MA: Harvard University Press, 1926), 1178a2–1178a7.

21. This is far more extreme, note, even than constructing a person's genome from scratch: here we are determining both genotype and phenotype.

22. Nonheteronomy is a weaker condition than autonomy, as commonly understood: People are not ordinarily autonomous or self-determining in the basic nature they start with, which is just an accident of no one's choosing, but for the same reason, neither are they heteronomous.

23. Perhaps authenticity isn't quite the right rubric for this concern since it seems to implicate us in speaking of being true to an "original" that neither exists nor has determinate form. But as just noted, the problem with soulmaking seems closely analogous to that of soulscrambling. It may be most accurate to say only that a kind of heteronomy is at stake, and this in turn bears on the *value* of an individual's authenticity, so that (say) a replicant from *Blade Runner* might be fully authentic, but only in a second-rate manner, with a diminished capacity for flourishing. To keep things simple I set this question aside here as it may not matter from a practical standpoint.

24. I usually omit this qualification for convenience.

25. Note, however, that similar-seeming concerns might arise with interventions targeting physical characteristics, say with the aim of promoting athletic ability. Whether these involve person-level characteristics is not entirely clear.

26. Confusion may arise over the fact that just about any personal characteristic, including having cystic fibrosis, can become part of a person's self-conception or identity, in one sense of that term. I do not elaborate here but do not think that notion of identity is relevant to the present discussion. Roughly, our discussion concerns psychological analogues of the "soul" (e.g., personality, character) and not (or not in the first instance) mere self-descriptions.

27. Cf. Levy, "Enhancing Authenticity."

28. See, for example, Peter Kramer, *Listening to Prozac* (New York: Penguin, 1993).

29. This sort of thought is familiar from Sartre and other existentialists; see also Levy, "Enhancing Authenticity."

30. For helpful discussion, see Parens, *Shaping Ourselves*; Levy, "Enhancing Authenticity."

31. Though, as noted previously, even they may tacitly rely on some notion of authenticity, say through an unacknowledged commitment to ideals of self-fulfillment.

32. Indeed, those values may be dispositive for policymakers deciding what's best for the people holding them, even if the values are ultimately mistaken (Daniel M. Haybron and Valerie Tiberius, "Well-Being Policy: What Standard of Well-Being?" *Journal of the American Philosophical Association* 1, no. 4 (2015): 712–733).

3

The Dismal Fate of Flourishing in Public Policy Bioethics

A Sociological Explanation

John H. Evans

There has been a long-standing ethical norm against modifying the germline of the human species for any reason. This is written into law throughout most of Europe and is also the centerpiece of the Oviedo convention.[1] The development of CRISPR technology, which could apparently modify human germ cells with ease, seemed to have caught the world by surprise. A group of prominent scientists immediately called for a temporary moratorium on using gene editing technology to "edit" the genes of human embryos and organized a three-day international summit to examine the safety and ethical issues.[2] After this 2015 summit the organizing committee, comprising ten scientists and two bioethicists, released a statement.[3]

They called for the continuation of "basic and preclinical" research on editing human sperm, eggs, and embryos as long as those entities were destroyed and not implanted in a woman. They reiterated the social consensus that somatic gene editing for disease is morally acceptable and should be treated like any other experimental medical treatment.

Without explicitly saying so, they argued against the idea of taking the germline to be an ethical line in the sand. They did, though, identify six issues of concern with germline modifications of humans. The first four were variations on risk or harms that our present lack of knowledge could cause, but, the authors of the statement implied, with advancing knowledge these concerns could soon be overcome. The fifth concern was that enhancements to subsets of the population could "exacerbate social inequalities or be used coercively." The sixth seemed to be a vague gesture in a catch-all phrase toward what the committee did not ultimately pursue at the summit: "the moral and ethical considerations in purposefully altering human evolution."[4] Everything besides relieving individual suffering, respecting the self-determination of persons, and avoiding social inequality is vaguely placed into "moral and ethical considerations."

The statement's authors went on to say that the clinical use of germline gene editing should not be done "unless and until" the "safety and efficacy issues have been resolved" and there is "broad societal consensus about the appropriateness of the proposed application." Again, in contrast to previous consensus against any germline modification, this presumes that some germline applications will be acceptable and others not, and that the germline is not morally significant. They supported these presumptions by noting that "as scientific knowledge advances and societal views evolve, the clinical use of germline editing should be revisited on a regular basis."

As is now common in these sorts of discussions, the group did not claim to be making decisions, but rather called for public debate. Again, as is also common, no specifics were offered regarding how that public debate could impact what actually happens with this technology. They invoked the "need for an ongoing forum," saying that the "international community should strive to establish norms concerning acceptable uses of human germline editing . . . in order to discourage unacceptable activities while advancing human health and welfare." In other words, human germline gene editing should go forward but should distinguish between the acceptable forms, which promote health, and the unacceptable forms, which, we are invited to infer, promote enhancement.

For those of us who believe that the public's values should influence which technologies are developed, it is deeply troubling that the organizing committee, after only a handful of short presentations on ethics at the summit, concluded that the traditional ban on germline modification—written into law in most of Europe—should be overturned. However, this result should not be a surprise and perhaps seemed almost natural to most people in the audience. In fact, any other conclusion would indeed have been illogical when the ends or goals that are allowed into the debate are limited to relieving individual suffering, respecting the self-determination of persons, and avoiding social inequality. Some readers may know that bioethicists tend to speak more of "principles" than of "ends." What I just called the end that is relieving suffering is closely related to the principle of *beneficence* (or doing good) and to its ethical cousin, *nonmaleficence*, which refers to avoiding doing harm. The end that is respecting the self-determination of persons is closely related to the principle of *autonomy*, and the end that is avoiding social inequality is closely related to the principle of *justice*. It is important to recognize, however, that each of these four principles represents what these bioethicists took to be a noncontroversial end or goal, something they thought that most human beings, across cultures, would endorse. This use of these three ends (or four principles, if you distinguish doing good and avoiding harm) is consistent with the dominant form of reason in contemporary public bioethics, which I will call a "thin" form of ethics. What was largely excluded from the summit is what I will call a "thick" form of ethics.

For the purposes of this chapter, by the word *thick* I mean a debate that is *about* the ends or goals that we should or should not pursue by means of a technology, with the ends and the means being considered together. A thick debate is about the ends or purposes that remain after we have dispensed with the ends (autonomy, beneficence, and justice) that are usually privileged; it is a debate about the more controversial end that is human well-being or flourishing. A thin debate assumes that the list of ends deserving public endorsement is fixed and relatively short and also assumes that the most pressing policy question is whether a given means at hand, like gene editing technologies, will maximize those ends.[5] The 2015 summit was thin because it largely presumed that the only relevant ends were beneficence, nonmaleficence, and autonomy—with a bit of justice (avoiding inequality) thrown in—and the question was how to promote gene editing without violating those ends. With only those ends in the discussion, however, it is difficult to argue against germline interventions as a whole, so it is no surprise that the summit leaders' conclusion seemed quite sensible by the conclusion of their gathering. The normalization of these thin debates in public bioethics poses a large challenge to the effort to foster a conversation about flourishing.

We should then ask, If there was a public debate about flourishing, what ends would that public identify that they think would be relevant to a debate about gene editing? Because professionals in this debate over the last 50 years or so have tended to forgo discussion of ends other than the ones articulated by the authors of the summit statement, we do not actually have a firm handle on which ends the public would identify. We do, however, have limited social science research suggesting that, in addition to the ends that are autonomy, beneficence, nonmaleficence, and justice, the public also values keeping humans natural and respecting the inherent value of all humans. (The research shows that by that latter phrase, the public is referring to more than what is captured by, e.g., autonomy.) More on these in material that follows, but yes, the now six ends in the list would contradict each other at least at points. For example, humans might suffer less if people disregarded naturalness and just optimized genetic changes to reduce physical suffering. These contradictions are, in my view, the messy reality of the public's values, and navigating them is the work of a thick public debate.

I should, of course, go one step more abstract and contextualize this public bioethical debate itself. The structure of the debate as having ends and means in relation to a genetic technology is only one possible way that biotechnology could be discussed. For example, one could question the focus on technology itself and ask whether addressing certain social structures, such as pollution and poverty, could have a greater impact on flourishing than any use of gene editing. In this volume, Dorothy Roberts (Chapter 14), Jackie Leach Scully (Chapter 10), and Rosemarie Garland-Thomson (Chapter 1) all ask variants of this more rad-ical question. I stick to the more limited and pragmatic public bioethical debate, while acknowledging that it is not the only possible debate and recognizing that it even serves as a bulwark against more radical critique.

The Reason to Want a Thick Debate

The reason to want a thicker debate in public bioethics is, as the adjective *thicker* is supposed to convey, that the current thin debate fails to reflect all that really matters to most people. I agree with the tradition of thinking associated with Jürgen Habermas, which worries that the "system" (institutions governed by thin ethics) is taking over the "life-world" (governed by thick ethics).[6] The life-world is the public sphere, the location of free debate about ends, unencumbered by the bias introduced by debates that presume only a narrow range of ends. The ability to have a substantively rational debate about our ends in the life-world has be-come limited due to this take-over.

The effect of this takeover is that if certain ends or values are assumed, you cannot then have a societal debate about what our collective ends or values should be. Without a debate about our goals, we are enslaved to our means. The problem with not debating ends was evocatively put by Leon Kass, who is politi-cally conservative. Articulating a perspective that is similar to the one articulated by politically liberal critics of technology such as Jacques Ellul, Kass wrote to the first government bioethics commission to examine human genetic engineering in 1982, rejecting that commission's thin assumptions:

> For to begin with "technology" . . . is to continue to give first place to power and derivative place to ends or goods or "values." It is of the essence of the modern view of technique . . . that it is neutral with regard to the uses to which it is put. Yet the human agents who practice or support science are not themselves neu-tral regarding the ends. Everybody acts on some notion, even if only implicit, of what they regard to be a good or worthy human life, for themselves or for their communities. The disjunction between the human view of the human and the modern technical view—"Now I have bricks, what can I do with them?"—is a deep cause of our problems with technology and with the relation between sci-ence and human affairs generally.[7]

That is, in a healthy public sphere, the summit I described at the beginning of this chapter would have started with a thick debate about our ends or goals, rather than simply assuming a few institutionalized ends and then proceeding to evaluate our means—gene editing technology—in relation to those ends. Large swaths of the public want to engage in discussion that includes more than those institutionalized ends. They want to engage in debate that allows for discussion of the end that in this volume is being called "flourishing." This desire suggests that the four ends that currently dominate the debate, while portrayed as either universal or somehow natural, are actually only the ends that are promoted by a particular group in society with power, such as scientists.

One end that is largely excluded from this debate is that all humans should be considered to have equal worth or value, regardless of their capacities. This is often what is meant by the term *dignity*.[8] Note that this is different from the autonomy (and justice) that was gestured to at the summit. The end that is autonomy enables us to respect human beings' choices. The end that is dignity enables us to respect what human beings are, independent of what they choose or can do. (For more on the concept of dignity, see Gaymon Bennett's Chapter 16.)

You can tell when someone has dignity in mind in these debates because they describe the problem with eugenics differently than do adherents of the thin debate. In the thin debate, eugenic practices are a problem if they are unequally available to citizens, but not if they teach us that different human beings have different human worth or value. For someone who invokes a value like dignity, even eugenic practices undertaken autonomously can be a problem insofar as they teach that people's moral worth is a function of what someone will be able to do or how they will appear, based on our interpretation of their genome. Hence, the concern of disability scholars is that the public is learning that people with some genetic profiles are worth less than people with others.[9] That people with disabilities could thereby lose, for example, access to certain services—the thin concern—is different from the thicker concern about the perception of the worth or value of people with disabilities.

No study has specifically investigated whether the public agrees dignity should be an end in relationship to human genetics. But, in a highly relevant and classic study, the authors wrote that "the belief in the equal worth and dignity of all human beings also underlies the modern welfare state," and that "this assumption of the equality of human worth is so deeply ingrained in American political culture as to be axiomatic for most people." They cited a survey where 78% agreed that "teaching children that all people are really equal . . . recognizes that all people are equally worthy and deserve equal treatment" and another that showed that 98% of the public agreed that "everyone in America should have equal opportunities to get ahead."[10] In a study focused on what the range of religious people in the United States thought about reproductive genetic technologies, I found that a central way that respondents organized their ethics was around the idea of dignity and equality of treatment.[11] I think that the public would like an end like dignity, at least as I am defining it, included in these debates.

Another end that the public likely would like to promote in these debates is "keeping humans natural." Obviously the word *natural* incites controversy among philosophers (see Gregory Kaebnick's Chapter 6 in this volume), but by it I refer simply to the way that humans "are," as a result of evolution. By keeping humans natural, I refer to the often-invoked desire to eschew the use of genetic technologies in changing the way that humans are. That is, on such a view, the flourishing of human beings entails appreciating and affirming the way we have come to be. It entails exercising caution in departing from what some call the "givenness" of our way of being.

This view concerning the value of affirming the way that we, absent direct human intervention, have evolved to be is in evidence in numerous studies that showed the public's great support for the use of germline modification to treat diseases—and its weak support for "enhancements."[12] Of course, what a disease is also is controversial among philosophers, but most people think of it as a negatively impactful deviation from "normality," or from "natural" or "species-typical" functioning. So, if there were no other concerns with germline modification (which there are), I suspect that Americans would generally favor germline modification to return people to genetic normalcy: to natural or species-typical functioning. For example, they would approve of removing a gene for Huntington's disease and giving the recipient the functional version of the gene that the vast majority of the public has. That highly technological change is still natural in that most humans have the "normal" version, and these humans evolved with little human intervention. Creating some genetic sequence that no human has ever had, even if it would "only" improve health, would be seen as enhancement and thus unnatural. So, using germline modification to pursue even this health-related end might create ethical concern in some, but we will not know because the grounds for articulating that concern have been ruled out of bounds in the public debate.

I have no doubt that there are other ends that many members of the public would use in their evaluation of human applications of gene editing. But, the main point is that we know little about what those ends or values are because we have set up our public debate to exclude the discussion of ends beyond the thin ones like autonomy.

Why Is the Debate about Gene Editing Thin?

The summit was thin, as is most of contemporary public bioethics. Showing how we got to this point will show a positive path forward, or at least reveal the magnitude of the problem, so a brief history of American public bioethical debate is in order.

The Original Thick Debate

During the 1960s, scientists had many meetings to discuss emerging technologies, such as human genetic engineering, that seemed to have profound moral implications. It was an era of questioning a wide range of ends, not just the means. Where are we taking ourselves with our new technological abilities? was the central theme. As one participant at a conference noted, "Although [medicine's] foundations have become more rational, its practice . . . is said to have become more remote and indifferent to human values, and once again medicine has been forced to remind itself that it is often the human factors that are determinant." The point of the conference was "not simply the question of the survival or the extinction of [humankind], but *what kind* of survival? A future of what *nature*?"[13]

Theologians, speaking in a secular register, as well as others with a thick orientation, soon entered this debate about *which* ends we should pursue with our newfound technological abilities. They were asking questions and using language that was surely not used at the summit and that is ever more difficult for us to imagine hearing in the public square today. In 1972, Leon Kass remarked about human cloning: "For man is the watershed which divides the world into those things that belong to nature and those that are made by men. To lay one's hands on human generation is to take a major step toward making man himself simply another of the man-made things."[14] That is, this technology would turn us into objects, which would violate our dignity. Daniel Callahan, cofounder of The Hastings Center, responded to Kass by asking "whether man's humanity can survive" the new technologies. He noted that scientists probably "believe that their work is both praiseworthy and intensively human. To seek knowledge is human. To improve man's lot is human. To make things, even human beings, is human." Holding in mind his own thought and taking seriously Kass's, Callahan called for further debate over "some general, comprehensive, and universal norms for 'the human.'"[15] This thick questioning was soon marginalized.

The theologians and their allies were questioning where the scientists were going with technologies like human genetic engineering, and the public began to pay attention, soon generating the attention of elected officials. But the debate quickly became thin when the bureaucratic state, which implicitly demands that arguments be thin, became its primary audience.

The emergence of a thin form of ethical argumentation called *principlism*, which would come to dominate mainstream bioethics, emerged out of the first federal bioethics commission, which first met in 1974. The commission was mandated to "identify the basic ethical principles which should underlie the conduct of biomedical and behavioral research involving human subjects" and "develop guidelines which should be followed in such research to assure that it is conducted in accord with such principles."[16] In other words, they were to create the ethical system for bioethics that could be useful for the bureaucratic state.

The commission called attention to three primary principles—or what previously I called "ends"—that were "among those generally accepted in our cultural tradition": respect for persons, beneficence, and justice. These three undergirded the practices of informed consent, risk-benefit analysis, and the selection of research subjects, respectively.[17] These principles were later given the force of law for research conducted with federal money. After promotion of a closely related system in a prominent textbook,[18] principlism came to be the dominant form of ethical argumentation in all debates that involved bioethical policy. The textbook arranged the ends into the form that will be familiar to some readers today, defining respect for persons as autonomy and splitting beneficence into two ends: beneficence and nonmaleficence. Two observers went so far as to say that "by establishing itself as the state-sanctioned authority for converting discussions of good and bad in American medical science into a common language and concepts, the bioethics of principlism achieved the status of an ascendant political currency with global potential."[19] These few principles became established as *the* ends or purposes, which would inform future debate—and would not need to be questioned. The debate had been thinned. These are roughly the ends used at the summit that I discussed at the beginning of this chapter.

Why the Bureaucratic State Prefers Thin Ethics

Whenever discussing an ethical issue as it relates to policy formation, the bureaucratic state prefers thin ethics and excludes the sort of thick ethics that would allow for a substantive discussion of flourishing. Even the few government ethics commissions that discussed the idea of flourishing, such as the commission of President George W. Bush, did not actually get the discussion to the point of defining it. The overarching reason for the state's preference for thin ethics is that American citizens do not trust government. Historian Theodore Porter wrote that in other countries government officials are "trusted to exercise judgment wisely and fairly. In the United States, they are expected to follow rules."[20] They are not trusted to exercise discretion. This is because, put simply, it is part of the US political culture not to trust authority, especially government authority, and the authority of bureaucrats in particular. Trust that individuals in government have the proper moral orientation to guide policymaking is low, especially given the diversity of moral views in the country.

This lack of trust in government to exercise moral judgment, combined with a need for moral judgments that apply universally to all citizens, helps to explain the thinness of the few ends that are forwarded by principlism and that were admitted into the CRISPR debate at the 2015 summit. In the words of the designers of principlism, it represents "the common morality." Beauchamp and Childress, in arguing against classical forms of justification from philosophy, wrote that "if we could be confident that some abstract moral theory was a better source for codes and policies than the common morality, we could work constructively on practical and policy questions by progressively specifying the norms of that theory. At present, we have no such theory." They continued that they "cannot reasonably expect that an inherently contestable moral theory will be better for practical decision making and policy development than the morality that serves as our common heritage."[21]

With common morality, the unelected official is portrayed as simply applying the values of the people, not using their own morality or the morality of a particular group with power. I can imagine nothing that would outrage the American public more than being told that an unelected government official used their own morality to decide which values or ends should be pursued by means of publicly funded medical research.

A second reason for the bureaucratic preference for a thin ethics is that it is more calculable and thus more transparent to the citizens. With only four fixed ends, all of the complications of ethical debate can be translated into a very simple discussion, the moral equivalent of a stripped-down pidgin language. Moreover, the weighing and balancing of preset principles such as beneficence and nonmaleficence (benefits and risks)—notice the simple decision-making rule—is purportedly more transparent. Like the allure of cost-benefit analysis, the public can feel that it understands the decision being made on its behalf, thereby giving the decision legitimacy. And, all of this ethical content feeds into bureaucracies, which also need to create standardized rules.[22] In fact, Albert Jonsen later concluded that the principles, which had become part of public law, had "met the need of public-policy makers for a clear and simple statement of the ethical basis for regulation of research."[23]

We can also see why the bureaucratic state would prefer the particular ends that are institutionalized in this debate. The principles of bioethics are simultaneously portrayed as the ethics to apply to science *and* the principles of the liberal democratic state *and* the basis of American law. Put simply, in liberal democracies people can pursue their own conception of a good life (autonomy) as long as it does not harm anyone else (nonmaleficence). Thus, thinking of two of the primary ends to pursue as autonomy and nonmaleficence (e.g., promoting health) fits well with American law. Having an end that is thicker than autonomy and nonmaleficence is said not to fit with American law and policy.

A challenge for a debate about flourishing is then that any new end that is successfully introduced into the debate about gene editing will probably be challenged for not fitting with the supposed limitations of American law and policy.

Since people are said to have autonomy, and thus can determine their own notion of flourishing, any imposition of a set of ends that are not portrayed as universal (as principlism is purported to be) will be seen as paternalistic. I simply say to this point that, with the exception of some pure libertarians, of which there are very few in the United States, *people who claim that you are being paternalistic because you are advocating a particular version of flourishing actually have their own particular version of flourishing that they are promoting but not owning.* For example, there is nothing more paternalistic than an institutional review board, which stops potential research subjects from voluntarily engaging in experiments simply because the government thinks that they should not put themselves at too much risk. Believe it or not, there was a time when volunteers put themselves at great bodily risk to test medical treatments because they felt they had a religious reason to do so. Today, though, that particular conception of flourishing is not allowed.[24] We now see some of the structural impediments to moving forward with a thicker debate about flourishing. One particular conception of flourishing is so triumphant that we can no longer see it as particular.

Thinning as the Result of Regulatory Capture by Scientists

Besides the supposed articulation with American law, there is another reason that debate is limited to these few particular established ends. Returning to bioethics, the very idea of public bioethics is—or at least was when the field started— that it is *not* the scientific community. The premise was that scientists needed ethical guidance, and they were to get it from an independent public bioethical debate. That is, after all, why these elite scientists call for "ethical summits" over issues like gene editing in the first place instead of just deciding the ethics themselves. Public bioethical debate is then a type of soft regulation of science, where scientists violate the ethical consensus at their peril. However, while public bioethics and bioethicists were somewhat independent of science in the founding years—when they actually clashed with the interests of the scientific and medical community—over the years public bioethics and bioethicists have lost their independence from science.

Historians have come to the conclusion that despite bioethics' self-perception and perhaps early history of being a soft regulator of science and medicine, the professions have never been in serious competition. I concur with historian Charles Rosenberg that bioethics has

> not only questioned authority; it has in the past quarter-century helped constitute and legitimate it. As a condition of its acceptance, bioethics has taken up residence in the belly of the medical whale; although thinking of itself as still

autonomous, the bioethical enterprise has developed a complex and symbiotic relationship with this host organism. Bioethics is no longer (if it ever was) a free-floating, oppositional, and socially critical reform movement.[25]

Early bioethics enterprises were outside the belly of the medical whale. The Hastings Center, arguably the first bioethics center, was and remains free-standing, unrelated to any university or medical school. The Kennedy Institute of Ethics at Georgetown University, founded in the same era, was more associated with the philosophy and theology departments than the medical school.[26] Now bioethics centers are largely part of medical schools and often dependent on them for their funding. Moreover, all of these centers are dependent on grant income, and the granting entities, such as the National Institutes of Health, are controlled by scientists, so scientists get to define the important questions. If the arguments of bioethicists ever strayed far from the interests of the medical/scientific profession, the medical/scientific profession would have already tried to kill off bioethics instead of letting it live in (or close by) its house.

Moreover, the ends that are dominant in the current thin debate were not concocted by bioethicists but are actually the ends that physicians and scientists have (largely) come up with themselves. For example, beneficence and nonmaleficence—doing good and avoiding harm—have always been central to medicine as embodied in strictures like "first do no harm." The original conflict between science and the nascent bioethics profession was not over the content of the principles, but rather about which profession would get to use its discretion in applying them. My conclusion about the early days of the nascent bioethics profession is that bioethicists forced the scientists and physicians to clarify and rigorously apply the practices like obtaining the consent of experimental subjects that had already supposedly been put in place by the scientists.[27] The principles behind the procedures were not controversial. That is, the ends and the thin ethics used by the bioethics profession—on display at the 2015 summit—*are* the ethics endorsed by the medical/scientific profession. Mainstream bioethics finds it hard to escape the thinness of the current debate because mainstream bioethics grew out of the valorization of thinness.

What Is to Be Done?

Clearly, for our public debate to be healthy, we need to create space for the articulation of concerns that are thin *and* those that are thick. First, we need a thick debate to determine what the public thinks human flourishing *is*. Then, we need to have the inevitably and necessarily thin policy-relevant debate about how the ends identified in the thick debate could be implemented, or at least honored.

The problem at present is that there is only the thin debate proceeding with assumed and not debated ends.

A truly open thick debate would probably need to occur outside the aegis of both the scientific and mainstream bioethics communities, as they are impervious to the critique described previously. Simply showing that public bioethics has a bias toward thinness, as academics have long done, does not seem to change anything. I have elsewhere called for not so much a debate about ends but rather for social science research that would determine the ends held by the public that are relevant for a particular technology. These ends—the true public morality on an issue—could then be used as input for policymaking.[28] However, it seems unrealistic that the scientific and medical community will follow the public's ends willingly. What is needed is an independent institution dedicated to ethics, science, and medicine that can conduct a parallel ethical deliberation about ends to move forward with gene editing. This chapter is one step in that direction.

Notes

1. Motoko Araki and Tetsuya Ishii, "International Regulatory Landscape and Integration of Corrective Genome Editing into In Vitro Fertilization," *Reproductive Biology and Endocrinology* 12, no. 108 (2014): 1–12.
2. David Baltimore, Paul Berg, Michael Botchan, Dana Carroll, R. Alta Charo, George Church, Jacob E. Corn, et al., "A Prudent Path Forward for Genomic Engineering and Germline Gene Modification," *Science* 348, no. 6230 (2015): 36–38.
3. "On Human Gene Editing: International Summit Statement." Distributed at International Summit on Human Gene Editing: A Global Discussion, Washington, DC, December 3, 2015.
4. "Summit Statement," 2015.
5. For more detail on thick and thin, see John H. Evans, *Playing God? Human Genetic Engineering and the Rationalization of Public Bioethical Debate* (Chicago: University of Chicago Press, 2002), 13–21.
6. Jürgen Habermas, *The Theory of Communicative Action, Vol. 2, Lifeworld and System: A Critique of Functionalist Reason* (Boston: Beacon Press, 1987); Jurgen Habermas, *The Structural Transformation of the Public Sphere* (Cambridge, MA: MIT Press, 1989).
7. Quotations in original. Letter, Kass to Alexander Capron, April 7, 1981. President's Commission archives, Georgetown University.
8. Daniel P. Sulmasy, "Dignity and Bioethics: History, Theory, and Selected Applications," in *Human Dignity and Bioethics* (Washington, DC: President's Council on Bioethics, 2008), 472–473; Roberto Andorno, "Human Dignity and the UNESCO Declaration on the Human Genome," in *Ethics, Law and Society, Volume I.*, ed. Jennifer Gunning and Soren Holm (Burlington, VT: Ashgate, 2005), 74–75.

9. Jackie Leach Scully, "Towards a Bioethics of Disability and Impairment," in *Handbook of Genetics and Society: Mapping the New Genomic Era*, ed. Paul Atkinson, Peter Glasner, and Margaret Lock (London: Routledge, 2009), 367–381.

10. Herbert McClosky and John Zaller, *The American Ethos: Public Attitudes Toward Capitalism and Democracy* (Cambridge, MA: Harvard University Press, 1984), 62, 65, 66, 83.

11. John H. Evans, *Contested Reproduction: Genetic Technologies, Religion, and Public Debate* (Chicago: University of Chicago Press, 2010), ch. 5.

12. Evans, *Contested Reproduction*, 54.

13. Emphases in original. Cited in Albert R. Jonsen, *The Birth of Bioethics* (New York: Oxford University Press, 1998), 13.

14. Leon R Kass, "New Beginnings in Life," in *The New Genetics and the Future of Man*, ed. Michael Hamilton (Grand Rapids, MI: Eerdmans, 1972), 54.

15. Daniel Callahan, "New Beginnings in Life: A Philosopher's Response," in Hamilton, *New Genetics*, 97–99.

16. Cited in Albert R. Jonsen, "Foreword," in *A Matter of Principles? Ferment in US Bioethics*, ed. Edwin R. DuBose, Ronald P. Hamel, and Laurence J. O'Connell (Valley Forge, PA: Trinity Press International, 1994), xiv.

17. National Commission for the Protection of Human Subjects of Biomedical and Behavioral Research, *The Belmont Report: Ethical Principles and Guidelines for the Protection of Human Subjects of Research* (Washington, DC: Government Printing Office, 1978).

18. Tom L. Beauchamp and James F. Childress, *Principles of Biomedical Ethics*, 6th ed. (New York: Oxford University Press, 2009).

19. Brian Salter and Charlotte Salter, "Bioethics and the Global Moral Economy: The Cultural Politics of Human Embryonic Stem Cell Science," *Science, Technology and Human Values* 32, no. 5 (2007): 561.

20. Theodore M. Porter, *Trust in Numbers: The Pursuit of Objectivity in Science and Public Life* (Princeton, NJ: Princeton University Press, 1995), 195.

21. Beauchamp and Childress, *Biomedical Ethics*, 388–389.

22. Charles Perrow, *Complex Organizations: A Critical Essay*, 3rd ed. (New York: Random House, 1986), ch. 1.

23. Jonsen, "Foreword," xvi.

24. Laura Stark, *Behind Closed Doors: IRBs and the Making of Ethical Research* (Chicago: University of Chicago Press, 2012).

25. Charles E. Rosenberg, "Meanings, Policies, and Medicine: On the Bioethical Enterprise and History," *Daedalus* 128, no. 4 (1999): 37–38.

26. Jonsen, *Birth of Bioethics*, 22–24.

27. Stark, *Behind Closed Doors*.

28. John H. Evans, *The History and Future of Bioethics: A Sociological View* (New York: NY: Oxford University Press, 2012).

PART II
THE VALUE OF ACCEPTANCE

4

Editing the Best of All Possible Worlds

Michael Hauskeller[1]

When in 2013 the CRISPR interference technique was introduced to the world as a new, easy-to-use, and powerful method for "editing" the genomes of mice and men,[2] it quickly captured the cultural imagination and rekindled waning hopes and fears that we will soon be able to manipulate the human genome any way we please.[3] Talk about gene (or genome) editing has since, in the public sphere, widely replaced the more familiar one about genetic "engineering." The editing metaphor suggests that the genome is not the finished product but rather like the draft of a text that requires for completion the helping hand of an expert reader and corrector before it can be released to the world.

In the modern sense of the word, editing a text not only means publishing it but also removing errors and making other changes that render it more presentable to a target audience prior to publication. The purpose of editing is to make a text presentable. Gene editing has a similar purpose. It is interposed between the writing (the genetic "code") and the publication (the organism that eventually results from its coding). In text editing, the editing process removes obvious mistakes and generally aims to make the text more readable before it goes to press. Beyond the obvious mistakes (the typos and grammatical errors), which need to be corrected to create a common ground of communication between the author and the reader, lies the gray zone: where changes are possible, perhaps desirable to increase clarity, readability, and indeed beauty, but are not strictly necessary. Here the editor has to tread carefully. They not only need to grasp the author's intention and help it become more transparent, which requires its alignment with the normal, the established conventions of writing in a certain language, but *also* need to make sure that the author's voice (unique way of expressing a point) does not get lost or distorted in the process. A good editor does not completely rewrite a text so that it better reflects his or her own views. Instead, they merely help it become what the author meant it to be, recognizing the fact that there are many different ways to express an idea and many different ideas to express.

When it comes to gene editing, we can also identify the obvious mistakes and distinguish them from, as it were, questions of style, where it is not immediately clear what is right and what is wrong, better or worse. And here, in this gray area,

I suggest, the aspiring gene editor also ought to respect the voice of nature (for more, see Gregory Kaebnick's Chapter 6 in this volume) as the original author of the text. The gene editor must recognize the fact that we are not all the same, or laid out to be the same, that there are many different ways of living a good life and being a valuable member of the human community. The good gene editor does not attempt to subject all human output to their own standards of correctness or their own ideals of what a truly good human life might require. Instead, they respect both the value of normality and the twin values of diversity and otherness without trying to enforce them. Some degree of normality is helpful because it promotes an individual's smooth integration into a community, without which a good human life is very difficult to achieve. At the same time, diversity and otherness make our lives rich, strong, and interesting.

Editing Dilemmas

If gene editing is to be used to select for certain traits that are deemed desirable and against others that are deemed undesirable, then somebody needs to decide which traits to select for and which to select against. However, it is far from obvious which criteria should be used to determine what is desirable and what not. The safest, most innocuous option would seem to be to concentrate on genes that we are confident are causally connected to certain devastating defects, disorders, diseases, and disabilities (the typos and grammatical errors of the genetic text) and can thus be understood as in some way seriously debilitating.

There are high hopes that the CRISPR technique will allow for better targeted somatic gene therapy, promising successful treatment of HIV/AIDS, hemophilia, sickle cell anemia, and cancer. That this is desirable is largely uncontested. Far more controversial is whether we should also use the technology to alter the human germline to eradicate diseases such as cystic fibrosis, Huntington's chorea, or Tay-Sachs disease.[4] In those cases, we would still be fixing obvious mistakes, but not only for the benefit of one particular individual, but also for the benefit of everyone who inherits that individual's genetics. The cure would then reach beyond the individual to benefit all future generations. The problem is that we can never foresee all the effects that the intended cure will produce, and we may become aware of unintended effects only after several generations, when it is too late to do anything about them. In theory, of course, genes that have been edited out may also be edited back in again, but in practice this might turn out to be extremely difficult. To dispel worries about germline editing and to ensure that somatic cell therapy can continue unhindered, some scientists working in the field have urged that the scientific community agree on a voluntary worldwide moratorium on human germline modification.[5]

Such an agreement is unlikely. Even though human germline modification is banned or at least discouraged in many countries, first attempts to edit the genomes of human embryos to treat genetic defects have already been reported,[6] and in the United Kingdom, where modifications of the human germline for reproductive purposes are prohibited (with the exception of mitochondrial replacement), a research team at London's Francis Crick Institute applied in 2015 for a license to do the same in order to study early human development (and thus not for therapeutic use).[7] Moreover, not everyone shares the view that human germline modification for reproductive use should be prevented. Thus Julian Savulescu and colleagues have argued that, on the contrary, we even have a *moral obligation* to continue research in germline modification and to try to use it to eradicate genetic birth defects. This would, after all, very likely prevent countless deaths. The supposed risks can and should be ignored, first because all new technologies have unpredictable effects and second because the expected benefits far outweigh the expected harms.[8]

The Enhancement Argument

The reason why the benefits are thought to be so great that it is worth taking all the risk of inadvertently bringing about new and perhaps serious harms on future generations is that the existing harm that we allow to continue if we forgo the possibility of human germline modification is deemed much more severe than commonly acknowledged. Savulescu and colleagues have a very expansive understanding of what should count as a genetic birth defect, which includes fundamental aspects of our common human nature. Thus aging is understood (and in fact redefined) as a fatal genetic disease that "kills 30 million every year and disables many more," as a consequence of which our alleged moral obligation extends to using germline gene editing to delay or turn off aging.[9] But this is only the beginning and simply what is perceived as the most urgent task (since we definitely are going to *die* if we don't do anything about it).

Generally, our alleged moral obligation to press on with germline editing extends to practically everything that could conceivably be improved. Savulescu claimed that we have a moral obligation to overcome our limitations, including our moral limitations, and if we need to edit the human genome to achieve that, then so be it.[10] Since humans are "unfit for complete freedom," they need rules and regulations, but they should not be too restrictive. What should be prohibited are merely changes that are clearly harmful, namely, those that undermine or diminish the "all-purpose goods" of intelligence, impulse control, self-control, empathy, and the willingness to self-sacrifice. But otherwise parents should be free to edit their children's genomes any way they like. This might be eugenics,

Savulescu conceded, but since it is of the liberal kind, there is nothing really to worry about.

And Savulescu is not the only bioethicist who thinks that and who is open to the new eugenic ideology. Thus John Harris has argued pretty much along the same lines that we have to escape our "fragile nature,"[11] that the United Nations Educational, Scientific, and Cultural Organization's (UNESCO's) commitment to the preservation of the existing human genome as the common heritage of humanity is "absurd" and "nonsense," and that the only duty that is relevant when it comes to the possibility of germline editing is the duty "to create the best possible child."[12]

This is more than just a plea to use germline editing for the purpose of human enhancement in addition to therapy. The argument derives its persuasiveness from the implied redefinition[13] of enhancement *as* therapy. We are told that there is more at stake here than just the life quality of some individuals who are unfortunate enough to suffer from a disease that could possibly be cured through a genetic intervention. Instead, it is humanity as a whole that is supposed to be in need of a cure, and the only conceivable cure consists in a complete rewrite of the muddled and really quite unpublishable text that is our human genome. The argument benefits from the fact that what counts as a disease or a disability is often contentious and clearly subject to interpretation and to change. It also echoes the zeitgeist.

There is an increased tendency today to identify the defective and debilitating with the *suboptimal*, so that virtually *any* trait that could conceivably be improved or enhanced is seen as defective with respect to the envisaged enhancement. (As one blogger put it,[14] not using gene editing to enhance our children would be tantamount to "condemning[15] a child to a substandard future.") We are now quite willing to view and treat aging as a disease, love as an addiction that compromises well-being,[16] our common moral psychology and our cognitive apparatus as corrupted by various biases and distortions,[17] and, as a result of all this, basically the whole human condition as the ultimate, all-encompassing disease.

The public attitude toward what we are has changed accordingly. There is an increased understanding that we, as a species, are simply not good enough. This leads to a situation where it is no longer the recognition of a disease that justifies the search for a cure, but the (actual or potential) availability of a supposed cure that proves the existence of the disease. Yet if the mere possibility of an improvement beyond what is normal and healthy according to current human standards brings about a moral obligation to provide said improvement, as Savulescu and Harris have argued, then we have a problem. Possibilities are by their very nature endless. Whatever abilities we have, they are always *limited*, so that they are always accompanied by some ability that we lack, in respect to which we would then have to consider ourselves as disabled and in need of (genetic) cure. This means that we are compelled to regard our lives as *never* quite good enough, which strikes me not only as incoherent, but perhaps more importantly as detrimental to the possibility of living a good life.

Which Lives Are Good?

One necessary condition of a good life is the ability to see the good in what one has got and in what there is. Yet if our outlook is such that no matter what we have and how much we have, no matter what we find (in ourselves or our children), it is never quite good enough, then this in itself poses a serious obstacle to our having a good life. In order to live a good life we need to be able to accept, and indeed embrace, our life as good enough. That does not mean that we have to accept *any* life as good, that there is *never* any scope for improvement, but simply that focusing exclusively on our limitations, on what we do *not* have and can*not* do—which drives us on and on, further away from ourselves—inevitably deflects our attention from what we *do* have and what we *can* do. It directs our attention constantly away from the actual present (and the opportunities it provides us) to a possible future. The point is not that one should *only* live in the present and *never* aspire to anything else, but that one should not, by default, depreciate present goods by comparing them to an ever-greater imagined future good. It is a mistake to think that our lives can always be better, irrespective of how good they may appear to us.

It is also a mistake to think that limitations are per se bad. We can only ever be one particular thing, one person and not many, which implies that there are always many things that we are not. Every ability that we have is bought with a plethora of abilities that we lack (i.e., with, if you want to call it that, disabilities). On the other hand, every limitation is an opportunity. It gives shape and direction to our lives. It grounds our being. We should, then, not concern ourselves with what we are not, but with what we are, and all the great and wonderful things that we can do and achieve with what we are. As Sartre supposedly once said, "Freedom is what you do with what has been done to you,"[18] which I understand as making the point that limitations (our given nature) and freedom are not opposites, but complements.

This is why, in contrast with Harris, I find the UNESCO's insistence on the importance of protecting the human genome as our common heritage not ridiculous at all, but on the contrary eminently sensible: "We are human because of the interplay of many biological, historical, and cultural determinants, which preserve the feeling of our fundamental unity and nourish the richness of our diversity. This is why the human genome is one of the premises of freedom itself and not simply raw material to manipulate at leisure."[19]

Clearly there are terrible diseases out there, diseases that make it very difficult, if not impossible, for those who suffer from them to live a good life. If there is a good chance that gene editing will allow us to cure those diseases or prevent them from occurring, then we should certainly explore that possibility if (!) there is no viable alternative and we can be reasonably sure that it is safe and in the long run will not do more damage than good. But to try to go beyond that, by editing our children's genomes with the intent of overcoming humanity's limitations or of creating the best possible child is a fool's errand, even if it is deemed safe. It has been claimed that "beyond safety, no good reasons for restricting germline editing research have been identified,"[20] and in a way that is true. But "safety" can and should be interpreted to mean different things.

Germline editing may be regarded unsafe if it leads to other horrible diseases or fatal weaknesses in a person's constitution, but even if we could rule this out, we may still find that it is unsafe in the sense that its use for nontherapeutic purposes endangers our (or our children's) chances of living a good life. The effectiveness and relative accuracy of the CRISPR technique as a new tool for gene editing has raised such high hopes because it makes the intervention seemingly safer, in the narrow sense. But it is precisely this accuracy that also increases the danger, in the broader sense. A gun that is not working properly is a dangerous tool because you never know whether it actually does what you intend it to do. But while a gun that is working properly can for this reason indeed not only be safer, but also even *more* dangerous in the hands of someone whose intentions are bad. We tend to forget that it is not only unintended consequences that we have to fear, but also, and perhaps even more so, the *intended* ones. Those intentions do not even have to be bad. As history has taught us (or should have taught us), even if the intentions are good, even if all that someone desires who has been given the power to change the world is a better life for everyone, the outcome of their intervention may well in important respects be worse than the situation they intend to remedy. The road to hell really is paved with good intentions.

Take for instance Savulescu's all-purpose goods, which he believes we should both protect and develop: intelligence, impulse control, self-control, empathy, and the willingness to self-sacrifice. We certainly value those properties, and we appreciate them in ourselves and in others. It is also quite clear that most of us can conceivably be better in each or some of these areas: smarter, more in charge of our emotions, more controlled, more compassionate, more willing to sacrifice ourselves for the greater good or other people. Yet if we improved in all of those areas, would that also make our lives better?

It seems to me that this is rather unlikely. Aristotle was right to think that we do best when we steer clear of the extremes. It is never good to have too much or too little of anything. Virtue (and accordingly, happiness) lies somewhere in-between. It is true that diminished mental capacities may deprive us of some of the goods that the world has to offer. Equally, if we have no or little control over our emotions and actions, we are likely to mess up our lives, and if we think only of ourselves and do not care at all about anyone or anything else, then we can never experience the joy of sharing, of living with others in mutual recognition and support. However, we can also be too smart for our own good, too much in control, and too willing to turn the other cheek and to sacrifice our own good for some supposed greater good. All in good measure is the recipe for a life well lived. It is also the recipe for a good person. Balance is key, not only for the individual, but also for human society as a whole. Some are more courageous than others, some are more thoughtful, some are smarter, some have a rich imagination, some are more decisive, some are more gentle, some are more handsome, some are taller, some are shorter, some are abled, some are differently abled. Not everyone has to live up to the same ideal. As soon as that is expected, things usually start going wrong.

Even the best of dreams, and perhaps *especially* the best of them, have a tendency to turn into nightmares once they become reality. In Ira Levin's underrated, almost half a century old novel *This Perfect Day*, everyone is very much the same.[21] All aggression and all selfishness have been edited out. Everyone is well educated and busy working for the common good. Everyone also looks very much the same, tall and handsome. Chip, however, the novel's hero, has one distinctive feature: While everyone else's eyes are brown, he has one green eye, which never bothered him. He likes it, he says. But Wei, the leader of the invisible government that rules over a united, peaceful, and thoroughly synchronized world, tells him that he shouldn't: "If nothing could be done about it, then you would be justified in accepting it. But an imperfection that can be remedied? That we must *never* accept."[22] He has always dreamed, he says, of a universe united in perfection, "a universe of the gentle, the helpful, the loving, the unselfish."[23] Naturally, people had, and still have, to be helped to get there (since they are, as Savulescu put it, "unfit for complete freedom"), by chemical treatment first, and eventually by genetic engineering, but that is surely a price worth paying for the creation of a better world.

If Levin's Wei had the CRISPR technique at his disposal, he would not hesitate to use it to create and maintain his universe united in perfection. His reasoning is completely in line with that of those who, like Savulescu and Harris, urge us to embrace germline editing in order to make the world a better place. Yet this better place is one in which supposed imperfections cannot be tolerated, where it is unacceptable for anyone to be "substandard." There is no room for diversity, no encouragement or incentive to honor what Parens (2015) called "different ways of being."[24] There is no room for otherness in a world in which everyone

I encounter is just another version of myself, another me, perfect perhaps (in a fashion), but also, since everyone is, completely exchangeable. But encountering otherness is important not only because it lends an element of surprise and challenge to our lives, but also because it saves us from our existential solitude.

Editorial Obligations

The best possible child that Harris claims we have a moral obligation to create is a myth. There is no such thing as *the* best possible child, as there is no such thing as *the* best possible human. Instead, for every parent their own child can and should be the best possible child. They should never be seen as "substandard" or "suboptimal," which they inevitably will be once we start fiddling with their genes (or worse, very deliberately and accurately editing them) in order to optimize them. Every single child can be seen as the best possible child without necessarily being thought to be better than other children. *The best possible child* is an absolute superlative, not a relative (comparative) one. If we have a duty toward our children, then it is not to create them as the best possible ones, but to treat them as if they could not have been created any better than they are. This is not just a matter of acceptance. We can and should do more than merely *accept* our children as what they are. We should positively *cherish* them for it.

When Leibniz, to justify the ways of God in the eyes of men, praised this world as the best of all possible worlds (for which he was justly ridiculed by Voltaire), he still showed more sense than the would-be gene editors of today who are so intent to rid us of all limitations and to have us create only the best possible children. Leibniz at least understood that the world hangs together: that the best things in life never come without a price, that the freedom to do good requires the freedom to do evil, that light requires darkness to shine, that there is no good in a vacuum.

This might not be the best of all possible worlds, surely not, but it is doubtful that we can make it better by imprinting our own ideals of what makes a good human into the genomes of our children. There is no best possible child (in the comparative sense). Instead, there are many different ways of being good. And if we want to live a good life ourselves, if we want to flourish as human beings and want our children to flourish as well, we need to, perhaps more than anything else, recognize the multiple realizability of the good.

However, it is also important to recognize that the pursuit of happiness is most likely to succeed not in the extraordinary, the larger than life and better than human and beyond average, but in the ordinary life, which has enough scope and depth to provide us with all the happiness that a human life can possibly have. It is, in fact, good to be normal.[25] I find this insight beautifully expressed in the British poet Philip Larkin's "Born Yesterday,"[26] which he wrote for his friend Kingsley Amis's daughter, Sally, on the occasion of her birth. Perhaps, he said, she will grow up to be beautiful and loved, in which case she is a lucky girl, but this is not what he wished her. Instead, he wished her to be average because that is where human happiness is most likely to be found: "May you be ordinary;/ Have, like other women,/ An average of talents:/ Not ugly, not good-looking,/ Nothing uncustomary/ To pull you off your balance,/ That, unworkable itself,/ Stops all the rest from working./ In fact, may you be dull—/ If that is what a skilled,/ Vigilant, flexible,/ Unemphasised, enthralled/ Catching of happiness is called."

Notes

1. I am grateful to my wife and fellow philosopher Teodora Manea for urging me to reflect on the meaning of the word *editing*; to those who commented on, and thus helped improve, an earlier version of this chapter, especially David Seamon, Maurizio Balistreri, Michael Morrison, and Brian D. Earp, who took part in an online discussion of the chapter; and to the participants of the Gene Editing and Human Flourishing workshop at The Hastings Center.
2. Le Cong, F. Ann Ran, David Cox, Shuailiang Lin, Robert Barretto, Naomi Habib, Patrick D. Hsu, et al., "Multiplex Genome Engineering Using CRISPR/Cas Systems," *Science* 339, no. 6121 (February 15, 2013): 819–823.
3. Jonathan Rockoff, "Why Gene-Editing Technology Has Scientists Excited," *The Wall Street Journal*, June 28, 2015. http://www.wsj.com/articles/why-gene-editing-technology-has-scientists-excited-1434985998
4. It should be remembered, though, that couples whose offspring are likely to inherit the disease do of course always have the option not to reproduce or to use preimplantation genetic diagnosis (PGD) to make sure that their offspring do not carry the disease. Germline editing is only necessary to prevent inheritable disease if we assume that every prospective parent has the right to a genetically related child, which is certainly contentious (cf. Rob Sparrow's Chapter 11, this volume). It can even be argued that there is a duty to adopt that trumps the desire to have a genetically related child (Tina Rulli, "Preferring a Genetically-Related Child," *Journal of Moral Philosophy* 13, no. 6 (2014): 669–698).
5. Edward Lanphier, Fyodor Urnov, Sarah Ehlen Haecker, Michael Werner, and Joanna Smolenski, "Don't Edit the Human Germ Line," *Nature* 519 (March 26, 2015): 410–411.
6. Puping Liang, Yanwen Xu, Xiya Zhang, Chenhui Ding, Rui Huang, Zhen Zhang, Jie Lv, et al., "CRISPR/Cas9-Mediated Gene Editing in Human Tripronuclear Zygotes," *Protein and Cell* 6, no. 5 (2015): 363–372.
7. Daniel Cressey, Alison Abbott, and Heidi Ledford, "UK Scientists Apply for License to Edit Genes in Human Embryos," *Nature News*, September 18, 2015.

8. Julian Savulescu and Ingmar Persson, *Unfit for the Future. The Need for Moral Enhancement* (Oxford: Oxford University Press, 2012).

9. Julian Savulescu, Jonathan Pugh, Thomas Douglas, and Christopher Gyngall, "The Moral Imperative to Continue Gene Editing Research on Human Embryos," *Protein Cell* 6, no. 7 (2015): 478.

10. Julian Savulescu, "As a Species, We Have a Moral Obligation to Enhance Ourselves," TED interview, February 19, 2014. http://ideas.ted.com/the-ethics-of-genetically-enhanced-monkey-slaves/

11. John Harris, "Why Human Gene Editing Must Not Be Stopped," *The Guardian*, December 2, 2015. https://www.theguardian.com/science/2015/dec/02/why-human-gene-editing-must-not-be-stopped

12. This in turn echoes Savulescu's principle of procreative beneficence (Julian Savulescu, "Procreative Beneficence: Why We Should Select the Best Children," *Bioethics* 15, no. 5–6 (2001): 413–426).

13. A *persuasive* redefinition in Charles Stevenson's sense (Charles Leslie Stevenson, "Persuasive Definitions," *Mind* 47, no. 87 (1938): 331–350)

14. Stan Erickson, Blog home page, https://aeon.co/users/stan-erickson.

15. It is the word *condemnation* that strongly suggests the essential defectiveness of any "substandard" condition.

16. James Burkett and Larry Young, "The Behavioral, Anatomical and Pharmacological Parallels between Social Attachment, Love and Addiction," *Psychopharmacology* 224, no. 1 (2012): 1–26; Brian D. Earp, Olga A. Wudarczyk, Bennett Foddy, and Julian Savulescu, "Addicted to Love: What Is Love Addiction and When Should It Be Treated?" *Philosophy, Psychiatry, and Psychology* 24, no. 1 (2017): 77–92. Earp et al. review the literature that suggests love is an addiction and discuss the implications this might have for the need to treat certain kinds of love. Although they do not claim that all love compromises well-being (and even suggest that we should review our assessment of addictions in general as inherently bad) and should therefore be treated, their argument nonetheless encourages us to see love itself as an addiction, and it is easy to conclude that we would be much better off without it.

17. Savulescu and Persson, *Unfit for the Future*.

18. The quotation is probably apocryphal, but even if Sartre never wrote this, it is still well said.

19. International Bioethics Committee, *Report of the International Bioethics Committee on Updating Its Reflections on the Human Genome and Human Rights*, October 2, 2015, 4, http://unesdoc.unesco.org/images/0023/002332/233258E.pdf

20. Christopher Gyngall, Thomas Douglas, and Julian Savulescu, "Editing the Germline—A Time for Reason, Not Emotion," *Oxford University's Practical Ethics Blog*, March 31, 2015, http://blog.practicalethics.ox.ac.uk/2015/03/editing-the-germline-a-time-for-reason-not-emotion/

21. Ira Levin, *This Perfect Day* (1970; repr., London: Corsair, 2014).

22. Emphasis in original, Levin, *Perfect Day*, 309. It should be noted that there is no obvious reason why brown eyes should be regarded as more perfect than green eyes. So

the presumed imperfection is likely to consist in the divergence from the norm. It is not brown eyes that are perfect, but conformity that is.

23. Levin, *Perfect Day*, 309.

24. Erik Parens, *Shaping Our Selves: On Technology, Flourishing, and a Habit of Thinking* (Oxford: Oxford University Press, 2014). I am not suggesting that germline gene editing for enhancement purposes (to create the "best possible child") would necessarily lead to a complete loss of diversity. I am less concerned with what gene editing will or will not accomplish, but more with what we *want* it to accomplish. It is the idea of how we need to be in order to have a good life with which I am concerned here. Consequently, I am not citing Levin to show that gene editing is likely to result in a world where everyone is the same, but mainly to show that even supposed all-purpose goods may not be so good anymore when they are enhanced to perfection.

25. I do not mean to suggest that we don't need the extraordinary. Of course we do. The point that I am trying to make here is rather that we don't *all* have to be extraordinary to live good, fulfilling lives. Geniuses and poets and remarkable creators certainly enrich our lives. But our lives wouldn't be better if we were *all* geniuses and poets and remarkable creators and the extraordinary became the new ordinary. We would lose out if there were no extraordinary people around, but we do not necessarily lose out by being rather ordinary ourselves. It is in fact the common (ordinary) mixture of variation and sameness whose importance I wish to emphasize. We don't have to become more equal (by subjecting ourselves, or being subjected to, a regime of presumed optimization) or more diversified (by allowing everyone to edit away to their heart's desire). There is great value in both the seemingly (but actually quite extraordinary) ordinary and in the (ordinary) extraordinary.

26. Philip Larkin, *Collected Poems*, (New York: Farrar, Straus & Giroux, 2003) 54.

5

Daoism, Flourishing, and Gene Editing

Richard Kim[1]

Given the potentially powerful effects of gene editing for human lives, it seems reasonable to reflect on the issue from a variety of scientific, moral, cultural, and religious perspectives to help us deploy this technology with a clear eye to all its possible implications. Given the global impact genetic modification will likely have, an inquiry seriously engaging with the values and ideals of non-Western cultures and societies will be helpful to achieve the sort of balanced understanding that will enable a proper evaluation.

The focus of this chapter is on one of the oldest, richest, and most influential moral traditions that arose in early China: Daoism. One key feature of Daoism, shared by other great philosophical traditions of early China such as Confucianism and Mohism, is its practical orientation. Although the Daoist texts represent a number of intriguing philosophical positions, they ultimately aim at helping readers achieve human fulfillment. Like the great eudaemonist traditions of the West such as Stoicism or Aristotelianism (see Daniel Haybron's Chapter 2, this volume), at the heart of the Daoist philosophical tradition is the attainment of flourishing or well-being. (I use these terms interchangeably.) This chapter examines the account of well-being found in the Daoist classic, the *Zhuangzi*, and highlights some insights that can be fruitfully explored in the context of the ethics of gene editing. My thesis is that from the perspective of Zhuangzi's conception of human flourishing, we have reasons to think we should reject the use of genetic modification technology. In this chapter, I do not attempt to settle whether, all things considered, those reasons are strong enough to support the rejection of any one form or use, much less all, of gene editing.

Gene editing technologies can be aimed at a variety of purposes, including what bioethicists refer to as "therapy" and "enhancement." Giubilini and Sanyal defined enhancement as "biomedical interventions to improve human capacities, performances, dispositions, and well-being beyond the traditional scope of therapeutic medicine."[2] Therapy, on the other hand, is understood as the restoration of human capacities to their normal or characteristic function.[3] This chapter explores reasons to think we should reject the use of human genetic modification technologies generally, when put to both enhancement and therapeutic ends. Because the therapeutic use of gene editing, at least for somatic engineering, is widely accepted, Zhuangzi's views will strike most readers as extreme (and perhaps unhelpful) in deepening our ethical understanding of the topic of gene editing.[4] But even if a wholesale endorsement of Zhuangzi's views is unlikely, there are elements of his thinking that merit careful consideration and can draw attention to possible negative consequences of deploying human gene editing technologies.

Zhuangzi's primary goal was not to build a coherent ethical system or uncover a set of fundamental moral principles. In line with many of the Hellenistic philosophers like the Stoics and Epicureans, Zhuangzi sought to reshape the reader's fundamental beliefs and attitudes in ways that advance their achievement of "the good life." Like Wittgenstein, we can see Zhuangzi as carrying out a form of philosophical therapy, although unlike Wittgenstein, his main goal was not to untangle or dissolve philosophical issues but to instill in the readers a fresh set of perspectives that can counter our common psychological propensity toward anxiety. In the next section I discuss the notion of the "heavenly perspective," which Zhuangzi believed offers an important tool for sustaining an attitude of detachment and equanimity. (As we will see, this concept is unconnected to an appeal to God or deities.) We also explore what I call the *virtue of spontaneity* that Zhuangzi took as an important feature of human flourishing. Finally, I draw on Zhuangzi's views about the human good to identify some possible reasons against the use of genetic modification technologies.

Zhuangzi's Account of Flourishing: Heavenly Perspective and the Virtue of Spontaneity

The *Zhuangzi*, like the other classical Daoist text the *Daodejing*, is generally believed to be the work of more than one author, integrating ideas from multiple sources. Nevertheless, the text as a whole presents a substantive vision of what matters in life and the sorts of dispositions and attitudes we should cultivate to obtain a life that goes well for us. The goal of this section is to highlight the core elements of Zhuangzi's conception of well-being.[5] Given the text's complexity and rich history, I am by no means offering a definitive interpretation. Nevertheless, I believe the discussion that follows captures key aspects of Zhuangzi's philosophical vision.

One of the central features of the positive vision of human flourishing advanced by Zhuangzi is freedom from the ordinary concerns that are constitutive of the struggle and anxiety permeating day-to-day life:

> Sweating and laboring to the end of his days and never seeing his accomplishments, utterly exhausting himself and never knowing where to look

for rest—can you help pitying him? I'm not dead yet! he says, but what good
is that? His body decays, his mind follows it—can you deny that this is a great
sorrow? Man's life has always been a muddle like this.[6]

Zhuangzi offered a diagnosis of the ills that trouble us: moving without pause or
rest from one task to another, we are so preoccupied with everyday affairs that
our minds are incapable of finding genuine rest. This is a common psychological
state that will resonate with most of us.

As Zhuangzi observed, our psychological disturbances are often the product
of our inability to satisfy our numerous and ever-expanding set of desires. Of
course, one way of resolving this predicament would be to find a way of satisfying all of our desires, but that is clearly a practically (perhaps even logically)
impossible task. Rather, Zhuangzi suggested we need to cultivate a different perspective, one that builds and sustains a kind of equanimity that can shield us
from the psychological pressures that afflict our minds. This perspective, which
recent scholars, including Justin Tiwald and Philip J. Ivanhoe, have labeled the
"heavenly perspective," offers a vantage point from which value distinctions and
categories fade away, and every event is considered simply a part of the grand
process of change: "Whether you point to a little stalk or a great pillar, a leper or
the beautiful Xishi, things ribald and shady, or things grotesque and strange, the
Way makes them all into one."[7] (I explain the Daoist notion of "the Way" in material that follows.)

To help understand this perspective, Justin Tiwald suggested reflecting on
a "broad, panoramic, view of the universe over the fullness of time, and how
human value distinctions, pretenses to knowledge, and absolutism must seem
from that perspective."[8] As I discuss further in this chapter, Zhuangzi was not
advocating the heavenly perspective as the only proper way of seeing the world,
but calling attention to its practical advantages. For example, the heavenly perspective loosens our confidence in the truth of our judgments concerning what
is valuable or good, thereby allowing us to become more receptive to new ideas.[9]

> Hold on to all that you have received from Heaven, but do not think you have
> gotten anything. Be empty, that is all. The Perfect Man uses his mind like a
> mirror—going after nothing, welcoming nothing, responding but not storing.
> Therefore he can win out over things and not hurt himself.[10]

Being able to detach ourselves from our preconceived judgments and values, we
place ourselves in a position of receptivity, cultivating an open-minded attitude.
The heavenly perspective protects us from prematurely blocking off worthwhile
considerations that may strike us as unappealing or even ludicrous. Another advantage is that by admitting the fallibility of our judgments, we are less anxious

about being in error and can detach ourselves from the kind of intellectual pride that is often the source of much personal frustration, as well as fruitless bickering.

Looking to help the readers cultivate the proper frame of mind to grasp the heavenly perspective, Zhuangzi concocted a combination of (at times outlandish) parables and rhetorical questions:

> Now let me ask *you* some questions. If a man sleeps in a damp place, his back aches and he ends up half paralyzed, but is this true of a loach? If he lives in a tree, he is terrified and shakes with fright, but is this true of a monkey? Of these three creatures, then, which one knows the proper place to live? Men eat the flesh of grass-fed and grain-fed animals, deer eat grass, centipedes find snakes tasty, and hawks and falcons relish mice. Of these four, which knows how food ought to taste? Monkeys pair with monkeys, deer go out with deer, and fish play around with fish. Men claim that Maoqiang and Lady Li were beautiful; but if fish saw them, they would dive to the bottom of the stream; if birds saw them, they would fly away; and if deer saw them, they would break into a run. Of these four, which knows how to fix the standard of beauty for the world? The way I see it, the rules of benevolence and righteousness, and the paths of right and wrong all are hopelessly snarled and jumbled. How could I know anything about such discriminations?[11]

The primary function of these questions is to help the reader recognize that while our value judgments about beauty, welfare, or morality may seem indubitable to us (from both an individual and species-level point of view), they arise out of our own necessarily limited perspective. Indeed, from the perspective of every creature, what appears good or beautiful will seem obvious, and it is all too natural for us to move from what we find appealing to universal claims about what is absolutely good or beautiful, a significant mistake in Zhuangzi's eyes. Coming to recognize the degree to which our evaluative judgments vary depending on the particular perspective from which the judgment is made will make us less dogmatic in our stance and enable us to flexibly employ a wider range of considerations to resolve intellectual and practical challenges. Consider the following allegory:

> When the monkey trainer was handing out acorns, he said, "You get three in the morning and four at night." This made all the monkeys furious. "Well, then," he said, "you get four in the morning and three at night." The monkeys were all delighted. There was no change in the reality behind the words, and yet the monkeys responded with joy and anger. Let them, if they want to. So the sage harmonizes with both right and wrong and rests in Heaven the Equalizer. This is called walking two roads.[12]

We can imagine a less amenable monkey trainer stubbornly sticking to his plan to give three acorns in the morning and four at night, remarking with exasperation, "What difference does it make if they get four now and three later?" As it turns out, there is a significant difference from the monkeys' point of view, recognized by the astute trainer who simply adjusted to their preferences. Commenting on this passage, Thomas Merton described Zhuangzi's normative vision as "at home on two levels: that of the divine and invisible [D]ao that has no name, and that of ordinary, simple, everyday existence."[13] As Merton went on to explain, despite initial appearances, Zhuangzi wasn't suggesting that we permanently stay within the heavenly perspective, detaching ourselves from every human desire and end. Rather, Zhuangzi was suggesting that we should seek to live well in the world *as it is* and to harmonize both the heavenly and human perspectives.[14] On this picture, we continue to strive for the realization of certain goals, while recognizing that from the cosmic perspective our ends will appear insignificant. In a number of passages, Zhuangzi offered examples of Daoist exemplars that occupied simple, ordinary roles in society—butcher, woodcarver, ferry guide—that find a way of achieving the highest levels of perfection in their craft, while at the same time having their hearts set on following the Way, the Daoist path for achieving the best, most flourishing life. These so-called skill stories reveal Zhuangzi's paradoxical attitude that one must cultivate an attitude of detachment from, and skepticism toward, what we tend to value, at the same time manifesting excellence in one's ordinary work.[15]

An important element of Zhuangzi's conception of the flourishing life, as exemplified in the skillful practices of the Daoist masters, is living according to certain natural, spontaneous, or nonrational tendencies that allow one to move along the path of life with dexterity and tranquility, resulting in both interpersonal and intrapersonal harmony. Consider this description of the psychological state of the master butcher Cook Ding as he cuts up an ox: "And now—now I go at it by spirit and don't look with my eyes. Perception and understanding have come to a stop, and spirit moves where it wants. I go along with the natural makeup, strike in the big hollows, guide the knife through the big openings, and follow things as they are."[16] We can read the butcher's "flow"-like activity (to borrow from Mihaly Csikszentmihalyi) metaphorically, referring to the way that our lives, when going exceedingly well, also seem to be carried along by a certain element of smoothness and effortlessness, where everything just seems to hang together properly, allowing us to live with balance and ease. I refer to the disposition that allows one to move forward in life with flow and tranquility through those nonrational spontaneous drives or inclinations identified by Zhuangzi as the *virtue of spontaneity*.[17] The development and maintenance of this virtue is one of the core features of the Zhuangzian conception of human flourishing.

As scholars have noted, Zhuangzi's choice of exemplars for articulating the best human lives were often those who are deemed least worthy of respect in early China: butchers, criminals, and those who are physically disfigured. Through these examples, Zhuangzi suggested that the range of lives that can go well is much broader than what most would think. As Philip Ivanhoe noted, "By calling into question established notions about what constitutes the good and the worthy, he illuminated forgotten corners of human dignity. . . . All are part of the great dao and each has dignity and worth in itself."[18] This is in stark contrast to the prevailing attitudes about human worth in early China, which were closely bound with hierarchy and roles. In Zhuangzi's eyes the cultivation of the heavenly perspective allows one to see past culturally constructed norms and values and appreciate a sense of oneness that ties together all things, processes, and change. In a variety of passages we see Zhuangzi endorsing skepticism toward much of what we ordinarily value and accepting all events as simply the unfolding of the natural pattern set by heaven.

While cultivating a receptive, *let it be* attitude may be an effective mindset for daily life, one might worry that when confronting tragic events such an attitude may be out of place. In one well-known passage, when Zhuangzi's wife dies, his friend Huizi comes to visit only to find him singing in a cheerful mood. Huizi chastises him for his callousness, and Zhuangzi responds:

> When she first died, do you think I didn't grieve like anyone else? But I looked back to her beginning and the time before she was born. Not only the time before she was born, but the time before she had a body. Not only the time before she had a body, but the time before she had a spirit. In the midst of jumble of wonder and mystery, a change took place and she had a spirit. Another change and she had a body. Another change and she was born. Now there's been another change she's dead. It's just like progression of the four seasons: spring, summer, fall, winter.[19]

One might initially find Zhuangzi's comparison of the death of a loved one with a change in season as perverse. But as we see in the passage, even Zhuangzi underwent an initial period of grief. In line with his practical and therapeutic aims, we can interpret Zhuangzi as primarily seeking to offer a way to move past the experience of grief by taking on the heavenly perspective from which life and death appear as both necessary and inevitable events that are charged with "wonder and mystery." In Zhuangzi's eyes, life and death were mysteries that lie beyond the scope of our rational capacity. By framing such events as part of the ineffable processes of the natural world, Zhuangzi believed that his readers would find comfort that can ease the pain of loss and enable us to move forward with our lives. The Zhuangzian spirit is at home in a more intuition-driven, less rationally focused way of life that finds consolation in the fact that many of life's most important experiences elude our rational grasp.

The conception of human flourishing that emerges from this discussion emphasizes the importance of cultivating an anxiety-free and open-minded attitude, with the ability to recognize that the importance we attach to our everyday affairs is, at least from a broader, cosmic perspective, insignificant. This perspective allows us to maintain equanimity in the face of challenges and to prevent ourselves from obsession with any particular goal, as well as suggesting that what most think of as meritorious, admirable, or ignoble are often the result of mere societal conventions and norms and do not match what is truly good from the perspective of the *dao*: the proper path that leads to the most flourishing life. Additionally, through the cultivation of the virtue of spontaneity, one leads a less rationally driven, more unencumbered life that moves with the grain of one's natural drives and inclinations.

But as noted, Zhuangzi was not claiming that we should aim to abandon our human perspective and extricate ourselves from all desires. As the stories of the Daoist exemplars reveal, those whose lives best exemplify the Daoist vision of well-being live fairly ordinary, simple lives that conform to basic cultural mores. But, in carrying out their ordinary tasks, they demonstrate excellence, and it is through their skillfulness that they discover a way to accord with the dao. The Daoist image of flourishing isn't that of a solitary hermit, but of someone living at peace in the world, according to one's natural impulses, harmonizing with both nature and other people. In Zhuangzi's view, much of what we think of as essential or important to our happiness—wealth, good looks, advanced technology—tends to distract us from a more enduring, deeper kind of joy that is achieved by a simplified life that is attuned to our more basic, natural promptings.

To summarize the discussion, let me identify two central elements of Zhuangzi's conception of flourishing:

I. *Heavenly Perspective.* This perspective prevents narrow-minded obsessions over trivial matters by allowing us to see events and people from a wider, more cosmic point of view. It allows us to face difficulties with equanimity and also to see that the values and norms we endorse are not timeless truths, but a product of culture and society, resulting in open-mindedness and receptivity toward finding value and worth in things and people that otherwise would have been neglected.

II. *Virtue of Spontaneity.* This virtue allows us to live according to the spontaneous inclinations rooted in our nature, which Zhuangzi believed will free us from our attachments to worldly goods and enable us to be at peace with ourselves and others. Because this form of life is best achieved when one is relatively free from worldly attachment—as exemplified by the Daoist sages like Cook Ding—it is marked by simplicity.

The Ethics of Gene Editing: Lessons from Zhuangzi

How might the use of genetic modification technologies affect the possibility of achieving the sort of life that Zhuangzi believed is best for us? Applying the values and ideas of an ancient Chinese thinker to a contemporary moral issue is bound to be messy, but it is possible to identify some considerations relevant to the ethics of gene editing. Given Zhuangzi's focus on the cultivation of the heavenly perspective and the virtue of spontaneity, I suggest that we at least have reason to think genetic modification would conflict with the account of human well-being proposed by Zhuangzi. The relevant question for our purposes is, How might the use of gene editing technology affect the sorts of dispositions and attitudes that Zhuangzi saw as essential for obtaining well-being?

One of the best-known objections to human genetic modification has been the way that such technologies strengthen what Michael Sandel called our "drive to mastery," thereby undercutting the "enlarged human sympathies that an openness to the unbidden can cultivate."[20] Sandel's core idea was that these technologies ultimately discourage the cultivation of certain values and dispositions, especially the disposition to accept with humility and gratitude human beings as they are, which can foster a sense of solidarity with all people. In a similar spirit, Michael Hauskeller comments in this volume, "There is no best possible child (in the comparative sense). Instead there are many different ways of being good. And if we want to live a good life ourselves, if we want to flourish as human beings and want our children to flourish as well, we need to, perhaps more than anything else, recognize the multiple realizability of the good (p. 67 in Chapter 4)."[21]

There are significant elements of Sandel's and Hauskeller's normative outlook that I think Zhuangzi would find congenial, for example, accepting people as they are and recognizing the dignity and worth inherent in everyone. By becoming increasingly focused on finding ways to improve human nature and design human beings, we seem to go directly against the flexible, open-minded attitude that Zhuangzi thought was so crucial for flourishing. Take, for example, the attitude expressed by parents who hope to apply genetic technology to produce in their children traits such as a certain height, eye color, or level of intelligence.[22] For Zhuangzi, the common assumption underlying this kind of use of genetic technology—that we have a sufficient understanding of which human traits are better than others—was dubious, particularly from the heavenly perspective. For Zhuangzi, much of our understanding concerning which human traits are more or less valuable is the result of cultural influences that far too often deter us from *really seeing* the true worth of things—that is, their true worth according to the perspective of heaven. At the very least, we should be far less confident about the extent to which we possess such knowledge. Besides Zhuangzi's skepticism regarding our ability to correctly grasp values, there are other reasons why Zhuangzi would disapprove of the use of genetic modification technologies. I identify three next.

The first reason is that increasing the use of enhancement technologies would undermine the kinds of attitudes toward ourselves and the world that Zhuangzi thought were essential for living well. So, where Zhuangzi would take "wonder and mystery" to be the natural and intuitive responses to the birth of our children and the genetic qualities they possess, pervasive use of genetic technology could lead us to see birth as the product of human agency.

This is not an assessment shared by everyone. For example, Allen Buchanan has argued that even the rampant use of genetic enhancement technology would still leave many things outside human control.[23] Moreover, as Buchanan also argued, not all human interventions in the processes of nature are bad: we cut out tumors, develop minds through education and learning, and grow genetically modified crops that yield greater quantities of healthier food. While these are legitimate points, they don't completely address the concern that by increasing our manipulation of the most profound and mysterious human events such as birth and death, we promote the disposition to seek greater control over nature—a disposition that lies in tension with the more detached attitude of the heavenly perspective.[24]

The second reason is that it isn't clear whether altering the human genome would, on the whole, be beneficial for us. On Zhuangzi's view, the requirements for living flourishing lives are much lower than people generally tend to think. A fairly simple life, as long as one cultivates the sorts of attitude we've identified, is sufficient for a high level of flourishing. There is empirical research that seems to support this point. In a study on life satisfaction levels by Ed Diener and Martin Seligman, the life satisfaction levels of the *Forbes* magazine's "richest Americans" were equal to the life satisfaction levels of the Pennsylvania Amish and the Inughuit (Inuit people in Northern Greenland), even though the lives of the Amish and Inughuit rank much lower in economic freedom.[25]

More important, Zhuangzi suggested that by increasing our options for the variety of goods that science generates, our lives are actually made worse—our minds are saturated with more expansive desires, which in turn cause greater frustration. Again, contemporary empirical research suggests that Zhuangzi was onto something. Studies of the Old Order Amish of Pennsylvania showed that their rate of nonmanic depression or "common cold depression" occurred at roughly between one-fifth and one-tenth of the depression rate among the citizens of Baltimore.[26] This suggests that even though our lives have much greater freedom in choosing from a range of economic goods compared to the Amish, in terms of subjective well-being, we may be doing a fair bit worse. Of course, to make the warranted judgment that city-dwelling Americans are overall doing worse than the Amish would require investigating the well-being of both populations as well as a variety of other factors. And while many of us may have fleeting thoughts about *how wonderful and free it must feel to live like that*—few of us would seriously consider joining the Amish community. One recent, notable exception is Matthew Secich, who was a sous chef at a world-renowned restaurant but decided after years of deep unhappiness to join the Amish community with his wife and family. Describing his current, radically simpler life, he commented:

> This is far better. You can hear the clock tick. . . . I truly believe God has his destiny for all things. From once upon a time being a four-star chef, to playing with meat in the backwoods, that was all God's plan. I feel so blessed to be here.[27]

It's almost as if Secich was following a prescription suggested by Zhuangzi over two millennia ago: "Be content with this time and dwell in this order, and then neither sorrow nor joy can touch you. In ancient times this was called the 'freeing of the bound.' There are those who cannot free themselves because they are bound by things. But nothing can ever win against Heaven—that's the way it's always been."[28]

The third reason Zhuangzi would take issue with the use of genetic technology draws on Zhuangzi's view that the heavenly perspective opens us up to see the dignity and worth that are present in lives that are too quickly dismissed by society. Because genetic enhancement, as scholars like Michael Sandel, Adrienne Asch, and Edmund Pellegrino have noted, may promote the sort of mindset that led to programs of eugenics in the early twentieth century—sharply demarcating what counts as desirable and undesirable traits in human beings; it could also decrease our capacity to appreciate just those kinds of lives that Zhuangzi saw as carrying the potential to flourish, including those who live with extremely unusual physical deformities.[29] In her powerful reflection on disability in this volume, Rosemarie Garland-Thomson (Chapter 1) comments on the increasing drive toward removing all forms of genetic anomalies:

> People like the four of us have long been the "bad news" of lying-in hospitals, delivery rooms, neonatal units, and prenatal imaging and testing—unexpected arrivals delivered by the Black Stork. In the swiftly developing world of genetic engineering, however, people like us are identifiable, legible in our distinctiveness and rarity, much earlier in the trajectory of medicalized human procreation than in the past. Detecting disability through selective testing is

carried out now at all developmental stages of human reproduction, from the gametic to the embryonic to the fetal to the neonatal. Germline interventions would seek to prevent people with rare diseases and congenital disabilities from coming into being. This pruning of human variation at the genetic level proceeds with little considerations of our perspectives as people who live out these genetic narratives. Enthusiasts about genetic engineering cite facts against us such as those described by the Global Burden of Disease Project, which calculates our supposed collective costs without accounting for our contributions. We are a vanishing tribe, those of us now detectable earlier and earlier in the process of human procreation. We are now often culled out before the traits that embryonic and fetal testing reveal are brought into being in a lived life.[30]

The march toward eradicating every genetic aberration has muted the voices of those who actually live with such conditions. Not only are we increasingly unable to appreciate the contributions that those with disabilities make to society, but also we now question whether such people should even exist. Consider this comment by the bioethicist Dena Davis:

> In my own mind I can discern a subtle shift in the way in which I view people with certain anomalies. Twenty years ago, seeing a woman in the supermarket with a child who has Down syndrome, my immediate reactions were sympathy and a sense that that woman could be me. Now that testing for Down syndrome is virtually universal in the United States, when I see such a mother and child I am more likely to wonder why she didn't get tested.[31]

One aspect of the shift in Davis's attitude is that now, with advanced understanding of genetic screening, there shouldn't even exist people with "anomalies" at all. What is strikingly absent in the thoughts and attitudes of those like Davis is the perspective of those who actually carry those anomalies, which frequently tells a very different story about what their lives are like. As Garland-Thomson describes in Chapter 1 of this volume:

> Living in a world not built for us and in a community where the majority of members understand themselves and are understood by others as being more fortunate, advantaged, better, more able, or healthier than we are has been an opportunity. From that place where we have lived our lives, many of us have developed a vibrant resourcefulness, interdependence, an alternative knowledge base, and a consciousness sometimes perceptible only in the recesses of our being, all of which have served us well.[32]

Zhuangzi tells a story of a man named Ziqi who discovered a large tree that he deemed worthless: "He saw that the smaller limbs were gnarled and twisted, unfit for beams or rafters, and looking down, he saw that the trunk was pitted and rotten and could not be used for coffins. . . . It turns out to be a completely unusable tree."[33] But in a flash of Daoist insight Ziqi realized that these anomalies had contributed to the tree's flourishing: "Aha!—it is this unusableness that the Holy Man Makes use of!"[34]

The crucial point Zhuangzi and Garland-Thomson highlighted is that without adequate reflection on the perspective of the disabled we will fail to appreciate how disabilities may serve as sources of prudential value. But the ability to recognize this fact is contingent on having a proper outlook, marked by the kind of open-mindedness and acceptance that Zhuangzi advocated throughout the text.

Conclusion

The point of this chapter was not to offer decisive reasons against the use of genetic modification technologies, but rather to draw attention to certain values and perspectives that Zhuangzi took as essential for human flourishing and that appear to be in tension with genome modification. Many contemporary readers—just like many thinkers in Zhuangzi's own time—will find Zhuangzi's conception of well-being, with its focus on detachment, heavenly perspective, and spontaneity, too narrow and implausible. There are two points to note in response. The first is that even if Zhuangzi's vision seems too radical for us, there are aspects of that vision, such as the abilities to shift perspectives, to detach oneself from particular ends, and to flow with the nonrational intuitive inclinations of our nature, that many will find appealing. The second point is that, given Zhuangzi's deep and enduring influence on the some of the best minds of the East, we have reason to believe he may be a resource to help us to examine some of our most basic—and therefore least analyzed—assumptions. Through deep and sympathetic engagement with profound thinkers of other cultures like Zhuangzi, we are less likely to become imprisoned by the particular values of our society and culture and more likely to extend our understanding of the possibilities for leading good human lives.

Notes

1. I thank Josephine Johnston and Erik Parens for all their helpful comments. This work was supported by funding from the John Templeton Foundation.

2. Alberto Giubilini and Segar Sanyal, "The Ethics of Human Enhancement," *Philosophy Compass* 10, no. 4 (2015): 233–243.

3. Norman Daniels, "Normal Functioning and the Treatment-Enhancement Distinction," *Cambridge Quarterly of Healthcare Ethics* 9, no. 3 (2000): 309–322.

4. Briefly, somatic engineering alters somatic cells and would not result in changes that would be inherited by one's offspring. Germline engineering, which alters germ cells, would result in changes that would be passed down to one's offspring. The latter technology is generally considered as more ethically problematic.

5. I acknowledge that the text attributed to Zhuangzi is drawn from multiple sources and is the product of more than one thinker. But since there is a general consensus that Zhuangzi was a historical figure who espoused the basic ideas attributed to him, for convenience I refer to ideas of the text as "Zhuangzi's views."

6. All translations of the *Zhuangzi*, unless noted otherwise, are from Burton Watson, trans., *The Complete Works of Zhuangzi* (New York: Columbia University Press, 1968), 33.

7. Watson, *Zhuangzi*, 11.

8. Justin Tiwald, "Well-Being and Daoism," in *The Routledge Handbook of the Philosophy of Well-Being*, ed. Guy Fletcher (London: Routledge, 2016), 62. I am greatly indebted to Tiwald's essay for many of the ideas explored in this chapter.

9. Tiwald, "Well-Being."

10. Watson, *Zhuangzi*, 59.

11. Watson, *Zhuangzi*, 15.

12. Watson, *Zhuangzi*, 11.

13. Thomas Merton, *The Way of Chuang Tzu*, 2nd ed. (New York: New Direction Publishing, 2010), 32.

14. For Western scholars, it may be helpful to contrast the heavenly and human perspectives with what Thomas Nagel called the "subjective" and "objective" points of view. See Thomas Nagel, *The View from Nowhere* (Oxford: Oxford University Press, 1986). While there are certainly notable differences, one common feature is that as we move back to a more cosmic point of view, what matters to us will gradually appear as less significant. But while, as I understand it, Nagel's inquiry was more conceptually and theoretically oriented, Zhuangzi employed the heavenly perspective for practical ends that he took to offer significant prudential benefits.

15. For philosophical discussions of the skillful stories and their role in Zhuangzi's thought, see *Essays on Skepticism, Relativism, and Ethics in the Zhuangzi*, ed. Paul Kjellberg and Philip J. Ivanhoe (Albany: SUNY Press, 1996).

16. Watson, *Zhuangzi*, 19.

17. The concept of "spontaneity" is complicated, and more discussion is needed than I can offer here. Here I mean to employ it within the context of the Daoist worldview, which suggests that there are certain "natural" inclinations, emotions, and attitudes that are in tune with the Dao or Nature. For his account of "flow," see Mihaly Csikszentmihalyi, *Flow: The Psychology of Optimal Experience* (New York: Harper and Row, 1990).

18. Philip J. Ivanhoe, "Was Zhuangzi a Relativist?" in Kjellberg and Ivanhoe, *Essays on Skepticism*, 206–207.

19. Watson, *Zhuangzi*, 140–141.

20. Michael Sandel, *The Case Against Perfection: Ethics in the Age of Genetic Engineering* (Cambridge, MA: Harvard University Press, 2007), 47.

21. See Michael Hauskeller, "Editing the Best of All Possible Worlds," Chapter 4, this volume.

22. There are important empirical questions about what is genuinely within the realm of practical possibility with regard to genetic technology, and we should not exaggerate what can realistically be achieved by it.

23. Allen Buchanan, "Enhancement and the Ethics of Development," *Kennedy Institute of Ethics Journal* 18, no. 1 (2008): 1–34.

24. But whether the changes of nature through human enhancement are of overall benefit to human beings would require us to ask whether the benefits conferred by such enhancement outweigh the loss incurred by it. This, however, is at least in part an empirical issue since we would need to know what the real psychological consequences of pursuing such technology would be.

25. Ed Diener and Martin E. P. Seligman, "Beyond Money: Toward an Economy of Well-Being," *Psychological Science in the Public Interest* 5, no. 1 (2004): 1–31.

26. Martin Seligman, "Why Is There So Much Depression Today? The Waxing of the Individual and the Waning of the Commons," in *Contemporary Psychological Approaches to Depression Theory, Research, and Treatment*, ed. Rick E. Ingram (New York: Plenum Press, 1990), 1–9.

27. Abigail Curtis, "Former Big-City Chef Turns Amish, Makes Charcuterie in Rural Maine," *Bangor Daily News*, January 13, 2016, http://bangordailynews.com/2016/01/13/homestead/former-big-city-chef-turns-amish-makes-charcuterie-in-rural-maine/

28. Watson, *Zhuangzi*, 48.

29. Michael Sandel, *The Case Against Perfection*, 63–83; Leon Kass, "Defending Human Dignity," in *Human Dignity and Bioethics: Essays Commissioned by the President's Council on Bioethics*, ed. Pellegrino Edmund D., Adam Schulman, and Thomas W. Merrill (Washington, DC: The President's Council on Bioethics, 2008), 301; Edmund Pellegrino, "The Lived Experience of Human Dignity," in Kass, *Human Dignity and Bioethics*, 515.

30. Rosemarie Garland-Thomson, "Welcoming the Unexpected," Chapter 1, this volume, XX–XX.

31. Dena S. Davis, *Genetic Dilemmas: Reproductive Technology, Parental Choices, and Children's Futures*, 2nd ed. (Oxford: Oxford University Press, 2010), 19.

32. Garland-Thomson, "Welcoming the Unexpected," XX.

33. Watson, *Zhuangzi*, 31.

34. Watson, *Zhuangzi*, 31.

6

Can We Care about Nature?

Gregory E. Kaebnick

I once asked one of my daughters, Rebecca, then only a child, whether she would like to have stuff done to her that would let her live way past when people usually die. "Maybe you could live five hundred years!" I proposed. "Maybe more!" I assumed she would go for it. Hannah, my younger daughter, at that time very much wanted wings, and great longevity seemed an even easier request. But Rebecca was aghast: "No way!" Maybe her reaction shouldn't have surprised me; she was deep into the Harry Potter series by then, and one of the recurring themes in those books is the value of accepting mortality. But, she seemed to cast about a little when I asked her why not. She frowned: "It would just be unnatural."

Rebecca's reaction is a central theme in the responses people have to the prospect of human enhancement and beyond enhancement to the genetic modification of humans, especially when traits that have long been taken to mark the parameters of who we are—that seem to be core parts of human nature—appear to be up for grabs. But finding the right words to express that reaction, and explaining why or how it should affect decisions about developing and using genetic technologies, has not been easy. Often enough, the view is expressed just as Rebecca, age ten or so, expressed it: in very blunt and forceful language. Modifying DNA is said to be "unnatural," "against nature," or an instance of "playing God." And just as often, this reaction is the subject of ridicule. It is derided as an unsophisticated "yuck" reaction, as a merely emotional sense of disgust or fear of change, or as reflecting a knee-jerk distrust of science.

I want to defend Rebecca's underlying impulses about human nature, but not (bless her) how she expressed it. I think there are different ways of expressing the concern about nature, and different ways of invoking that concern when contemplating decisions about genetic technologies, but they are not all the same and do not all stand or fall together. The quickest and most common, those that jump first to mind, use terms like *unnatural*, but I argue that these are not the most helpful. Rather than speak of what goes against nature, we do better to speak of what goes against our moral preferences for the relationship we aim to have with nature. The question is not whether we must conform to nature, but how much we want to preserve nature.

Making sense of Rebecca's view of the ideal human relationship to nature does not mean that other views are taken off the table, though. On this moral issue, there may be no one right view, and other views certainly have their *own* adherents. As a society, the policy goal may not be to enforce any particular view but to avoid eliminating important views to figure out how to allow incompatible ideas to coexist.

Nature and Human Flourishing

Before defending my daughter, however, I should say something about how the human relationship to nature relates to human flourishing, which in this volume is the central moral concept. I believe that some understanding of the human relationship to nature is on the one hand implicated in our ideas about human flourishing (understanding that concept, in keeping with the other chapters in this volume, as a life of engagement in meaningful activities) but is on the other hand a complement or perhaps even a corrective to them.

The relationship to nature is implicated in the idea of human flourishing because a person's relationship to nature can be part of what counts as flourishing for that person. The relationship with nature is, at least for many people, a meaning-giving aspect of life. Perhaps this is easiest to see in our relationship to nature *outside* ourselves—the natural environment, the world around us. We may find meaning in activities that seek to improve nature: clearing the land and building communities, farming and gardening, controlling or suppressing things that cause disease or other harms to humans. And we may also (many of us, anyway) find meaning in activities that cherish or honor the world as we humans found it: protecting *from* our improvements the wild plants and animals that inherited the world with us and preserving natural phenomena ranging from ecosystems to awe-inspiring rock formations to the deep darkness of the night sky filled from horizon to horizon with the Milky Way. Both of these kinds of activities may be important for one and the same person, moreover. This person's ideal relationship to nature, that is, may involve a mixture of remaking and accepting nature.

I believe similar things can be said about our relationship to nature *within* us, which means the nature of our own bodies, as we find them, and (extrapolating from the diversity of bodies) some understanding of what is typical for humans overall as a species. We certainly often seek to improve ourselves, and flourishing consists in good measure in pursuing those improvements. Yet in some way limiting our self-improvement projects to the bodies we were given—becoming "who we are through the bodies we have," as Rosemarie Garland-Thomson puts it in Chapter 1 of this volume—is important for many people. As Daniel Haybron points out in Chapter 2 of this volume, the kind of account of human flourishing that this volume accepts tends "to accord an individual's 'given' nature special status, as something to be honored or respected." Although we are the kinds of creatures who ponder our own identity, appearance, and behaviors and work deliberately to improve them, many of us, at least, suppose that our improvements should somehow be improvements of what we were originally given, rather than transformations into somebody else altogether. Again, there is a complex balance to be struck. Athletes, at least if they stick to the ideal advanced by many sports governing bodies, are often seen as exemplars of this balance insofar as they seek to refine and perfect their talents yet refine and perfect *only their* talents, eschewing interventions that would seem to replace their given nature with some other given nature. The idea of hewing to our own nature is therefore closely related to the idea of authenticity (which Haybron explores at length). Perhaps, in fact, it is best understood as just another way of putting the same point—a variant that tends to emphasize language about nature instead of language about the "true self" or "who one really is."

But while the relationship to nature is implicated in the idea of human flourishing, the alternative language it provides also enriches and complicates our understanding of what's morally at stake in human flourishing, and it may even serve as a corrective. To speak of finding value in the natural world is to suggest that our own flourishing may not be the only thing that we humans value. The kinds of activities usually seen as constituting human flourishing make demands on the world around us, and a preservationist stance toward nature tends to lead toward curbing those demands. It leads toward deciding against the larger house, the exotic vacation, and the extra four hundred years of life that I dangled in front of Rebecca.

There is, of course, a way to read "human flourishing" so that it encompasses *all* moral considerations. To really do well as a human, one might say, we ought to do all the things that good humans do. So understood, human flourishing becomes just a heading for all of morality, and to speak of "true human flourishing" is like talking about pursuing "the good" or "doing what's right." But there's another way of reading human flourishing that refers to a subset of morality, and arguably, talk of human flourishing always tends to highlight that subset. It tends to emphasize what is good *for the person*. (Haybron's overview of various kinds of accounts of human flourishing brings this feature out.) Insofar as it does, the language of the value of nature differs from the language of human flourishing—and likewise from the language of authenticity, with its emphasis on the true self. It highlights a slightly different set of moral considerations. To take a preservationist stance toward nature as an ideal is precisely to look beyond the question, "What is best for me?"

The inevitable emphasis on personal matters is one reason not to read human flourishing so that it encompasses all other moral considerations. There are some other reasons as well. Reading it that way may suggest that the subsidiary moral considerations fit together rather neatly, with no real conflict between them once we have carefully thought everything out. If the bases of moral judgment are multiple and sometimes conflicting, then putting human flourishing at the top of the list may be somewhat misleading, at least until it's proven that everything comes down to human flourishing.

Rather than strictly emphasizing the flourishing of the self, thinking about nature and our relationship to it is also what gives the treatment-enhancement distinction whatever moral weight it has. That distinction is meant to be between interventions to make a person well versus interventions to make a person "better than well." The idea that there is such a thing as a given nature is necessary first just to make sense of "well"; we need to be able to talk simultaneously about some general understanding of what humans are like as a species and about how individuals happen to find themselves in the world, perhaps very happily being different from whatever is species-typical. The idea that a given nature is something to honor or respect can help make wellness *good*. Michael Hauskeller points out in Chapter 4 of this volume that a "necessary condition of a good life is the ability to see the good in what one has got and in what there is." If we limit our moral touchstones to the idea of human flourishing, however, it will be tempting to say that if an enhancement is really an enhancement—if it genuinely makes a life better—then it has to be a good thing to do. If we accord some value to the nature we happen to have been given, then we can more easily say, with Hauskeller, that what we have got is good, and that we're okay with getting old and dying and don't mind not being the smartest person who ever lived. Wings are not needed (sorry, four-year-old Hannah).

For me, cosmetic surgery sometimes helps bring out the different moral emphases of human flourishing and "the relationship to nature," in a way that gives some substance to the treatment-enhancement distinction. It may well be, for a given man, that a finer nose or stronger jawline would be an enhancement and help him to flourish, if only by giving him more confidence in a room and freeing him from self-doubt to pursue his goals. Perhaps it's enough of an enhancement that it's even worth doing. Yet one might still have misgivings about it, and that residue of misgivings suggests a sense that acceptance or honor is owed to one's given nature.

Nature as Rulebook or Nature as Something We Care About

There are many reasons to be wary about "the human relationship to nature," however. The idea is a kind of conceptual thicket, and in trying to explain what we might mean by it and why we might care about it, we must work through a series of conceptual junctures: forks in a road through the thicket, as it were, where we can choose between different understandings. Each fork is connected to something problematic about Rebecca's declaration, "It would just be unnatural!" and the choice of routes is an opportunity to rethink the problem.

The first fork in the road has to do with who's in charge. On the one hand, we might think of nature as a moral rulebook, showing us right and wrong, but on the other hand, we might think of nature as one of the many things that we humans, drawing on our own resources, care about morally.

The idea that nature is a source of moral guidance is the human relationship to nature that's posited in natural law theory, according to which (to give a rough, thumbnail account) fundamental moral principles can be discerned in nature by a properly thoughtful and sensitive person. There is a long and rich philosophical and theological pedigree to this idea. It has been central to Catholic moral thought, especially to prohibitions against human sexual behaviors that (Catholic theologians have argued) violate the reproductive purpose of human sexuality. It has also been used to justify certain traditional relations between the sexes, on grounds that men are by nature the proper leaders of families. It has also been deemed to justify social structures in which some categories of people are subservient to others.

Because of these uses, the idea that nature provides moral guidance has come under withering philosophical fire. One of the most scathing and frequently quoted fusillades is an essay that John Stuart Mill wrote toward the end of his life to clear away some religious beliefs that he thought stood in the way of moral progress: "Man necessarily obeys the laws of nature, or, in other words, the properties of things, but does not necessarily *guide* himself by them. . . . In sober truth, nearly all the things which men are hanged or imprisoned for doing to one another are nature's everyday performances."[1]

Whatever one thinks about natural law theory, there is another and very different way of thinking about the human relationship to nature, and Mill himself (in another place) suggested it: "Nor is there much satisfaction in contemplating the world with nothing left to the spontaneous activity of Nature; with every rood of land brought into cultivation . . . ; every flowering waste or natural pasture ploughed up, . . . and scarcely a place left where a wild shrub or flower could grow without being eradicated in the name of improved agriculture."[2] In the relationship Mill presupposed here, it is not nature that is in command of humans, but humans in command of nature, and nature has become, not a source, but an object of moral concern. It is (just) a thing that we humans care about deeply.

The Value of Nature: Like a Physical Fact or Like a Social Phenomenon

Mill's desire not to turn all of the natural world into a farm sounds like a lot of contemporary environmentalism. But a second fork in the road must now be pondered. There are different ways of explaining *why* people should value nature. One possibility is that people are simply recognizing the truth: Nature has value, and it would have value even if people failed to see that it does. Alternatively, the value found in nature could be understood as a social phenomenon, perhaps as a social *truth*, but in any event as an aspect of human ways of being in and responding to the world.

The first position—that the value of nature is more like a physical fact than a social phenomenon—would be a powerful reason for valuing nature, but it depends on a lot of strong claims that are not easily explained or defended. It requires that values are real, independent features of the world around us, perceived by the mind rather than by any sensory process, but somehow part of the cosmic order. When critics of environmentalism, or of the claim that altering human bodies is "against nature," argue that valuing nature seems to be "mystical" or "religious," it is a view like this that they have in mind. If the position is to be put on a secular basis, then a convincing explanation is needed of how it works.

Another problem with this position is that it seems likely to drive a wedge *between* humans and nature, turning them into things that are fundamentally different from each other. If something has value just by being on the natural side of the cosmic order and that value is destroyed whenever humans alter it and make it artificial, then humans are apparently radically different from nature. In the cosmic order, they lie elsewhere; they are the antinature, annihilating nature wherever they find it in the way that antimatter annihilates matter. Presumably, human *bodies* are part of nature, and it is the human mind that lies elsewhere. A long tradition in Western philosophy, with René Descartes front and center, takes this view of mind and body (and nature). The view is known as dualism because it holds that the physical world and the mental world are dual realms of reality, somehow linked to each other but fundamentally independent of each other. The challenge for dualism, of course, is that it also seems rather complicated and mysterious—mystical to its critics, anyway, and probably in need of some pretty good explanation.

The alternative road at this fork has us saying—admitting, perhaps—that moral values are always constructs of human thought and culture. If we go this way, our walking companion is David Hume, who argued that all moral judgments are matters of what he called "sentiment." Sentiments are emotions, which might suggest that moral judgments are not to be taken seriously, that they are whimsical, capricious, or idiosyncratic. That is not where Hume is taking us, however. Moral sentiments can be deeply held, settled positions, and if they are deeply held, then we can expect them to be carefully considered, shaped by reason, learning, and dialogue with others.[3]

This explanation puts all the different categories of things mentioned—values, humans, mind, and nature itself—into a single pot. The value of nature does not stand apart from the rest of our values, and humans do not stand apart from nature. The distinction between humans and nature is not like that between angels and Earth but more like that between organisms and environment. Unlike other organisms, though, humans create systems of thought and culture. We develop a sense of self, and we make judgments about how we want to be related to each other and to our world. As a result, our relationship to the environment is not the same as the relationship other organisms have to the environment: Beavers are also great environmental engineers, but unlike beavers, we humans can *see ourselves as* different from the environment, and we can therefore set standards for our relationship to the environment.

These standards can take different forms. On the one hand, we can celebrate our difference from nature. We can value our ability to create systems of thought and culture, understand and gain mastery over our environment, clear pastures and build cities, and so on. As already noted, to stand in such a relationship to nature can be seen as an aspect of human flourishing; in a way, it celebrates uniquely *human* flourishing. On the other hand, perhaps simultaneously, we can celebrate our being *in* nature, cherishing it and seeking to live with it. We can look at the universe and recognize that we are but creatures within it. And that relationship, that of being parts of a larger whole of life and activity, even our position within it—of being shifted off center and standing in awe of a large reality—may provide a kind of grounding, a sense of place and identity, and may be a matter of great importance to us. It may be part of what gives life meaning and structure for us. This relationship to nature also can be seen as an aspect of human flourishing.

Is Nature Inviolable, or Do We Aim for a Kind of Balance?

So in what ways might we reasonably decide to change nature, and in what ways will we aim for restraint? Such decisions will depend on many considerations.

First, if moral values are many and stand in tension with each other, then a preservationist ideal about the human relationship to nature would be but part of a larger range of moral concerns against which it would have to be balanced, and in fact, it might not be as clear and compelling as some other moral concerns. The values of beneficence, liberty, and justice must also be honored. (It is worth pointing out that this kind of balancing may make sense only if we understand the value of nature in the way described previously. It's because we put the value of nature in the same large pot as all our other values that we are able to stir it in with these values. The goal is to get the overall recipe right. If nature is a source of all moral guidance, or if nature imposes value on us from outside, as it were, then it is likely to impose absolute requirements. Making trade-offs with other requirements is harder to explain and harder to do.)

Setting such balancing considerations aside for the moment, though, even the very idea of "nature"—and "against nature" or "aligning with nature"—can be taken in different directions, with different implications for how we might aim for restraint in our relationship to nature. Here's a third fork. On the one hand, we might hold that there are certain hard, bright lines that we may not cross; perhaps some things in nature are *inviolable*. The foremost candidates for bright lines seem to be some of the things that give the living world its shape: organisms' genomes, for example, or the evolutionary processes by which genomes were formed. On the other hand, we might take a more holistic or organic approach and say that the limits are not bright lines but a matter of shades and degrees: How far do we want to go in remaking the world, and to what extent do we want to cherish it as we find it?

The holistic approach is the most plausible way of understanding environmentalism's "preservationist" or "conservationist" sentiment. The object of concern in preservationism and conservationism tends to be molar rather than molecular, ecological rather than atomistic. It's about places, populations, and systems. It's hard to see, then, why sequences of DNA would be considered inviolable. Why ever would we focus our attention on a string of molecules, and why would we insist on their inviolability? It's just hard to see why we'd care about genomes or any other specific thing in nature in quite that way. We might see our stance toward genomes or evolutionary processes as specially important because it is *symbolic* of our overall human relationship to nature and because they provide footholds, places where we can stand as we try to slow down our overall incursion in nature, but even so, inviolability seems a stretch. A claim of genomic inviolability seems to fit better with the view that the value of nature is part of the cosmic order; that position inclines us to the view that nature has a conceptual and moral structure. For many natural law theorists, this structure was the Great Chain of Being, which put humans atop the natural world (and some humans atop others). Each thing takes its place in the chain because its "essence"—its true internal nature—puts it there. The idea that genomes are the most important is a residue of this idea of essences.

Taking an ecological or systemic focus lets us say that altering genes is not bad in itself, that the issue is rather with how gene editing is used. Gene editing might be used in ways that harm natural systems, or it might be more or less neutral, or—in principle—it could even be used to protect or restore nature. That is, one could dismiss the claim that gene editing itself is against nature and focus on the larger effects on natural systems: on species, ecosystems, and (in the case of human gene editing) human bodies and behavior. If we value a preservationist relationship to nature, then we may well be more inclined to accommodate and accept the world as it is and ourselves as we are. For now, the impact of such a stance is limited as there isn't all that much gene editing to be done, but as the tools become more powerful—and if we can gain a better understanding of what the genes do and how changing them can change our bodies and behaviors— then perhaps there will be more to think about. Conceivably, some significant features of human life as we know it could be revisable, not only our life spans, but also our social and moral traits, cognitive skills, and aesthetic appreciation and humor. Behavioral phenomena that undergird our fundamental values could be in question. Moral agency itself might, someday, prove alterable.

There will be lots of room for debate, of course, about which alterations should be unattractive to a preservationist-minded person and which would be fine, even attractive. It is hard to say what preserving "the world as it is" means, given how long humans have been altering the world, but identifying "we humans as we are" is harder yet. Human nature is not fixed. It always *takes form*, and the form it takes is a function to some extent of human creativity. Collectively, we invent social systems and conventions that channel and shape human formation; individually, we may set out (sometimes accepting collective systems and conventions, sometimes in deliberate opposition to them) to *discover* who we are, to make ourselves better, to reinvent ourselves. Part of human nature is precisely to engage in such creativity—"Art is man's nature," as Edmund Burke summarized it. Human nature encompasses creativity, and creativity expands and complicates human nature.

Personal Ideals Versus Societal Obligations

I have been defending Rebecca's resistance to dramatically changing human nature by trying to say more clearly what she might have been thinking about, drawing a series of distinctions between different things she might have meant, setting some positions aside as too strong, too hard to defend, or too absolutist and suggesting that others are plausible and attractive. "It's unnatural" and "It's against nature!" do not strike me as quite right—not flatly wrong, but misleading and unhelpful. They connote that nature tells us what to do, that the proper behavior toward nature is a matter of moral truth, and that bright, inviolable lines outline acceptable behavior toward nature, when we might do better to think of nature as (merely) within the realm of things we care about within the great welter of sometimes-conflicting human values, and about which we have deeply felt but not sharply delineated preferences. This way of discussing nature brings nature down to earth, as it were, and makes it manageable, even if very complicated. It's hardly surprising that ten-year-old Rebecca—and all the rest of us, for that matter—have to work hard to say what it is that's at stake. The difficulty of talking about "nature," together with the difficulties of discussing values, means that there can be no easy way forward.

There is, unfortunately, one final set of difficulties—with yet more forks in the road. How can Rebecca's concern be addressed in the public sphere? What are the right governmental policies? One difficulty is that—as already noted—an ideal about nature is but part of a much larger set of moral concerns alongside which, and sometimes against which, it must be considered, and it seems likely to be inherently limited compared to moral concerns that have to do with fundamental aspects of human society and relationships with each other. Concerns about fairness and individual liberty might be vital to any liberal society, for example.

Another difficulty is that bringing talk about nature down to earth may have limited it. When we confronted the question concerning why people should adopt a preservationist relationship to nature, the answer was not that *everyone should*, but that *people reasonably may*. When people adopt it, they see it as imposing obligations on them, and they may also hope that other people adopt it and accept the same obligations, but they might not see it as something all people *must* accept on pain of irrationality or unreasonableness. It might be more like a personal or social *ideal* than an out-and-out public moral obligation. What would Rebecca have said if I'd asked her, not whether she wanted to live until she was five hundred, but whether other people should be allowed to? I'm imagining that she might have been unsure whether her strong feelings about what *she* found acceptable could translate into enforceable rules for everybody, and if she tried to do so, she might have tried to draw on other moral resources than merely an ideal about the human relationship to nature. (To argue for universal limits, she might have appealed to concerns about fairness; to argue against them, she might have appealed to concerns about liberty.)

These different ways of thinking about the moral stakes might have different implications for public policy. If moral views about the human relationship to nature are inherently personal, then when we make public policy about them, the goal might be to ensure that people who hold those views—assuming enough people hold them to be socially significant—are able to live by them. That might already be the goal in much environmental law, at least that which has to do with preservationism as opposed to public health: Government imposes some general constraints (to protect endangered species, say), but the overall spirit is to physically set aside some places for preservationists while permitting very nonpreservationist activities in other places. It describes the status of rules against biotechnological enhancement in sports; those rules are adopted and enforced by nongovernmental organizations, and other private organizations could (and do) set up quite different rules, if they wish. It could be one rationale for mandatory labeling of foods that contain genetically modified organisms (GMOs); people sometimes express their sense of self through their food choices, and if they wanted to avoid GMOs because they saw doing so as a way of honoring their sense of the relationship they want to have with nature, labels would help them do so.

I don't know what kinds of policies could support this goal—or even whether the goal is achievable at all—if we ever have genetic enhancements that let people live to be five hundred. Creating national parks, having different weightlifting leagues, and labeling foods are a far cry from envisioning a society with some people who live into their nineties and some people who live into their four hundred nineties. But that is perhaps the challenge that now confronts us.

Notes

1. J. S. Mill, "Nature," in *Essential Works of John Stuart Mill*, ed. Max Lerner (New York: Bantam Books, 1961), 374, 381.
2. J. S. Mill, *The Principles of Political Economy*, vol. 2 (London: Parke, 1848), 311, quoted in D. Wiggins, "Nature, Respect for Nature, and the Human Scale of Values," *Proceedings of the Aristotelian Society* 100 (2000), 1–32.
3. G. E. Kaebnick, *Humans in Nature: The World as We Find It and the World as We Create It* (New York: Oxford University Press, 2015).

PART III

IS CONTROL THE KEY
TO FLOURISHING?

7

Do More Choices Lead
to More Flourishing?

Sheena Iyengar and Tucker Kuman[1]

Let's take a trip to the genetic supermarket.[2]

Casey and Taylor are a young couple hoping to start a family. They live in a future where editing embryos has become a normal and accepted part of life. Clinics across the country offer free and equal access to gene editing technologies that are safe to use and perform entirely without error.

> Scenario 1: The baby is conceived and carried to term, and Casey and Taylor do not consider gene editing.
>
> Scenario 2: Casey and Taylor go to a local reproduction clinic where they can have an embryo gene edited according to their preferences. They are asked to choose from among a handful of trait categories, which offer roughly five to ten options per trait. For eye color, for example, there is a choice of brown, blue, green, hazel, gray, or amber. The face can be oval, oblong, square, diamond, or heart shaped. For personality, parents can specify whether they want their child to be more serious, cheerful, calm, logical, or obedient. After making their selections, Casey and Taylor leave the clinic. Nine months later, their baby is born.
>
> Scenario 3: Casey and Taylor go to a reproduction clinic in a nearby city where highly specialized gene editing procedures allow for an abundance of options—close to a hundred for each trait. For eye color, they can choose the exact shade of brown or blue or green they would like from a virtual color wheel of gradients. For height, they can tweak the length of the torso in relation to that of the legs. For facial shape, they can specify the prominence of the cheekbones, the size of the nose, and the droop of the earlobes to within a millimeter. For personality, they are offered varying strengths of attributes like cheerfulness, from cautiously optimistic to vivaciously bubbly or even Pollyannaish. After making their selections, Casey and Taylor leave the clinic. Nine months later, their baby is born.

Each of us may have an opinion about which of these scenarios is, for them, to be preferred. The first is familiar—it describes the way humans have had children for millennia. But Scenarios 2 and 3 propose situations in which parents exert an unprecedented degree of control over the physical and mental characteristics of the child or children they plan to bring into the world. As Erik Parens and Josephine Johnston remind us in their introduction to this volume, the startling complexity of gene interactions behind human traits renders it unlikely that future parents will encounter quite the same kinds of options for traits like personality that comprise Casey and Taylor's choice set. Nevertheless, the hypothetical arc of this couple's experience serves to illustrate the plain fact that gene editing technologies, as they undergo continual refinement and innovation, portend an inevitable *general* kind of change: exponential growth in the *number* of choices available to parents in the procedures of human creation and enhancement.

Having more choices to make and think about might readily be viewed as an improvement over our Scenario 1 status quo. After all, with this increased power to choose comes the freedom to enact our desires and, the hope is, circumvent the accidents of nature and chance. Our limits, according to this perspective, extend only as far as our wills. But are we right to think that more choices necessarily equate to more freedom and better outcomes? Do more choices always lead to more flourishing?

From casual conversation to national constitutions, it is commonplace to recur to the idea of choice as a metonymy for freedom or a fundamental human right. Since the Enlightenment, a familiar story goes, the modern worldview in the West has maintained an overwhelming respect for self-determination, for the ideal of a life chosen for and by oneself, which at least in the United States continues to underpin our philosophical, political, and economic lives.

Moreover, as several contributors to this volume make clear, unswerving belief in the good of choice—and specifically the good of *more* of it—has a history in bioethical debates. In Chapter 3 in this volume, John Evans analyzes the tendency among bioethicists to rally around the ethically "thin" principle of autonomy (that is, individuals' right to self-determination) as a justification for letting the gene editing chips fall where they may. Evans argues that such a principle is not, however, as abstract and value neutral as it's often made out to be. Jackie Leach Scully alludes in Chapter 10 of this volume to similar strains of reasoning when she writes of armchair bioethicists who presume that "more choice means greater reproductive freedom, which is good because it contributes to maximizing personal liberty and therefore also maximizes personal autonomy, *which is good in itself*" (italics added). Critics of this logic urge us to affirm values beyond personal autonomy and control; indeed, further considerations swim into view as we ponder and reflect: Scully shares, for example, evidence from her empirical research in which nonexpert participants not only exhibit enthusiasm "about the benefits of choice" but also go on to express, at greater length, their qualms and hesitation, feeling that choices in reproductive science are distinctive for being "morally problematic."

In the aisles of the genetic supermarket, our moral hesitation collides with our faith in choice and its benefits. Doubts arise because choosing the basic form of a life is not just *any* choice: Can we truly imagine that future parents might, like Casey and Taylor in their alternative universe, walk into the doctor's office with much the same attitude they bring to the car dealership today, seeking a customizable child? It seems outrageous to suggest an equivalence between choosing a jam, a job, or a luxury sedan and choosing a human life. Yet even mundane choices such as those just listed have something vitally important to teach us about what may be considered one of life's most consequential decisions; it is precisely because of the far-reaching significance of Casey and Taylor's task that it becomes all the more urgent to consider how best to support and enable their decision. For what if it *is* the case that the best way of doing so is to provide Casey and Taylor with as many choices as the technology can feasibly allow?

We cannot peer into our future, or Casey and Taylor's, with absolute certainty, but we can make a prediction on the basis of choices people have made and do regularly make. To better understand the stakes and nuances of choice-making, we turn in this chapter to research by social scientists investigating the psychology behind our decisions. As one might expect, a large body of research shows that the freedom to choose indeed poses undeniable benefits to individuals and society at large, serving as a practical vehicle for self-expression. But as we shall also see, studies in social psychology have shown that the availability of more or fewer choices can pose problems when we misunderstand the psychological constraints on individuals' agency or ignore the common pitfalls to which individual choice-makers across all sorts of contexts fall prey.

Turning to this body of literature, we can begin to disentangle the complicated act of making a choice from the supposed freedom such an act represents. In doing so we hope to draw out insights relevant to the problems posed by gene editing in order to reflect on how we think about and treat choice in this context and to assess what increased numbers of choices may or may not serve to achieve. Whatever excitement or anxiety the prospect of "engineering" our future may inspire, it must be appropriately tempered with an appreciation and respect for how individuals recognize choices and how we choose.

Choice Overload and the Trouble with Our Preferences

Choice Overload

Suppose you are in Casey and Taylor's shoes. Faced with the opportunity to select the traits of your future child, how many options would you want to choose from? Recall that in Scenario 2, Casey and Taylor have five to ten options per trait. In Scenario 3, they have a hundred. In which case would you predict yourself, as the agent behind this momentous decision, to be best off?

For many, even those hesitant about the prospect, it will perhaps seem safest to elect for Scenario 3: with more to choose from, you increase the odds of coming on the right and best option, of discovering a perfect fit. As it turns out, however, one has to make a lot of assumptions in order to say with confidence that Scenario 3 would make us better off. We must assume that we have stable preferences; that those preferences are really ours and can be effectively expressed through our choices; and that the more options we have, the better able we are to enact our preferences—and thus the better off we will be. Studies in psychology have called each of these assumptions into question.

While it is true that more choices can allow for the creation of new opportunities, they also pose their fair share of costs. In a phenomenon psychologists call *choice overload*, human beings experience negative effects when forced to deal with more than a handful of choices. Across a range of contexts, research documents that once a choice set exceeds roughly twelve options, people experience exhaustion, confusion, and regret, turning them into tired, less effective, and unhappy choosers.[3]

Why should more choices—something commonly believed to be an unmitigated positive—sometimes lead to negative consequences? The adverse outcomes associated with an increased number of options have been linked to a wide variety of choosing situations in which individuals are tasked with making a selection, whether from mundane assortments of products, like jams and chocolates, to more consequential items such as funds for retirement savings, healthcare plans, and employment opportunities. In one famous example, people were more likely to buy jam at a store when there were only six types on display, as opposed to twenty-four, revealing a diminished ability to choose in the presence of increased options.[4] Similarly, individuals are less likely to put off signing up for a retirement savings program when there are few choices present and more likely to delay or neglect programs altogether when there are lots of options, despite the incredible difference it makes to one's later financial stability to invest as soon as possible.[5] In another investigation, researchers who tracked students during their undergraduate senior year found that those who had sought out more rather than fewer job prospects reported less satisfaction with their eventual employment outcome, even though such students also reported salaries that were on average 20 percent higher than their peers' salaries.[6] As such findings show, more choice can have the adverse effect of not only paralyzing our ability to choose, but also decreasing our later happiness with the choices we ultimately made.

Add to this the fact that humans bring a finite amount of mental energy to any given task: *ego depletion*, in psychology, refers to the fact that expending effort on one task means we have less energy to use for another task.[7] The extreme amount of effort required to evaluate multiple options at once, and then compare and contrast them on the basis of those evaluations, translates to a significant cognitive handicap. The exhaustion associated with making a series of choices has even been found to lead to a diminished immune system response.[8] In practice, we can only process so many comparisons simultaneously before we lose track of the relevant attributes.

To capture the way in which choice quantity affects our well-being, it has been proposed that choice satisfaction follows an inverted U curve: more choice improves our lives, but only up to a point. And beyond that point, dissatisfaction, confusion, and regret drag us down.[9] What the studies investigating choice overload revealed, in other words, is that the benefits of an increasing number of choices are subject to diminishing marginal returns; perhaps more profoundly, it teaches us that simply having more choices, whether or not we use or want them, alters our experience of and subsequent feelings toward the choices we end up making. One study found that a chocolate selected from six options, rather than from thirty, was more satisfying—no matter which chocolate was selected.[10] Does the sweetness of our lives grow harder to taste when a world of rich temptations beckons us to think ever more on the choices to come—or on the choices we didn't make?

Let's return to Casey and Taylor. Imagine they arrive at the clinic in Scenario 3 with a relatively concrete sense of which choices they plan to make. They begin the task of making their selections, but as they sort through the hundreds of options they begin to feel less certain about, say, just how light they want the hazel of the eyes to be and whether the gradation between two skin tones is so great that the one they choose makes a critical difference. After comparing dozens of different trait combinations, they will almost certainly grow exhausted, or perhaps confused, about which options they most prefer. Perhaps they feel increasingly intimidated by their sense of how much is riding on each decision, by their growing awareness of how these traits will impact their future child's likelihood of making friends, securing a good job, being well liked, and finding an ideal spouse, among endless other unforeseeable variables. Will hazel-colored eyes be out of fashion, viewed simply as this year's trend? Will such a choice turn out to mean nothing—or everything?

Weighing all of this, Casey and Taylor may finally decide they want to think about their choices for a bit longer and then leave the clinic without making a final selection. It may turn out, in the end, they are so overwhelmed by the number of possibilities and their potential consequences that they never end up making a choice, completely forgoing the decision to have a child or perhaps choosing to forgo gene editing entirely and have the child in the absence of such interventions. Alternatively, Casey and Taylor may, after sitting with and thinking through their options over a couple of weeks, eventually return to the clinic and make their final decision. But even if they do, we can imagine they might—faced with hundreds of options and exponentially more *combinations* of options—still be uncertain about whether the selections they've made are what they truly want or what is truly best for their child's future. Indeed, perhaps Casey and Taylor will, in the course of their child's life, come to reevaluate what they chose. After all, they could hardly keep it from their minds given how easily they might have chosen differently: What if they had instead gone with that *other* option, over which they had agonized for so long? And what might their feelings be toward their child as a result of such second-guessing and, potentially, regret?

The Trouble with Preferences

The human trouble with choice overload does not begin and end with our finite capacity to manage lots of options, as Casey and Taylor's hypothetical experience serves to hint. As our search for the best option becomes increasingly complicated, we not only lose track of which options we are comparing and how they compare, but can even, as some studies have shown, lose a sense of what our preferences are.[11] Thus when our options become too much to handle, our preferences, too, can get lost and confused amidst the onerous task of rank ordering. Another assumption we tend to bring to the act of making a selection is that we imagine our preferences will guide our choices: we survey the options, pick those in accordance with our supposed wants, and witness the result. That we have preferences and choose in accordance with them has been a long-standing assumption in the field of economics as well as psychology,[12] but this linear sequence of preference, choice, and outcome oversimplifies the picture.

When coming to a choice, we tend to think we'll know what we want, or believe that when we discover what we want, our preferences will be stable. Research has served to show, however, that our preferences are in many ways fluid and subject to environmental manipulation, changing not only over long durations but sometimes even from one moment to the next—often without our conscious awareness.[13] Beyond any unsettling implications this fact may hold for our conceptions of the self, the malleability of our preferences means we are susceptible to influences beyond our control when making choices. As we shall see, our minds are constantly trying to make sense of the world, and the way the world is structured is constantly affecting how and whether we make sense of it and what kind of sense we take away.

In one classic study, researchers showed lab participants pictures of two different women and asked them to choose which one they thought was more attractive.[14] But when subjects were later shown pictures of the woman they had earlier disregarded and explicitly asked why they chose her, on average 74% of participants failed to realize they had been tricked and offered explanations for why they had chosen the picture that was, in fact, not their original choice! The subjects' original preferences proved a poor guide when faced with a simple trick.

Although the researchers in this case deliberately fooled participants into thinking they had made a choice they had not, our preferences can be manipulated in more subtle ways even before we choose, simply as a function of how the choice environment is structured and the options are presented. For example, in a phenomenon psychologists refer to as *ordering effects,*[15] the options you encounter first or last or midway through the course of selection can impact the choice you make: reading through a list from beginning to end, people better remember the items that fall at the beginning or the end of a list. Imagine that in Casey and Taylor's clinic hazel and blue are the colors that are the first and last in the series of options for their child's eyes. Research suggests that we could see a pattern among parents attending that clinic, with more instances of hazel- and blue-colored eyes being chosen, in the same way that items at the top or bottom of a restaurant menu tend to dominate what people order.

In addition, seeing an option repeatedly can bias our memories, such that our positive feelings toward that option are enhanced, something known as the *mere exposure effect.*[16] Imagine that you see lots of other parents choosing green eyes for their children. Without your even being aware of it, this repeated exposure to one choice can subtly impact the one you choose. Clearly, in subtle yet substantial ways, our supposedly pure individual preferences are not the only things that go into the choices we end up making.

There are further ways in which the *framing* of information affects how and what we choose. Consider the following choices:

Imagine a country is threatened by new drug-resistant disease, which is predicted to kill its entire population of 600,000. Time is short, and two plans are proposed, each with its own set of risks. A panel of experts has offered the following estimates of each plan's success:
If Plan A is chosen, 200,000 people will definitely be saved.

If Plan B is chosen, there is a one-third probability that 600,000 people will be saved and a two-thirds probability that no one will be saved.
Which of the two plans would you choose?

Now consider that, instead of Plans A and B, you are choosing between Plans C and D:

If Plan C is chosen, 400,000 people are certain to die.
If Plan D is adopted, there is a one-third probability that nobody will die and a two-thirds probability that the entire population of 600,000 will definitely die.
Which of the two options would you choose?[17]

Sharp-eyed readers will have immediately realized something suspicious: Plans A and B are respectively identical to Plans C and D! The apparent difference between the choice of Plan A or B and the choice of Plan C or D has nothing to do with content, but everything to do with how information about the outcomes is framed. Although the risks outlined in Plans A/C and Plans B/D are respectively equivalent, Programs A/B emphasize lives saved, whereas C/D are concerned with lives lost.

As it turns out, this is not a trivial shift in emphasis. In an experiment from the 1970s, psychologists Daniel Kahneman and Amos Tversky presented a version of this problem to two different groups of participants, asking one group's members to choose between Plans A and B and the other's to choose between Plans C and D. The researchers found that group preferences radically diverged: while 72% of participants in the first group chose Plan A and 28% chose Plan B, only 22% in the second group chose Plan C, and 78% chose Plan D.[18]

Our minds are susceptible not only to what information says, but how it is said. Such framing effects have been shown to lead people to choose differently across situations even when, as illustrated, their options stay the same.[19] In particular, as Kahneman and Tversky demonstrated across multiple studies, we are significantly and systematically "loss averse."[20]

How information about our options is presented can cause certain options to dominate, such that it may become easier to choose in line with our preferences or such that we choose according to different criteria than we might have otherwise. As these examples highlight, choice-making occurs at a point of push and pull between the mind and the world where the effectiveness of our decisions is mediated by features of our environment.

This resultant mediation may not bode well for the choices we ultimately make. When our environment provides us with a lot of information, our inability to effectively navigate that information, coupled with our finite mental energy, leads to the consequences we explored previously. Individuals are more likely to delay making a choice, even when it goes against their best self-interest[21]; are more likely to become uncertain about their preferences or to switch their preferences[22]; are more likely to make errors and become confused; and are more likely to experience regret subsequent to having made the choice.[23]

Yet, despite the adverse effects we often suffer as a result of increasing choice quantity, most of us will elect to choose from more options, even when doing so is to our own detriment.[24] When it comes to choice, most of us end up drawn like moths to a flame, failing to learn even as contact has singed our wings.

Nudging toward Choice

What can be done to manage the challenges we encounter when making choices?

Likening defects in judgment to diseases whose discovery, as in medicine, is a "diagnostic task," Daniel Kahneman considered this very question and somewhat pessimistically concluded: "The short answer is that little can be achieved without a considerable investment of effort."[25] This attitude might, perhaps, push us to share the highly contentious view of one philosopher, who has proposed that our cognitive biases are precisely the kinds of human flaws that gene editing enhancements might serve to edit out of our species![26]

Others have concluded—also not uncontroversially—that it is the duty of institutions and governments to correct for our poor choices. Specifically, they recommend that such institutions devise choice architectures, "wise" interventions,[27] and "nudges," so-called because, rather than force an action perceived by the policymaker to be beneficial, they merely *nudge* the decision-maker toward it with a tendentiously designed choice environment while preserving choosers' autonomy to opt out.

When we begin considering nudges in the context of gene editing, and the potentially controversial choices such nudges may encourage, the specter of old-fashioned, top-down eugenics threatens to reemerge. Should we nudge? Who decides which nudges to implement? There is much in nudging to recommend it, not least the success of nudges in achieving policy objectives on a wide scale (e.g., countries whose organ donor consent status is considered affirmative by default exhibit significantly higher participation rates) and experimental studies showing how nudges can motivate individuals to make objectively healthier choices.[28] The argument in favor of nudges goes that in any case we *will* be nudged, this way or that, by consciously curated choice architecture or the accidental form in which our choosing experience unfolds in any given context.

Nevertheless, there is something about nudging that seems to leave us with a bad taste. The very questions of responsibility and freedom to which nudging gives rise demand closer attention, for we instinctually resent and resist the idea that someone who is not me can possibly know what is best for me personally. We want to be responsible for significant choices, like whether or how to use gene editing, that affect either those we care about or ourselves. This desire for control is, we would suggest, at the root of our desire for more choice in general.

Conclusion

Our intuitive love of choice as a means to freedom has been validated by decades of research in psychology, with studies revealing how choice promotes feelings of intrinsic motivation and personal control and is aligned with physical and mental well-being and life satisfaction.[29] It is because choice is so often a boon to both individuals and societies that we appear to have rational grounds for believing *more* choices are bound to enhance freedom. In the case of the individual, more options from which to choose suggest an increased likelihood that we will find something that perfectly matches our preferences. In the case of the collective, more choice appears to be more inclusive of diverse perspectives. It is a short step from the positive effects of having choices to the belief that choice is a pure good, on whose worth no cap should be placed.

But what is it we are truly valuing when we value "choice"? In treating choice not as an ideal, but instead as the combined acts of search, evaluation, and selection, we come away with a quite different picture of the outcomes we should expect of adding more choices to our lives. Even in circumstances where the freedom to choose appears to be vital, the provision of more choices is not always going to prove the best way of making good on that freedom. Our love of being free to choose should never be conflated with having countless options *from which* to choose. Because our language around choice permits such an easy slip in reasoning, we may end up in thrall to choice rather than masters of it.

As a culture of choosers, we have grown familiar with the experience of customizing our technology, our homes, and even our physical selves with the aid of cosmetics and plastic surgery. It is already easy to imagine ourselves blueprinting human looks and personality to requested specifications, with just a tweak to one gene here and another there: countless individuals have gone through the ritual of choosing new selves, thanks to a proliferation of virtual worlds, in the form of diversely crafted avatars of every size, shape, and hue imaginable, with personality profiles to match. Gene editing now stands to bring this choosing exercise—though assuredly a less fantastic version of it—into the real world.

The severe granularity of the options provided to Casey and Taylor should vividly illustrate the simple fact that, given the form these choices take today, and no matter what eventual form they will take in the future, their mere provision has consequences for how we cope with the act of choosing and relate to our final selections. Despite the fact that we have never faced choices similar in impact or kind to those that gene editing could provide, the pursuit and enactment of those choices will be subject to the same biases, confusions, and manipulations that affect other, more mundane, choices.

None of what we have discussed here is to dispute the obvious possibility that gene editing technologies can and will, when assessed in each individual application, afford us choices that could promote human flourishing, whether by remedying deleterious medical conditions or providing novel gene therapies. But our flourishing as *choosers*, of our children's futures and our own, will also be irrevocably shaped by the provision of such new choices. It is for precisely this reason that, in the same way we urgently compare and contrast options among which to choose, we should be prepared to interrogate with equal fervor what we stand to gain by the presence or absence of ever more choices in the creation of human life.

Notes

1. The authors would like to thank Francis Russo for his comments and assistance during the writing of this chapter.
2. The phrase *genetic supermarket* comes from Robert Nozick, *Anarchy, State, and Utopia* (New York: Basic Books, 1974), 315n.
3. A number of studies have investigated boundary conditions and moderators of the choice overload effect; for a review and critique of the extant literature, see Alexander Chernev, Ulf Böckenholt, and Joseph Goodman, "Choice Overload: A Conceptual Review and Meta-Analysis," *Journal of Consumer Psychology* 25, no. 2 (2015): 333–358.
4. Sheena Iyengar and Mark Lepper, "When Choice Is Demotivating: Can One Desire Too Much of a Good Thing?" *Journal of Personality and Social Psychology* 79, no. 6 (2000): 995–1006.
5. M. Kate Bundorf and Helena Szrek, "Choice Set Size and Decision Making: The Case of Medicare Part D Prescription Drug Plans," *Medical Decision Making* 30, no. 5 (2010): 582–593.
6. Sheena Iyengar, Rachael E. Wells, and Barry Schwartz, "Doing Better But Feeling Worse: Looking for the 'Best' Job Undermines Satisfaction," *Psychological Science* 17, no. 2 (2006): 143–150.

7. Roy Baumeister, Ellen Bratslavsky, Mark Muraven, and Dianne M. Tice, "Ego Depletion: Is the Active Self a Limited Resource?" *Journal of Personality and Social Psychology* 74, no. 5 (1998): 1252–1265.
8. Kathleen Vohs, Roy F. Baumeister, Jean M. Twenge, Brandon J. Schmeichel, and Dianne M. Tice, "Decision Fatigue Exhausts Self-Regulatory Resources" (unpublished manuscript, 2006).
9. Elena Reutskaja and Robin M. Hogarth, "Satisfaction in Choice as a Function of the Number of Alternatives: When 'Goods Satiate,'" *Psychology and Marketing* 26, no. 3 (2009): 197–203.
10. See Study 3 in Iyengar and Lepper, "When Choice Is Demotivating," 1000–1003.
11. Talie Sharot, Cristina Velasquez, and Raymond Dolan, "Do Decisions Shape Preference? Evidence from Blind Choice," *Psychological Science* 21, no. 9 (2010): 1231–1235.
12. For example, see the model of sequential rational choice in John R. Hauser and Birger Wernerfelt, "An Evaluation Cost Model of Consideration Sets," *The Journal of Consumer Research* 16, no. 4 (1990): 393–408.
13. Aiden Gregg, Beate Seibt, and Mahzarin R. Banaji, "Easier Done Than Undone: Asymmetry in the Malleability of Implicit Preferences," *Journal of Personality and Social Psychology* 90, no. 1 (2006): 1; Steve Hoeffler and Dan Ariely, "Constructing Stable Preferences: A Look into Dimensions of Experience and Their Impact on Preference Stability," *Journal of Consumer Psychology* 8, no. 2 (1999): 113–139.
14. Petter Johansson, Lars Hall, Sverker Sikström, and Andreas Olsson, "Failure to Detect Mismatches Between Intention and Outcome in a Simple Decision Task," *Science* 310, no. 5745 (2005): 116–119.
15. Jon Krosnick and Duane Alwin, "An Evaluation of a Cognitive Theory of Response-Order Effects in Survey Measurement," *Public Opinion Quarterly* 51, no. 2 (1987): 201–219.
16. Robert Bornstein and Paul D'Agostino, "Stimulus Recognition and the Mere Exposure Effect," *Journal of Personality and Social Psychology* 63, no. 4 (1992): 545.
17. This problem is adapted from Amos Tversky and Daniel Kahneman, "Rational Choice and the Framing of Decisions," *Journal of Business* 59, no. 4 (1986): S251–S278.
18. For an extended discussion of the results, see Tversky and Kahneman, "Rational Choice."
19. Irwin Levin, Sandra L. Schneider, and Gary J. Gaeth, "All Frames Are Not Created Equal: A Typology and Critical Analysis of Framing Effects," *Organizational Behavior and Human Decision Processes* 76, no. 2 (1998): 149–188.
20. Daniel Kahneman suggested that this particular cognitive bias is adaptive in nature, writing that the "asymmetry between the power of positive and negative expectations or experiences has an evolutionary history. Organisms that treat threats as more urgent than opportunities have a better chance to survive and reproduce"; Daniel Kahneman, *Thinking, Fast and Slow* (New York: Farrar, Straus and Giroux, 2011), 282. Subsequent investigations have borne out this speculation, documenting that loss aversion afflicts children as early as age five and is exhibited even in the responses

of capuchin monkeys to risky gambles; see William T. Harbaugh, Kate Krause, and Lise Vesterlund, "Risk Attitudes of Children and Adults: Choices Over Small and Large Probability Gains and Losses," *Experimental Economics* 5, no. 1 (2002): 53–84; M. Keith Chen, Venkat Lakshminarayanan, and Laurie R. Santos, "How Basic Are Behavioral Biases? Evidence from Capuchin Monkey Trading Behavior," *Journal of Political Economy* 114, no. 3 (2006): 517–537.

21. Sheena Sethi-Iyengar, Gur Huberman, and Wei Jiang. "How Much Choice Is Too Much? Contributions to 401(K) Retirement Plans," In *Pension Design and Structure: New Lessons From Behavioral Finance*, ed. Olivia S. Mitchell and Stephen P. Utkus (Oxford: Oxford University Press, 2004): 83–97.

22. George Loewenstein and David Schkade, "Wouldn't It Be Nice? Predicting Future Feelings," In *Well-Being: The Foundations of Hedonic Psychology*, ed. Daniel Kahneman and Edward Diener (New York: Russell Sage Foundation, 1999): 85–105.

23. Iyengar and Lepper, "When Choice Is Demotivating"; Barry Schwartz, "Self-Determination: The Tyranny of Freedom," *American Psychologist* 55, no.1 (2000): 79.

24. Iyengar and Lepper, "When Choice Is Demotivating"; Dan Ariely and Jonathan Levav, "Sequential Choice in Group Settings: Taking the Road Less Traveled and Less Enjoyed," *Journal of Consumer Research* 27, no. 3 (2000): 279–290.

25. Kahneman, *Thinking, Fast and Slow*, 417.

26. Allen Buchanan, *Better than Human: The Promise and Perils of Enhancing Ourselves* (Oxford: Oxford University Press, 2011), 188.

27. Gregory Walton, "The New Science of Wise Psychological Interventions," *Current Direction in Psychological Science* 23, no. 1 (2014): 73–82.

28. See Eric J. Johnson and Daniel Goldstein, "Do Defaults Save Lives?" *Science* 302, no. 5649 (2003): 1338–1339; Eran Dayan and Maya Bar-Hillel, "Nudge to Nobesity II: Menu Positions Influence Food Orders," *Judgment and Decision Making* 6, no. 4 (2011): 333–342; John Bohannon, "Government 'Nudges' Prove Their Worth," *Science* 352, no. 6289 (2016): 1042.

29. Ellen Langer, "The Illusion of Control," *Journal of Personality and Social Psychology* 32, no. 2 (1975): 311; Edward Deci and Richard Ryan, *Intrinsic Motivation* (New York: Wiley, 1975).

8

"Good Parents" Can Promote Their Own and Their Children's Flourishing

Josephine Johnston

Advances in genetic technology, including new methods for gene editing, promise to provide parents and prospective parents with more information about and more control over the genetic makeup of their children. Information and control are both highly prized in our culture, and both could offer substantial benefits to parents and children. Yet offers of information and control that promise to benefit children can quickly generate new parental responsibilities, morphing from opportunities to obligations, and raising the question whether refusing to use the technologies—in the case of gene editing, refusing to edit a prospective child's genes—might one day be considered inconsistent with being a "good parent." In this chapter, I explore the idea of the good parent and argue that our understandings of the good parent need to evolve so that they take parents' own flourishing into account. Only with this richer understanding of the nature and responsibilities of parenting can we adopt technologies like gene editing in ways that benefit both parents and children.

Advances in genomics already have, and will in the future continue to have, implications for those whose genes are the subject of analysis. In reproductive contexts, this includes the prospective parents whose genes were analyzed during carrier screening, the baby whose genome is sequenced at birth, or the child whose genome was sequenced while they were a fetus in utero. In the areas in which I research and write (ethics, law, and policy), my colleagues and I focus much of our attention on these individuals—the ones whose genes are analyzed or, in the case of gene editing, the ones whose genes would be altered. We seek to understand the impact of genomics on their health outcomes and their life experiences so that we can understand and develop recommendations about the use of these technologies in varying clinical, legal, or social contexts. We also address the impact of use of these technologies at the societal level, as seen in this volume in chapters by Maartje Schumer (Chapter 15), Robert Sparrow (Chapter 11), and others.

But these same technologies also have implications for the parents and prospective parents who are—or will soon be—asked to consider consenting to use of them in their children and future children. These individuals may not have their own genes analyzed or edited; they are not, as usually understood, the direct subjects of the technologies. Yet they will be asked to decide for others in the context of one of the most significant and intimate relationships that humans experience. The first parents offered gene editing of their gametes, embryos, fetuses, or children will be called on to make decisions that I did not have to make when I was a prospective parent and that I have not had to make since my child was born. As a result, their experience of parenting will be different: They will be offered control over one or more aspects of their child's or future child's genome that I was not offered, and whether they accept or decline use of the technology, they will have to make decisions about information and control that I simply did not face. While not the ones on whom the genetic technology would directly act, they will nonetheless be impacted and possibly even changed by it.

It is this ability for gene editing to impact parents and prospective parents that motivates my chapter. In particular, I am interested in how the very presence of this technology will interact with ideas about what good parenting requires of parents and prospective parents. Because this volume is responding primarily to advances in gene editing, I focus on those technologies. I note, however, that versions of my analysis can be applied to parental choices about whether and how to use other kinds of genetic technology, including many technologies that are widely available today, from carrier screening, to genetic testing of embryos, to prenatal testing, to the sequencing of newborns and children. In its focus, my chapter is tightly connected to several others in this volume, including Nicole A Vincent and Emma A. Jane's Chapter 9, in which they imagine the emergence of a parental responsibility to use gene editing technology, bolstered by uncritical assumptions about the relationship between flourishing and disease or disorder and backed by social pressure.

Gene Editing Technology Could Benefit
Future Children

Genomic technologies are thought by many in science and beyond to offer clinicians new ways to improve the health of individual patients and to give parents and prospective parents new opportunities to improve their child's health and well-being. Researchers investigating the use of sequencing technologies in newborns have, for instance, argued that even if not directly relevant to medical care, the results of genome sequencing could supply parents with information that can empower them to anticipate and address that child's future educational and behavioral challenges.[1] Although many scientists, researchers, and commentators remain cautious about the possible use of gene editing technologies in gametes, embryos, and fetuses, early research in this area emphasizes the benefit of eliminating serious diseases from families and, perhaps, from the human gene pool altogether. At the time of writing, several groups have reported using gene editing technologies in embryos to repair genes associated with beta thalassemia, a heart disorder called hypertrophic cardiomyopathy, and Marfan syndrome, which are lifelong and in some cases lethal conditions.[2] A scientist in China has reported the birth of babies whose genes were edited using CRISPR technologies with the aim of making them resistant to HIV.[3] In principle, the same kind of editing could be done for variants associated with everything from increased risk for some forms of cancer to some kinds of athletic ability.

Whether these uses of gene editing will be shown to be safe and effective enough to gain regulatory approval remains to be seen. Any application of the technology would certainly be limited by significant gaps in knowledge about the genetic basis for many common diseases, disorders, and other kinds of human traits (e.g., polygenic risk studies notwithstanding, performance on IQ tests, while known to be highly heritable, is still poorly understood at the level of individual genes[4]). Still, it is possible that gene editing technologies could one day be applied so that the future child is never at risk for particular diseases, so that the risk is greatly reduced, or so that they would be expected to be of slightly higher intelligence than they would have been had their genes not been edited, or slightly taller, or more athletic. If any of these kinds of gene edits can be made, those children will have access to improved health or to the supposed social advantage that is associated with the enhanced trait. If these benefits really are on offer, it will be very tempting to welcome gene editing technologies as enabling new ways to promote the welfare and social advantage of children, as providing exciting options for reducing suffering and advancing flourishing, as wonderful new choices for parents and prospective parents committed to the welfare of their children and future children. After all, what could be more constitutive of good parenting than promoting your child's health and chances for success, even if that child does not yet exist?

Germline Gene Editing Could Be an Available Choice and Will Focus on the Best Interests of Children

I want to back up here for a second to explain why I think that at least some parents and prospective parents are likely to have the choice to use gene editing in gametes, embryos, and fetuses. At the time of writing, these gene editing technologies are not available to prospective parents, and in fact because these uses could result in heritable genetic changes, such a use of the technology would be against the law in dozens of countries, including the United Kingdom, Canada, Brazil, Australia, and many European nations, and against national guidelines in many others.[5] Although not a federal crime in the United States, a long-standing ban on the use of federal money for research involving the creation of embryos for research or the destruction or endangerment of embryos means that US-based researchers interested in this area will have to use nonfederal funding sources for much of the research that would be needed to develop such interventions, making research in this area challenging to carry out (I note, though, that some US-based researchers are already managing to secure such funds).[6] More important, a provision first included in a 2015 federal budget law prohibits the Food and Drug Administration (FDA) from considering any application for a clinical study "in which a human embryo has been intentionally created or modified to include a heritable genetic modification."[7] As a result of this rider and existing FDA law, in the United States today no researcher, regardless of funding source, can transfer for gestation an embryo made using a gene-edited gamete or an embryo that itself has been altered using gene editing technologies. Together, these prohibitions and limitations prohibit use of heritable gene editing in many nations.

But if the techniques show significant promise, determined and well-resourced parents will work around those controls, just as they already do in order to access certain kinds of assisted reproductive services as well as mitochondrial replacement techniques (see, e.g., the 2016 case of an American doctor performing mitochondrial replacement in Mexico to avoid US regulation[8]). And if gene editing is shown to be safe and effective, even if only for one or two serious diseases, then the kinds of blanket prohibitions and restrictions currently in place will not hold. Jurisdictions currently holding restrictions against heritable genetic modifications will face compelling requests from scientists, clinicians, and families to revise their laws and regulations so that families carrying genes for serious diseases can use the technology in gametes, embryos, and fetuses (interventions with fetuses, while not always included when commentators speak of "germline modification," could result in some degree of modification in the resultant child's germ cells[9]). Once using the technology is legal, the decision whether to use it will very likely rest with parents and prospective parents. They will have the authority to make decisions about whether and in what ways to alter the genes of their children and future children.

How will they decide? Of course, no two decisions will be the same, and it is likely that many and varied considerations and influences will shape the decisions of individual parents. Yet, if patterns of decision-making about use of other genetic technologies in similar contexts are any indication, among these considerations will be ideas about what a good parent would do.

Research shows that the idea of the good parent is already at play in decisions about genomics—and that, as parents currently understand this idea, it requires them to maximize their use of the technology for the good of their children or future children. In one study, researchers at the Hospital for Sick Children in Toronto offered genome sequencing to children who had been referred to the hospital's genome clinic for conventional genetic testing. All parents who agreed to have their child's genome sequenced were informed that researchers would return to them news of any variant that is known to predict a childhood-onset disorder (these results would be returned to everyone). In addition, if they wished, parents could elect to learn whether their child carried gene variants associated with a number of medically actionable adult-onset diseases, and they could also learn whether they themselves carried those same variants. Most parents elected to learn the additional results about their children, even if they did not opt to learn the same information about themselves.[10] Researchers who interviewed parents about their decisions reported that many parents expressed ambivalence about learning this additional information, which they realized might enable them to prevent or prepare for unanticipated health vulnerabilities in the child but might also cause psychological distress, lead to insurance discrimination, and be difficult to make sense of. Yet they agreed to receive the additional results about their children because of "a perceived moral obligation to learn, to the extent possible, the full range of current and future risks for their children, no matter how unpleasant."[11] The researchers analogized this felt obligation to "inflicted insight," which refers to the phenomenon of research subjects gaining insight into their own flaws as a result of participating in an experiment. They named the felt obligation "inflicted ought." Parents felt this obligation even regarding information on their child's risk for adult-onset disorders, about which they as parents could not take action, and they felt the obligation to be very powerful: "Faced with this opportunity [to receive their child's adult onset results] parents felt they had no choice."[12]

This version of the good parent—this idea that good parents ought to know all they can about their child or future child's genome—is in the interests of the genetic testing companies. Indeed, it is already their message. Anne Wojcicki, the chief executive officer of 23andMe, told *The Observer* newspaper in 2016: "I tested my son as soon as he was born and I tested my daughter's amniotic fluid. . . . Genetic testing is a responsibility if you are having children."[13] A similar message is promoted in marketing materials for some of the new prenatal tests, which emphasize that "knowledge is empowering,"[14] and that the test offers "peace of mind."[15] In a study of Internet advertising of noninvasive prenatal tests, researchers in the United Kingdom found that a large number of websites used "persuasive and emotive language," including suggesting that using these prenatal tests relying on saliva or blood samples can save women from the decision "to risk amnio or CVS [chorionic villus sampling]," and contained "statements that were misleading, incomplete or conflicted with other information on the same website." As a result of these misleading statements, the authors concluded that "it should be mandatory for companies to clarify that no prenatal test can guarantee the health and wellbeing of a baby."[16]

This construction of good parenting as requiring maximal use of genomic technology is also consistent with the rhetoric of some very prominent scientists, who see universal use of genome sequencing as a welcome fait accompli. Francis Collins, an American geneticist who led the Human Genome Project and is currently the director of the US National Institutes of Health, wrote in 2010: "I am almost certain . . . that whole-genome sequencing will become part of newborn screening in the next few years. . . . It is likely that within a few decades people will look back on our current circumstances with a sense of disbelief that we screened for so few conditions."[17] Collins surely does not plan to force sequencing on anyone, but the benefits of it are so very clear to him that he assumes that sequencing is something that all parents will want.

This idea—that good parents choose to use genetic technologies to the maximum extent—rests on the notion that such use of the technology will benefit the child or the future child. While we can cleverly show how that idea is wrong in the case of prenatal testing—since a fetus cannot currently gain a medical advantage though prenatal testing, and there is much that it could lose—and while it is unclear how realistic that idea is in the case of sequencing results that show risk for something that cannot be clinically or otherwise acted on, the case that gene editing benefits the child or future child could be very strong indeed. After all, sequencing followed by editing could both secure the gestation of an embryo or fetus *and* "repair" its genes, whether to reduce the risk of heart disease, deafness, cancer, or HIV or to increase the chance that this potential future child will one day graduate from college.

So, if the technology works well (and I realize that's a big if), and if scientists and companies support the notion that use of a technology that promotes a child's welfare is not only consistent with good parenting, but also constitutive of it, might we not eventually—or even rather quickly—reach a point where utilizing the technology is not simply "a choice" or "an opportunity" for parents and prospective parents, not merely something that good parents *can* do to benefit their children, but a new responsibility of parenting, something that good parents ought to do? I'm not suggesting that using gene editing will be required by law, at least not initially (although some parental obligations, particularly around provision of medical treatments and including decisions about prenatal and delivery care, are backed by legal sanction[18]). But it might be required by (at least some) prospective parent's culture or social group; it could become a norm of parenting. These parents and prospective parents might feel, as the Toronto parents did, that they have no real choice about whether to agree to using the technology because using it will be synonymous with good parenting.

Discharging This New Responsibility Could Burden Parents

While gene editing could well benefit future children, it might not be an out-and-out boon for parents and prospective parents. At least in its earliest iterations, it is likely to be physically burdensome to women in particular. Right now, it would require prospective parents to refrain from procreating "the old-fashioned way" and to instead undergo in vitro fertilization (IVF), which involves medical testing, medically induced superovulation, and surgical egg extraction before embryos can be created in the lab, tested, edited, and then transferred to the woman's uterus for gestation. If pregnancy is not achieved or does not lead to a healthy birth, the process may need to be repeated. Significant physical discomfort and some health risks accompany IVF,[19] yet the need for this process is rarely discussed in coverage of gene editing. In the future, it may be that, as Hank Greely predicted in his book *The End of Sex*,[20] sperm and egg can be generated from skin cells, requiring very few interventions on the prospective parents to generate dozens or even hundreds of embryos, which can then be tested and edited before being transferred for gestation. Yet even under Greely's so-called easy scenario, individuals will be obliged to avoid getting pregnant "naturally" (or whatever term will be ascribed to unassisted procreation), which itself will likely require some kind of medical intervention.

Use of gene editing might also come with a time burden. IVF takes many months from initiation of testing through egg development and retrieval, embryo creation and testing, and embryo transfer. In addition, clinicians will need to take time to discuss sequencing results and gene editing options and implications of various choices with prospective parents. Genomics will remain uncertain and complex for a long time to come (as Jason Vassy, the lead author of a 2017 study on the impact of whole-genome sequencing in primary care, put it: "It's misleading to equate advances in big data and genomic tools with similar strides in understanding how genetic variants impact health"[21]).

Understanding this complexity and making gene editing choices will likely be cognitively burdensome on clinicians and prospective parents alike. In 2015, the 1000 Genomes Project reported that "a typical genome" differs from the reference human genome at between 4.1 million and 5 million sites and "contains an estimated 2,100 to 2,500 structural variants . . . affecting ~20 million bases of sequence." [22] In this typical genome, about 2,000 of these structural variants are currently understood to be associated with complex traits, and more than two dozen of them are associated with rare diseases. Many will have variable pene-trance. In Chapter 7 in this volume, Sheena Iyengar and Tucker Kuman describe the cognitive burdens of expanded choice and encourage skepticism about the notion that more choice necessarily leads to more flourishing.

Utilizing the results—deciding what to edit and what not to edit, which risks to take and which to seek to avoid—could also be emotionally burdensome. We already know from multiple studies of decision-making around prenatal testing that the presence of variants, even those that are uncertain, generates worry in prospective parents.[23] If gene editing can repair these variants, it might alleviate the worry, but this same prenatal research indicated that worry can continue in prospective parents and parents, even after the "all clear" is given.[24] We also know from research on prenatal testing that prospective parents can be distressed by information they learn about themselves and their partners in the process of testing their fetuses. Sometimes they find out that they likely carry variants as-sociated with autism, cancer, schizophrenia, or early-onset Alzheimer's,[25] things people sometimes choose *not* to know about themselves.[26] Gene editing, because it would begin with sequencing, would turn up this same kind of potentially un-wanted or unexpected information.

Gene editing might also be financially burdensome to parents and prospective parents, yet be something they feel they ought to pay for. Costs would exceed the $12,000–$15,000 associated with one cycle of IVF,[27] and like IVF we might expect significant variation between and within nations about when access to the technology would be covered by national or medical insurance and when it would fall to individual parents to cover. Will paying for gene editing be an expected part of the cost of childrearing, much like the costs of childcare and college education?

Finally, some or all uses of gene editing technology in reproductive contexts[28] might conflict with prospective parents' identities or values, such that using the technology would require them to act against their values or deeply held beliefs. A version of this argument is documented in Jackie Leach Scully's Chapter 10, when she notes that for some discussants in her focus groups it is "wrong" for a prospective parent to seek significant control over their future child precisely because "too much control risks compromising a fundamental feature of parent-hood, one that parents benefit from as much as the future child." This objection to reproductive uses of genetics contains a parent-focused argument, one that seeks to protect the parent or prospective parents from undertaking actions that harm or compromise the parent as a person. One such values conflict could center on the nature of disability. A prospective parent who sees disability as thoroughly consistent with flourishing, as Rosemarie Garland-Thomson in Chapter 1 attests that it can be, could view the choice to edit a gene associated with disability as the adoption of a discriminatory or misguided view. To this parent, choosing to eliminate a gene for deafness would directly conflict with their understanding of deafness as a difference to be embraced not a disorder or fault to be repaired. Reproductive use of gene editing could also conflict with a prospective parent's understanding of the nature of parenting. For this prospective parent, the parenting role privileges acceptance over control, making them reluctant to use gene editing technologies because being a parent who knows this much about and exercises this much control over their child's genes conflicts with the kind of parent (person) they want to be. They might not see themselves as the "maker" or "fixer" of their child or children.

These burdens on parents, which are seldom acknowledged, will not be experienced by all parents and prospective parents, and they will not weigh equally on those who encounter them. But they will be very real for some, could fall disproportionately on women (especially the physical burden associated with preimplantation or in utero gene editing), the poor, the disabled, those with a history of genetic disease, and people with particular religious, moral, or political commitments. The reality of these burdens means that while using gene editing technologies might benefit children and future children, *doing so could negatively impact* the health and well-being of parents. Does that potential clash between the best interests of future children and the flourishing of prospective parents matter? In particular, does it matter for our understandings of good parenting? If we think that a good parent's sole obligation is to further the best interests of their children, then no. But if we think, as I seek to persuade you, that their flourishing matters, that good parents *also* need to take their own interests *as persons* into account in these decisions, then yes the burdens on parents are relevant to our understandings of good parenting in an age of gene editing.

Current Constructions of Good Parenting in the Face of Genomics Exclude Parental Well-Being

Of course, I am not the first to ask whether prospective parents should seek to control the genetic makeup of their future children. Arguments for and against parents and prospective parents seeking this kind of control have been made by a huge variety of scholars, including Adrienne Asch, Michael Sandel, Ronald Green, and Julian Savulescu, as well as authors represented in this collection, including Erik Parens, Robert Sparrow, and Michael Hauskeller. Among these scholars, there is no agreement about whether and how much a good parent uses genetic technologies; indeed, in this volume alone, Sparrow in Chapter 11 seems to be questioning the very same impulse that Hauskeller in Chapter 4 is commending. Those who do agree with each other can disagree about the circumstances under which use or refusal of reproductive genetics is justified and the ends to which those decisions should aim. But there seems to be agreement that the best interests of the child are constitutive of the obligations of parents and prospective parents: that good parents act in the best interests of their (prospective) child, with the disagreement being about how best to do this.

Ronald Green argued in 1997 that parents "should strive to give our children lives unimpaired by serious genetic (or congenital) disorders and we should take reasonable care to avoid doing so by inadvertence or neglect."[29] While Green didn't believe that this obligation stretched to include enhancements, Julian Savulescu did, arguing that "procreative beneficence" requires that parents "should select the child, of the possible children they could have, who is expected to have the best life,"[30] an obligation he has not yet fully extended to the use of gene editing technologies but that might easily be applied if safety issues can be addressed.[31] Baked into these arguments is a biopolitical understanding of the good life, the limitations of which are explored by Gaymon Bennett in Chapter 16 of this volume. For the purposes of my chapter, I note also that these arguments are premised on the idea that arguments for or against parents' use of genetic technology should be guided by whether that use could significantly reduce their child's or their future child's suffering and promote that child's flourishing. The flourishing of parents is not discussed.

Scholars who have raised concerns about parents' use of genetic technology are similarly focused on the well-being of children. Jürgen Habermas feared that the resultant child's freedom could be damaged by use of genetic technologies, as could the nature of that child's relationship to their parent.[32] Both Michael Sandel and Adrienne Ash, who urge parents to *attend to the true nature of good parenting*, tied that true nature to children's best interests by arguing that good parenting—real parenting—is about acceptance and openness, virtues or commitments that ensure the well-being of the individual child who will be born.[33]

I do not dispute the importance of the best interests of the child in our understandings of good parenting. This focus is probably accurate (it reflects how parents actually make many key decisions) and will often be appropriate (it is a reasonable rule of thumb in parental decision-making). But notice that parental well-being is completely missing from these understandings of what it means to be a good parent. Indeed, on these constructions, it might be selfish and therefore inconsistent with good parenting to even consider, let alone on occasion privilege, the well-being or flourishing of parents.

This characterization of the obligations of parents is not realistic or fair to parents. While I recognize that the flourishing of parents and the flourishing of children are frequently inseparable, asking parents to attend only to their child/children's interests to the exclusion of their own establishes a limitless responsibility that the vast majority of people will fail to discharge. Further, it is simply not fair to parents as persons to define the role of parent in such a way that individuals taking up that role must give up attending to their own interests and values or must always prioritize the interests of their child if there is a conflict between the two. Asking parents to adopt this understating of good parenting is akin to asking them to cease to understand themselves as persons.

Good Parents in Action

One result of the broader understanding of good parenting that I propose is that both the choice to use and the choice not to use gene editing technology could, depending on the circumstances, be consistent with being a good parent. This way of thinking about what a good prospective parent should consider makes legitimate a decision not only to find and seek to control some things, but also to leave some things to chance.

Practically, this approach means that prospective parents and parents need a *real* choice about whether to be tested, what they are tested for (which means that routinization of genetic technologies in ways that obviate real choice as well as social pressure to use reprogenetic technologies will both need to be avoided), and whether and which genes to edit. By a "real choice," I mean that parents will need to be supported if they choose not to edit genetic differences in their child. Because the idea that parenting is only about the child's best interests or the child's flourishing is deeply ingrained in Western culture, along with the idea that considering parental interests or well-being is selfish and inappropriate, an attempt to broaden the concept of the good parent in the way that I am advocating will require some work. Some of that work can be undertaken by social institutions, including universities as imagined by Nicole A Vincent and Emma A. Jane in Chapter 9. The media and the arts can—indeed, already do—also play an important role in testing assumptions about flourishing and control, as evidenced by film and television projects like *Gattaca* and *Westworld* that question the wisdom of transhumanist futures.

Individual prospective parents may also need to be helped to reflect on their own values and interests, including what they care about and why, and to consider what a decision to edit or not to edit might mean for who they are as responsible actors with their own life stories. On that understanding, there is room not only for parents to use these technologies if they feel it will benefit their future child and is in line with their values, but also for them to set limits about how they use them, including limits on what or how much they seek to control. Clinicians, clergy, counselors, family, and friends can encourage this kind of nuanced self-examination.

Good prospective parents not only have responsibilities to future children, but also have obligations to themselves. The burdens that gene editing could place on them—including pressure to eschew their own values and act in ways that are inconsistent with their flourishing—are relevant considerations in their decisions about whether and how to use gene editing technologies. It is incumbent on us to recognize these burdens and to be open to supporting parents who act to protect their own flourishing.

Notes

1. Kathryn Asbury and Robert Plomin, *G Is for Genes: The Impact of Genetics on Education and Achievement* (Malden, MA: Wiley, 2013).

2. Puping Liang, Yanwen Xu, Xiya Zhang, Chenhui Ding, Rui Huang, Zhen Zhang, Jie Lv, et al. "CRISPR/Cas9-Mediated Gene Editing in Human Tripronuclear Zygotes." *Protein & Cell* 6, no. 5 (2015): 363–372; Hong Ma, Nuria Marti-Gutierrez, Sang-Wook Park, Jun Wu, Yeonmi Lee, Keiichiro Suzuki, Amy Koski, et al. "Correction of a Pathogenic Gene Mutation in Human Embryos," *Nature* 548, no. 7668 (2017): 413–419; Yanting Zeng, Jianan Li, Guanglei Li, Shisheng Huang, Wenxia Yu, Yu Zhang, Dunjin Chen, et al. "Correction of the Marfan Syndrome Pathogenic FBN1 Mutation by Base Editing in Human Cells and Heterozygous Embryos." *Molecular Therapy* 27, no. 11 (2018): 2631–2637.

3. Antonio Regalado. "EXCLUSIVE: Chinese scientists are creating CRISPR babies." *MIT Technology Review*, November 25, 2018, https://www.technologyreview.com/s/612458/exclusive-chinese-scientists-are-creating-crispr-babies.

4. Jonathan A. Plucker, and Amy L. Shelton, "General Intelligence (g): Overview of a Complex Construct and Its Implications for Genetics Research," *Hastings Center Report* 45, no. S1 (2015): S21–S24.

5. Motoko Araki and Tetsuya Ishii, "International Regulatory Landscape and Integration of Corrective Genome Editing into In Vitro Fertilization," *Reproductive Biology and Endocrinology* 12, no. 1 (2014): 108.

6. The original rider was at Section 128 of Public Law 104–199, which became law on January 26, 1996. The same rider has been included in subsequent appropriations bills.

7. Section 745, 59 Consolidated Appropriations Act of 2016, HR 2029, 114 Cong., 1st session (adopted December 18, 2015). The same section has been included in subsequent appropriations bills.

8. Sara Reardon, "Reports of 'Three-Parent Babies' Multiply," *Nature News*, October 19, 2016.

9. National Academies of Sciences, Engineering, Medicine, *Human Genome Editing: Science, Ethics, and Governance* (Washington, DC: National Academies Press, 2017) 82.

10. J. A. Anderson, M. S. Meyn, C. Shuman, R. Zlotnik Shaul, L. E. Mantella, M. J. Szego, S. Bowdin, N. Monfared, and R. Z. Hayeems, "Parents Perspectives on Whole Genome Sequencing for Their Children: Qualified Enthusiasm?" *Journal of Medical Ethics* 43, no. 8 (2016): 535–539.

11. Anderson et al., "Parents Perspectives," 537.

12. Anderson et al., "Parents Perspectives," 537.

13. Zoe Corbyn, "Genetic Testing Is a Responsibility If You're Having Children," *The Observer*, January 8, 2016.

14. Phrase used on Sequenom MaterniT21 website: https://www.sequenom.com/tests/reproductive-health/maternit21-plus%20.

15. Phrase used on Illumina website: https://www.illumina.com/clinical/reproductive-genetic-health/nipt.html.

16. Heather Skirton, Lesley Goldsmith, Leigh Jackson, Celine Lewis, and Lyn S. Chitty, "Non-invasive Prenatal Testing for Aneuploidy: a Systematic Review of Internet Advertising to Potential Users by Commercial Companies and Private Health Providers," *Prenatal Diagnosis* 35, no. 12 (2015): 1167–1175.

17. Francis Collins, *The Language of Life: DNA and the Revolution in Personalised Medicine* (London: Profile Books, 2010) 50.

18. Lawrence J. Nelson, Brian P. Buggy, and Carol J. Weil, "Forced Medical Treatment of Pregnant Women: Compelling Each to Live as Seems Good to the Rest," *The Hastings Law Journal* 37 (1985): 703.

19. Torbjörn Bergh and Örjan Lundkvist, "Clinical Complications during In-Vitro Fertilization Treatment," *Human Reproduction* 7, no. 5 (1992): 625–626.

20. Henry T. Greely, *The End of Sex and the Future of Human Reproduction* (Cambridge, MA: Harvard University Press, 2016).

21. Aggie Mika, "The Consequences of Sequencing Healthy People," *The Scientist*, June 27, 2017.

22. 1000 Genomes Project Consortium, "A Global Reference for Human Genetic Variation," *Nature* 526, no. 7571 (2015): 68.

23. Barbara A. Bernhardt, Danielle Soucier, Karen Hanson, Melissa S. Savage, Laird Jackson, and Ronald J. Wapner, "Women's Experiences Receiving Abnormal Prenatal Chromosomal Microarray Testing Results," *Genetics in Medicine* 15, no. 2 (2012): 139–145.

24. Theresa M. Marteau, Rachel Cook, Jane Kidd, Susan Michie, Marie Johnston, Joan Slack, and Robert W. Shaw, "The Psychological Effects of False-Positive Results in Prenatal Screening for Fetal Abnormality: A Prospective Study," *Prenatal Diagnosis* 12, no. 3 (1992): 205–214.

25. Bianchi, Diana W., Darya Chudova, Amy J. Sehnert, Sucheta Bhatt, Kathryn Murray, Tracy L. Prosen, Judy E. Garber et al. "Noninvasive prenatal testing and incidental detection of occult maternal malignancies." *JAMA* 314, no. 2 (2015): 162–169; Bianchi, Diana W. "Pregnancy: prepare for unexpected prenatal test results." *Nature News* 522, no. 7554 (2015): 29; Brison, Nathalie, Kris Van Den Bogaert, Luc Dehaspe, Jessica Me Van Den Oever, Katrien Janssens, Bettina Blaumeiser, Hilde Peeters et al.

"Accuracy and clinical value of maternal incidental findings during noninvasive pre-natal testing for fetal aneuploidies." *Genetics in Medicine* 19, no. 3 (2017): 306.

26. Flatau, Laura, Markus Reitt, Gunnar Duttge, Christian Lenk, Barbara Zoll, Wolfgang Poser, Alexandra Weber et al. "Genomic information and a person's right not to know: A closer look at variations in hypothetical informational preferences in a German sample." *PloS one* 13, no. 6 (2018): e0198249.

27. American Society for Reproductive Medicine, *White Paper: Access to Care Summit*, September 10–11, 2015, http://www.asrm.org/globalassets/asrm/asrm-content/news-and-publications/news-and-research/press-releases-and-bulletins/pdf/atcwhitepaper.pdf.

28. Chris Kaposy made a similar argument when he considered the possibility that ter-mination of a pregnancy because the fetus had Down syndrome could be understood as supporting or sharing certain neoliberal and capitalist political and economic values; see Chris Kaposy, *Choosing Down Syndrome: Ethics and New Prenatal Testing Technologies* (Cambridge, MA: MIT Press, 2018).

29. Ronald M. Green, "Parental Autonomy and the Obligation Not to Harm One's Child Genetically," *The Journal of Law, Medicine & Ethics* 25, no. 1 (1997): 5–15.

30. Julian Savulescu, "Procreative Beneficence: Why We Should Select the Best Children," *Bioethics* 15, no. 5–6 (2001): 413–426.

31. Savulescu, Julian, Jonathan Pugh, Thomas Douglas, and Christopher Gyngell. "The moral imperative to continue gene editing research on human embryos." *Protein & Cell* 6, no. 7 (2015): 476–479.

32. Jürgen Habermas, *The Future of Human Nature* (Cambridge, MA: Polity Press, 2003).

33. Adrienne Asch and Dorit Barlevy, "Disability and Genetics: A Disability Critique of Prenatal Testing and Pre-implantation Genetic Diagnosis (PGD)." *eLS* (2012) https://doi.org/10.1002/9780470015902.a0005212.pub2; Michael Sandel, "The Case Against Perfection," *The Atlantic* (April 2004): 1–11.

9

Parental Responsibility and Gene Editing

Nicole A Vincent[1] and Emma A. Jane

> They used to say that a child conceived in love has a greater chance of happiness. They don't say that anymore. I'll never understand what possessed my mother to put her faith in God's hands rather than those of her local geneticist. Ten fingers, ten toes, that's all that used to matter, but not now. Now, only seconds old, the exact time and cause of my death was already known.[2]
>
> —Vincent Freeman, *Gattaca*

Until recently, little could be done about genetic diseases and disorders like hemophilia, Huntington's disease, muscular dystrophy, phenylketonuria, and cystic fibrosis. But with the development of genetic screening and intervention technologies, this may change. Once such technologies become sufficiently safe, effective, and inexpensive, an *unavoidable* risk of conceiving a child with a serious genetic medical condition will become an *avoidable* risk.

When unavoidable risks strike and someone is harmed, we do not usually lay blame. That's just bad luck. But when people knowingly take easily avoidable serious risks with other people's lives, that's different. We call them "reckless" and "irresponsible," and not only do we blame them, but also sometimes we even punish them. Considerations such as these will likely raise two questions once genetic screening and intervention technologies become sufficiently safe, effective, and inexpensive:

1. Would prospective parents have a responsibility to use such technologies to ensure that their child is not born with an avoidable serious genetic disease or disorder?
2. Would prospective parents who don't avail themselves of such technologies be reckless and irresponsible because they would, in effect, be gambling with their future children's potential for a happy and flourishing existence?

As Josephine Johnston notes in Chapter 3 in this volume, parents of children who have undergone genetic testing already feel a very powerful obligation to learn about their children's genetic risks. Moreover, they feel this obligation even when they realize that there is nothing they can do about those risks, even though having such information is likely to be very distressing. Given this, we fully understand why some (and perhaps even many) people might answer yes to both of the questions, all the more so if gene editing technologies could enable them to reduce or even eliminate those risks. Indeed, we understand this on a deeply personal level because one of us (Emma) feels guilty even when her daughter gets a cold. She worries if there was something more she could and should have done to prevent her child getting so sick and miserable. Nevertheless, despite all this, in this chapter we answer both questions with a no. That is, in our view parents neither have a responsibility to use such technologies nor would they be reckless or irresponsible if they decided not to use them.

In part, our aversion to the idea that parents might have such a responsibility, and that parents who choose not to avail themselves of genetic screening and intervention technologies would be reckless and irresponsible, stems from sentiments not unlike what Josephine Johnston voices in Chapter 3 of this volume. Parents are already expected to do so much for their children that we are disinclined to weigh them down with yet more obligations. However, what we wish to focus on in this chapter is a different set of issues. Namely, we feel that the two questions we posed rest on some very dubious assumptions about the connection between flourishing and disease, and that those questions also frame this whole topic in a way that overlooks certain other important issues.

To bring these issues to the foreground, our discussion proceeds as follows: First, we argue that a range of social pressures, rather than a felt sense of parental moral obligation, is more likely to lead most, if not all, parents to use genetic screening and intervention technologies. Second, we highlight serious problems with the idea that less disease and disorder would necessarily result in greater flourishing. Third, we argue that if adequate attention is not given to how our choices are influenced by our own and others' prior choices, then over time nobody may even notice when our use of genetic screening and intervention technologies veers in directions we might not currently view as conducive to flourishing. In the penultimate section of this chapter, we propose that in order to navigate around this hazard, social institutions must be created that enable society to keep an eye on how genetic screening and intervention technologies are used, that promote a thick social dialogue (of the sort that John H. Evans describes in Chapter 3 in this volume) about our evolving views on what constitutes flourishing, and, where needed, that create a social milieu conducive to individual parents making better choices about their use of genetic screening and intervention technologies.

In a nutshell, our case is that no meaningful debate about parental responsibilities in relation to genetic screening and intervention technologies can take place until the right social institutions are created to oversee, evaluate, and control the social factors that influence individual people's decisions in undesirable ways. With this overview of the ensuing discussion, and where it will ultimately take us, we now proceed to our first point, foreshadowed in the preceding paragraph.

Why Eventually All Parents Will Feel the Pressure to Screen and Intervene

To see why a felt sense of moral obligation is not likely to be the most salient factor in shaping prospective parents' choices about the use of genetic screening and intervention technologies, consider some of the social pressures that we think are likely to arise and how those pressures are likely to influence individual parents' decisions. Although we obviously cannot predict the future with Cartesian certainty, here's how we think things will unfold.

Our sense is that initially, if given the option, at least some parents will choose to screen and intervene for precisely the sorts of reasons that we gestured at previously. That is, they will want to give their children the best possible start in life rather than taking avoidable risks with their welfare. However, such initial use of these technologies by *some* parents will gradually transform the social environment in which economic, competitive, and cooperative pressures will make *other* parents' choice not to screen and intervene increasingly untenable.

The genetic diseases and disorders we mentioned in the first paragraph of our chapter are all serious. And out of genuine care for their future children's welfare, we think that many parents will indeed freely choose to screen their zygotes and fix affected genes. Prevention is better than cure, so why wouldn't they take one more step—especially when they already go to such great lengths—and use genetic screening and intervention technologies to ensure their children are not born with serious genetic ailments?

But will society stop at treating only serious genetic diseases and disorders? Or might we eventually develop and use treatments for less serious ones too? For instance, genetic fixes that improve children's immunity to bacterial and viral infections, to forming alcohol and drug dependence, or to proneness to depression and other genetically mediated mental illnesses? Personally, we think that as a society we won't stop once all the "serious" conditions have been eradicated. With scientific, technological, and medical progress, we may eventually develop preventive treatments for a wide range of genetic conditions and susceptibilities.

And why wouldn't parents use the very same logic that warrants screening and intervention for *serious* genetic ailments to screen and intervene for *less serious* ones? Why take *any* avoidable risks, when the only "gain" is that your child might catch colds, become drug addicted, or be depressed? In our view, there is every reason to expect that parents will fortify their children against less serious genetically influenced medical conditions like these ones too, not just catastrophic ones: to avoid suffering from illness; to save the time, money, and effort involved in providing and undergoing medical treatments; and to avoid the not-infrequently nasty side effects of medical treatments.

So that's how we think things will go at the start. We don't think that all parents will necessarily choose to do these things initially, but we suspect some will—and not only to promote their future children's flourishing, but also to avoid unnecessary, costly, and unpleasant medical procedures. However, once *some* parents do this, their choices will start changing the social environment, and in this way these early adopters' decisions will start impacting what *other* parents feel they must do.

After all, the fewer children are born with such medical conditions, the less common these conditions will become. Due to economies of scale, this may raise the cost of treating these conditions. And that, in turn, will make the cost of the choice not to screen and intervene, and the economic pressure to do so, even greater.

There are also insurance implications. Insurance companies frequently charge different categories of clients different insurance premiums. Typically, people in higher risk categories pay higher premiums. Insurers also provide incentives (in the form of lower premiums) to clients who take active measures to reduce their risk factors. Thus, parents who do not use genetic screening and intervention technologies and their children are likely to pay higher insurance premiums, and parents who elect to use them and their children are likely to pay lower insurance premiums. Given the high cost of medical care, the prospect of reducing a family's health insurance bill may be incentive enough for parents to screen and intervene.

Now consider what life will increasingly be like for children whose parents did not screen and intervene in a society where competition and collaboration are the norm and where other children's parents did.

People who have medical conditions or susceptibilities to becoming sick may experience more downtimes at work. One reason why employers sometimes pay for their employees' annual flu shot is to prevent their employees from becoming ill and taking sick days. *You* might get a flu shot to avoid the yuckiness of getting sick, but the reason why your *employer* pays for it is because it makes good business sense. Also, people who are more robust against illness are likely to reap greater rewards at work. Those who don't get sick as often are likely to be more productive and have more impressive CVs (curriculum vitae). And those who have fewer medical expenses will have more resources (time, energy, and money) to devote to other things (e.g., family, relaxation, education, or just more work) that will benefit them even more. Thus, the greater the number of people whose parents go down the screening and intervention route, the more relatively disadvantaged will be those children whose parents did not. Life is competitive, and the stronger and more resilient our fellow citizens become by comparison to us, the more our vulnerabilities will disadvantage us in competitive contexts.

Finally, social life also involves collaboration, and children whose parents did not screen and intervene may increasingly not fit in as well into collaborative projects as children of parents who did. At present, we make room for the likelihood that work colleagues might become sick. Employers even grant employees annual sick leave, which tacitly acknowledges that we currently expect *everyone* to be sick from time to time. But how will attitudes change if falling ill becomes less common? Will we still set aside the same margins for people getting sick in our collaborative plans, even when people no longer get sick as often or for quite as long? Or will these margins gradually shrink in line with shrinking needs to accommodate illness? Might we become increasingly less tolerant of those who are prone to illness and inconvenience everyone else whenever they become ill? Will they eventually be viewed as too risky for collaboration, as imprudent gambles by employers?[3] As with everything else we've said in this section, we have no crystal ball or time machine, so we cannot predict anything for certain. But we do suspect that as disease, disorder, illness, and proneness to such things become less common, we will set aside increasingly smaller margins for sickness in our collaborative plans, and this will disadvantage those people whose parents did not screen and intervene.

In summary, in this section we argued that if some parents choose to screen and intervene, then parents who don't may disadvantage themselves and their children. Their lives may be harder and more expensive, and their children may increasingly suffer marginalization from being less competitive and less attractive as potential collaborators. Just like in the movie *Gattaca*, once some parents screen and intervene, eventually all parents will feel pressured to do so.

But perhaps you think this might not be bad. Wouldn't the world be better if genetic diseases, disorders, and susceptibilities to illness were eradicated? Wouldn't less disease and disorder necessarily equal more happiness and flourishing for everyone? Our succinct answer is, *Nope*. In the next section we elaborate.

Why Less Disease and Disorder Does Not Necessarily Equal More Happiness and Flourishing

In this section we make two claims. First, because the concepts of happiness and flourishing are so contested, we find it difficult to endorse any *universal* claim about how happiness and flourishing can be promoted. Second, since plenty of people with diseases and disorders lead flourishing lives, we also find the *specific* claim that preventing genetic diseases and disorders would result in more happiness and flourishing deeply problematic.

On the first point, you only have to ask around your university, workplace, or local ferret-racing chapter to realize that people have widely divergent ideas about what happiness or flourishing is or how we might get more of it. Some folks, for instance, subscribe to the idea that more of everything—more fitness, more career success, more money, more status, more speed—is the best way to feel good, and that feeling good is what happiness is all about. As Michael Hauskeller puts it in Chapter 4 in this volume, among those who endorse this kind of position, there appears to be the view "that we, as a species, are simply not good enough.... [They] identify the defective and debilitating with the *suboptimal*, so that virtually *any* trait that could conceivably be improved or enhanced is seen as defective" and in need of being fixed if flourishing is to be increased. Others, though, argue that simplicity, minimalism, slowness, an attitude of acceptance toward what we have, and altruistic rather than individualistic orientations are the key to cracking the happiness code. For instance, Richard Kim's Chapter 5 in this volume reports that on a Daoist approach "the requirements for living flourishing lives are much lower than people generally tend to think. A fairly simple life, as long as one cultivates [an attitude of acceptance towards how things are] is sufficient for a high level of flourishing."

Debates between proponents of such divergent views are not new. Ever since Aristotle coined the term *eudaimonia*,[4] the range of views has multiplied about what happiness or flourishing might be, and what kinds of behaviors, habits, outlooks, and so on might produce it.[5] When it comes to our personal views about flourishing, we are most persuaded by ideas from Buddhism. Striving for perfection fills us with dis-ease and anxiety, not calmness and contentment. Thus, rather than constantly trying to optimize everything about ourselves, we find it way more fulfilling to cultivate kindness and compassion, to make some peace with where we find ourselves in any given moment, and to calmly observe (rather than compulsively "shoe shop" through) all of the inevitable human cravings. Indeed, as Sheena Iyengar and Tucker Kuman's Chapter 7 in this volume demonstrates, having *fewer* rather than more options is, somewhat paradoxically, more conducive to happiness. Our own experiences also comport with a growing body of neuroscience and psychology research supporting the benefits of mindfulness and contemplative practice.[6] These findings do not suggest that "meditation = happiness," but that mindfulness practices can increase our ability to do things like concentrate, weather stress, and engage richly with our experiences.[7]

At the end of the day, however, our personal happiness experiments involve a sample size of $n = 2$. As such, we do not venture anything like a universal claim about the recipe required for flourishing. We do, however, voice our enthused agreement with Daniel Haybron's observation that happiness really is a "*paradigm* of unclarity" and "the Mother of all Swamps" because it involves wrestling with "some of the most rich, complex, nebulous, diaphanous, fluid, and evanescent phenomena known to humankind."[8] (Haybron's Chapter 2 in this volume does, however, offer a helpful map through at least one corner of this swamp.)

For the kinds of reasons mentioned, we are suspicious of *universal* claims about what happiness or flourishing might be or how they might be increased. At the same time, though, we are also highly critical of the *specific* claim that happiness and flourishing would necessarily be increased by preventing genetic diseases and disorders.

As we noted at the beginning of this section, countless examples demonstrate that the equation "less disease and disorder necessarily = more happiness and flourishing" just doesn't add up. For instance, the so-called disability paradox refers to the fact that many people with serious and persistent disabilities report experiencing a good or excellent quality of life.[9] A powerful illustration of this was offered by Heather Kirn Lanier in her very moving story about her belated realization that when she was pregnant she had "tried to make a SuperBaby" by eating organic food, taking supplements, staying away from microwave ovens, and so on.[10] And yet, five years after giving birth to a daughter with a chromosomal deletion syndrome, Lanier realized that her failure to make a SuperBaby "was a good failure, the very best of [her] many failures to date."

Bringing together the growing number and variety of such examples, and supported by a constantly expanding body of literature and scientific studies,[11] the disability rights movement has compellingly argued that the root problem is that society tends to pathologize ways of being that are not inherently problematic. The real handicap, they urge, is not a differently abled person's body, but the stigmatization, exclusion, ableist language, endless ignorant and discriminatory social practices, along with the construction of adverse and unaccommodating environments (e.g., buildings with no ramps but only stairs or the increasing reliance on screens with graphical user interfaces that create hurdles for people with visual impairments). In Chapter 1 in this volume, Rosemarie Garland-Thomson poignantly writes:

The limitations to our life projects due to blindness, deafness, weakness, and deformity are not inherent in the conditions themselves but exist largely because the world that we live in was built by and for hearing, sighted, walking, strong, and fully handed people. That we do not experience our way of being in the world as disadvantage, diminishment, or distress can be difficult to grasp for people who understand themselves as nondisabled. . . . The experience of minorities is always challenging for those in the majority to imagine. While disability can occasion suffering, living with disabilities is not necessarily a limitation, a reduction of future opportunities, or a predictor of distress or suffering. And the state of being we think of as perfect health or able-bodiedness is no guarantee of flourishing.

Our take-home message in this section is not that there is no such thing as happiness (because there are so many different views about what it is), that being sick mightn't make our lives go less well (because some people with disorders and disabilities evidently flourish), or even that *any* way of being is as good as *any other* way. We don't know if any of these things are true. Rather, given how contested the terrain of happiness and flourishing is, and given the evidence that plenty of people with diseases and disorders lead happy and flourishing lives when they are not subjected to discrimination, ignorance, and unaccommodating environments, the claim that less disease and disorder would necessarily produce more happiness and flourishing is very implausible.

Shifting Norms and the Need for a Normative Compass

There is, however, another problem with the idea that happiness and flourishing can be increased by using genetic screening and intervention to prevent diseases and disorders, and we think that this problem is potentially even scarier and more difficult to notice and grasp. Namely, by focusing on disease and disorder, we are likely to overlook (1) how genetic interventions will gradually reshape humanity over time, (2) how this will change what it takes for humans to flourish and (3) alter us as evaluators, and (4) how all of that will make it difficult to even assess whether the way we've changed ourselves is positive or negative.

Why think that we might overlook such things? Here are three reasons: Our first, and somewhat banal, observation is that humans get used to things. When we have it good for a while, we get used to that, and when things get less good, we complain. Not only about things we once complained about (bumping our head), but also about smaller things (too much goat's cheese in the salad). Just as people who are used to living in rough conditions can scoff at what the well-off see as problems, so too people in the future who will never even know the maladies we currently have might see what we now view as minor scuffs as mortal wounds.

Second, there's also the fact that these changes would happen gradually and in small increments. Not all parents will embrace genetic technologies right away. And only with adequate scientific progress will we develop ways to detect and prevent new diseases and disorders. Our point is that small and gradual changes tend to be insidious, and things that are insidious are generally difficult to notice.

Third, consider the distinction between the terms *treatment* and *enhancement*. What qualifies as enhancement rather than treatment is blurry, in good measure because how we classify the effect of a given intervention depends on what baseline we presuppose for what is "normal." Consider common analgesic medications like aspirin, ibuprofen, or acetaminophen (also called paracetamol). We typically think of these medications as *treatments*. But to people in a world where analgesics were unheard of, a pill that made pain disappear would be an *enhancement*. Their norm would be that some mornings you wake up with your head in a vice, feeling heavy and vague, and that is just how things roll. And the reason why we don't think that things need to roll that way—that it is normal to spend the day with your head in a vice—is precisely because pain medications have become so ubiquitous, a common feature of our lives. The baseline for what is "normal" shifts when what is inevitable and common becomes treatable and uncommon. The treatments we use rarefy conditions, and this rarefication reclassifies them from being common and *normal* to avoidable and *abnormal*.

Over time, medical interventions reposition and reshape the dividing line between treatment and enhancement by changing what is normal. Consequently, what we pick out on any given occasion as an instance of treatment is itself a product of what we previously chose to treat and made increasingly less common. This means that things we once thought of as enhancements will gradually migrate into the category of treatments, which is another important reason why we think that people are unlikely to notice when they start using genetic screening and intervention techniques in ways they might once have found objectionable, for instance, for what they once thought of as enhancement. And to be clear, our point is not that enhancement is bad and only treatment is good. Rather, our point is that if our current reasoning only warrants using genetic screening and intervention in some cases but not in others, then just by treating the former cases we will eventually alter what qualifies as normal, and with that some of the latter cases will be reclassified as diseases and disorders. Norms will shift with use of these technologies, so that new characteristics—perhaps smaller differences between people or perhaps qualitatively new features—will eventually be categorized as maladies and thus as legitimate targets for genetic screening and intervention.

These are some reasons why we think that people won't notice when humans start changing themselves in what we would currently view as increasingly radical ways. However, even if these changes are noticed, because genetic screening and intervention may change us as evaluators, we may no longer retain the ability to evaluate whether we have changed for better or for worse. The problem here has been described by Laurie Paul as one of "transformative choices,"[12] and there are a number of reasons why this problem impacts this chapter's topic. For one, it prevents humans of the current generation from being able to make reliable long-term plans for the advancement of humanity. If we don't know how the way we change our children will affect what changes they will see fit to make—after all, their decisions will be informed by values we do not yet possess and may not even quite understand—then this will diminish our ability to predict the future even further. For another, if we wish to consider the pros and cons of possible ways of altering ourselves, it's unclear whose evaluative frame we should use to decide precisely how to change ourselves. The one we have right now (i.e., prior to the genetic interventions and thus prior to our values being changed) or the one possessed by future people? Should our current views prevail about what disease, disorder, and flourishing look like, or should we defer to the views of our genetically modified descendants, that is, those who will be affected by our genetic meddling?

But in case we have lost you by now, or perhaps you think we have lost the plot, here are two important clarifications. What we are *not* saying is, "OMG if we gene edit we'll end up as dystopic creatures who plug themselves into walls to recharge their batteries instead of making and eating lovely dinners. Surely that's not going to be very flourish-y." What we *are* saying is, "If we go about using gene editing without all of us thinking really carefully about the potential long-term consequences, we'll end up who-knows-where. Maybe it will be a great place or maybe it won't be. Surely that would be a crazy gamble if what we are really interested in is everyone's flourishing."

These are difficult problems. But given what's at stake, we are not entitled to just throw our hands up in despair, hope for the best, and leave it up to chance how humans will shape themselves. Rather, we need a method to plan ahead, and in the next section we sketch out our thoughts on how this could be done.

The Responsibility of Social Institutions to Reflect on History and Foster Public Debate about Disease, Disorder, and Flourishing

Nonreflective decision-making around constructs like "disease," "disorder," and "flourishing," alongside use of genetic screening and intervention, can mean that nobody exercises any control over how humans evolve—because nobody even notices, and those who do have no way of deciding how to evaluate the changes. However, although our argument employs a slippery slope, our aim is not to be scaremongers because we honestly do not know where this process will lead. Rather, our aim is only to note that this way of deciding when to screen and intervene (i.e., when the target is classified as a *medical condition*) is a dodgy process. It is dodgy because it involves little forethought about how our use of such technologies may alter future views about what even qualifies as a genuine medical condition[13] and where that may eventually take us.

Against the backdrop of the predictive and evaluative challenges we just discussed, it is hard to know whether a given change would lead humanity toward or away from flourishing. One course of action might be to avoid getting on the slippery slope. If we decide, however, that the potential benefits of genetic technologies are too great to forgo, then to avoid slipping on that slope, we need a way to retain our normative compass. We need a way to remind ourselves of the views we once had, the reasons we once found compelling, why our views changed, and that our views may likely change again due to the interventions that we make.

However, we do not think *individual people* are equipped to keep track of how views and values change over time or to take others' and our previous and future views into account in our reasoning. Thus, from a public policy standpoint, if we have a commitment to using genetic technologies to promote human flourishing, our case is that we should set up the right social mechanisms to help us retain our bearings over time. That is, to literally set up *social institutions* that keep track of how our views and values—about disease, disorder, and flourishing— change and keep explicitly feeding these older views and values back into current debates, as well as to remind us that our choices will impact people's views in the future. Additionally, because we think that university professors and sages are just as prone to getting it wrong about happiness and flourishing as normal people—probably because they *are* just normal people—we need all the help we can get to acquire as rich and diverse a set of views on this topic as we can get.

Accordingly, to ensure this process is as broadly informed as possible, the public should be involved on an ongoing basis in reflection on what counts as disease, disorder, and flourishing and in evaluating the sorts of regulations (incentives, disincentives, requirements, and prohibitions) that will guide everyone toward making choices that are conducive to promoting our common conception of flourishing. (For a sobering discussion of existing hurdles to including the public in these discussions, and a compelling argument for why it is critically important to overcome these hurdles, see John H. Evans's Chapter 3 in this volume.) Don't get us wrong, though: A common conception of flourishing may still be difficult to secure and potentially even flawed. But at least if it is arrived at through an inclusive, reflective, and rigorous process like the one we recommend here, then we will be less likely to run into the sorts of problems that we alluded to previously.

Furthermore, we think that even if individual parents may sometimes feel convinced that they have a responsibility to use genetic technologies to promote their children's flourishing, at a collective level society may also have a responsibility to sometimes step in and override these decisions, especially when decisions made by a few people are likely to start creating social pressures that eventually push the rest of us into making choices we would rather avoid. This might sound like a decision to side either with society (and sacrifice individual liberty) or with individuals (and embrace the chaos of that slippery slope). However, this is a false dichotomy since there is no other thing called "society" against which its constituent individuals must be pitted. Rather, there is just us— we are the society—and together we should consider how temporally, technologically, and socially extended and mediated creatures like us should exercise self-control.

This is what it means for creatures like us to exercise our freedom in a responsible manner. To realize that the technologies we create and use, and the reasons we will see as *good* reasons in the future, are a product of the choices that we make today. Given that these things are under our control, to be responsible we must choose with our past and our future selves in mind, and not just with our present selves in mind. We must ask ourselves such questions as, What would I once have thought of the decision I'm now contemplating? and What decisions might my future self—the one I'm about to start creating—make, and do I really want to become that person? We should engage, as best we can, in debates with our past and future selves about what we have reason to do, what we have reason to want, leaving open the possibility that our current selves' views may turn out to be less compelling than our past or future selves' views.

Although this is admittedly only a sketch,[14] we hope it conveys the message that to retain our normative compass, we need to take ourselves seriously as creatures who perdure—who have a past and a future as well as a present—and that the choices we make on any given occasion should make sense when viewed from the perspective of the historical narratives that we will create through our actions.

Conclusion

The discussion in this chapter has important upshots for the two questions we posed at the start, namely whether parents have a responsibility to use such technologies and whether they would be reckless and irresponsible if they didn't.

The first upshot is that even putting these questions like that is unhelpful because it presents the notion of malady—of disease, disorder, and disability—as if it were static, which it simply is not. The second upshot is that this way of putting these questions implicitly pulls focus to the *now*, which fails to give due recognition to the transformative nature of our choices. Answering our questions without properly appreciating these two points could undermine our ability to even assess whether we are making ourselves better, worse, or just weirdly different over time. This is why, to avoid being reckless with our future when we make individual decisions, we need our social institutions to do things that we are simply not equipped to do as individuals. We need to create environments that help us make choices that are rational, especially when we keep in mind that the choices we now make will eventually create social pressures that might in turn make further choices (perhaps ones we would rather not make) rational in the future.

With these considerations in mind, we now offer the following answers to our questions: Parents should be allowed, though not required or prohibited, to use these technologies. What would be reckless, though, is if our social institutions did not regulate these technologies to create the right milieu for parents to make their choices. Parents have every reason to make decisions that are best for their children. However, because other people's decisions alter the environment in which we make our choices, and in this way they can alter what decision would be best for our children, the social institutions we create have a responsibility to foster an environment—through regulation and by encouraging public reflection—that conduces to all parents collectively making the best possible choices, rather than the best choices given what choices others have made. Our social institutions should create an environment that helps us to take into account how the social context we create through our individual choices can in turn influence our future decisions in unexpected and undesirable ways. Surely it is better to create the social context in which our present choices will take such matters into account, so that our future choices are not unintentionally constrained and pushed in directions we would rather avoid?

Notes

1. Nicole's work on this publication was made possible through the generous support of a grant from the John Templeton Foundation, via The Enhancing Life Project. The opinions expressed in this publication, though, are those of the authors and do not necessarily reflect the views of the John Templeton Foundation.
2. Andrew Niccol, dir. *Gattaca* (Culver City, CA: Columbia Pictures, 1997) film.

3. The same kind of discrimination already disadvantages women. Some employers view women as more risky prospects—as less reliable—than men because every month they menstruate, and there's the possibility that they might become pregnant, need maternity leave, or even decide to leave employment.

4. Richard Kraut, "Aristotle's Ethics." In *The Stanford Encyclopedia of Philosophy*. Stanford University, 1997–. Summer 2017 edition. Substantive content change Summer 2018. https://plato.stanford.edu/cgi-bin/encyclopedia/archinfo.cgi?entry=aristotle-ethics

5. For example, Stephanie M. Hare and Nicole A Vincent, "Happiness, Cerebroscopes and Incorrigibility: Prospects for Neuroeudaimonia," *Neuroethics* 9, no. 1 (2016): 69–84.

6. Jon Kabat-Zinn, *Wherever You Go, There You Are* (London: Piatkus, 2004); Jon Kabat-Zinn, *Full Catastrophe Living* (New York: Bantam Books, 2013); Daniel Seigel, *Mindsight* (London: Oneworld, 2011); Daniel Siegel, *Mind* (New York: Norton, 2017). Also see Sheena Iyengar and Tucker Kuman's Chapter 7 in this volume.

7. Steve Paulson, Richard Davidson, Amishi Jha, and Jon Kabat-Zinn, "Becoming Conscious: The Science of Mindfulness," *Annals of the New York Academy of Sciences* 1303 (2013): 87–104.

8. Daniel M. Haybron, *The Pursuit of Unhappiness: The Elusive Psychology of Well-Being* (Oxford: Oxford University Press), vii, emphasis in original.

9. Gary L. Albrecht and Patrick J. Devlieger, "The Disability Paradox: High Quality of Life against All Odds," *Social Science & Medicine* 48, no. 8 (April 1999): 977–988.

10. Heather Kirn Lanier, "Superbabies Don't Cry," *Vela*, April 2017, http://velamag.com/superbabies-dont-cry/.

11. Albrecht and Devlieger, "Disability Paradox."

12. Laurie Paul, *Transformative Experiences* (New York: Oxford University Press, 2014).

13. Relatedly, Nicole is reminded of what Mr. Panforte, her high school teacher, used to say when students who were absent the previous day rocked up with a doctor's certificate saying something to the effect that they missed classes because they had a medical condition. "*Life* is a medical condition!" Fair point, Mr. Panforte.

14. For a more detailed description of the sketch we offer in the following section, please see Nicole A Vincent and Emma A. Jane, "Cognitive Enhancement: A Social Experiment with Technology," in *New Perspectives on Technology in Society: Experimentation beyond the laboratory*, ed. Ibo van de Poel, Lotte Asveld, and Donna C. Mehos (Abingdon, England: Routledge), 125–148.

PART IV

BALANCING ACCEPTANCE AND CONTROL

10

Choice, Chance, and Acceptance

Jackie Leach Scully

Right from the start it was clear that the potential to use gene (or genome) editing technologies raises a set of profound philosophical questions about what we think of as "a good life" and what we are prepared to do to achieve it. Gene editing offers an effective route to deliberately modifying the human genetic makeup (the genotype), and so—to the extent that a particular genotype produces a particular body (or phenotype)—to shaping (although not determining)[1] the embodied physical and mental characteristics of people as well. Eventually, its advocates suggest, gene editing will enable societies to control the "kinds of people" that exist, at least in terms of those characteristics that are predominantly due to gene action.[2] So, there is an urgent need for a proper examination of how the ability to decide on the sorts of bodies that populate the world relates to a person's chances of experiencing a genuinely good life.

To many people the relationship seems obvious. Being able to rewrite genetic sequences could help us eliminate genetically influenced illnesses and impairments that can prevent people flourishing in their lives, and this clearly is a good. Rewriting the genome could also in principle extend to features that are not overtly disabling but are perceived by some people as flaws, and the discussion of gene editing also includes the possibility of enhancing/transforming the human species through more far-reaching interventions. I do not discuss either the removal of minor flaws or the road to radical enhancement here; challenges to those classes of intervention are not difficult to find. Rather, I address what I take to be the class of interventions that is harder to criticize: ones aimed "simply" at the removal of disability.[3]

Currently, genetic intervention against disease is primarily about prenatal identification of those genetic variants that are associated with impairment and offering parents the option of avoiding affected infants' births. The technologies to do that are prenatal diagnosis (PND) and more recently preimplantation genetic diagnosis (PGD). Both remain morally troubling to many people because they are so strongly linked to termination (in the case of PND) or selection against "disabled" embryos (for PGD). The intervention here is purely *eliminatory*, and their use raises the ethical question of whether the predicted disabling condition is bad enough that parents believe, and the society in which they live agrees, it's better[4] for an infant with the condition not be born—even if it means terminating the pregnancy or undergoing the physical, emotional, and financial burden of PGD.

Gene editing by contrast promises to give reproductive choice through *therapeutic and restorative* interventions. Rather than preventing the birth of persons with genetic impairments, the aim is to repair or remove the genetic sequences that are statistically associated with those impairments, so that an embryo (or even gamete) is "cured" of the condition, in a sense before ever actually having it. Gene editing could be used to alter the inherited genetic makeup of both the affected individual *and* that individual's descendants. Moreover, repair of the genome is morally more acceptable to most people than the eliminatory approaches of PND and PGD, so all other things being equal uptake of gene editing is likely to be higher. Taken together, these facts ground the claim that gene editing could effectively wipe out most genetic anomalies from the human genome and, eventually, from the lived experience of subsequent generations.

Many commentators in the gene editing debate have emphasized the necessity of pushing beyond important but relatively superficial ethical issues, about risks to the individual with a genetic disorder or the appropriate governance of the new technology, to engage with the kind of fundamental questions that contemporary bioethics often seems to sidestep: What does it mean to flourish as an individual and as a society, and in this particular case, to what extent can gene editing contribute to personal and societal flourishing. (This discussion is taken up in several chapters in this volume but particularly those by Bruce Jennings [Chapter 17], Michael Hauskeller [Chapter 4], and John Evans [Chapter 3]). For bioethicists, clinicians, healthcare policymakers, and affected families alike a central question then is, If it becomes possible to eradicate genetically influenced disability, whether through gene editing or any future development,[5] is this a step toward ensuring a good life for all, or not? Would anything be lost, and if so a loss to whom or to what? Put another way, is it possible to think of genetically influenced impairment as anything other than an overall harm: to the individual who experiences disability, to parents potentially engaged in reproductive choice, or to society as a whole?

I want to suggest that it is a mistake to think of impairment as never anything but an unambiguous harm, and that therefore it is not always obviously right to use technologies like gene editing with the aim of removing bodily differences. To make sense of this provocative claim, we need to reflect more generally on the value of control.

Removing Disability: The Value of Control

Genetically influenced disabilities come about most commonly through the inheritance of genetic variants that, originally, arose through random mutation.
Gene editing promises a way to control these previously uncontrollable vagaries
of the genome. Being able to eradicate genetically influenced disability is, in
many eyes, just another form of technological control over the intrinsically unpredictable natural world—although one that is historically unprecedented in its
scope and power (and some, like Bruce Jennings in Chapter 17 of this volume,
consider the capacity to manipulate life at the molecular level to be a "significant
discontinuity" with our past).

But both control itself and the value we place on it warrant careful
reexamination. Here I want to consider both the kind of control over biology
that gene editing offers in general and the kind of control we would gain specifically through the use of gene editing in the context of reproductive decisions.
First, I discuss how developed societies today treat the nexus of ideas relating
to control, including choice, chance, and acceptance. Then I look at some empirical data on the views of members of the UK public that offer an alternative
perspective for bioethical thinking about control in the context of reproductive
decision-making. From that, I sketch an argument about relationality, autonomy,
and parenthood that I think is both unexpected and conceptually fruitful.

In the contemporary world, choice is generally presented as an unquestioned
good[6] (although Sheena Iyengar and Tucker Kuman's Chapter 7 in this volume
draws on evidence from psychology to show that having more choice is, in terms
of decision-making and satisfaction with the outcome, not "an unmitigated positive"). One basic reason for this is the close link between *choice* and our ideas
about control and autonomy, both of which also tend to be treated as unalloyed
goods. To be a person in modernity is to be an autonomous agent, and to have
the capacity to be self-determining is fundamental to our picture of ourselves as
living well. An individual is an autonomous agent when she can and does make
independent *choices* about her life without coercion. In other words, making
choices is the primary way in which agency and autonomy are expressed or dis-
played. Making choices enables us to self-determine, that is, to exert control in
such a way that our lives go how we want them to, and to make free choices is also
to pursue and protect our own interests. Conversely, *not* to make choices is not to
be in control of our lives, to be at the mercy of others' choices about us or of the
not necessarily benevolent forces of the natural and social worlds. The rhetoric
of choice in health services, consumer rights, and so on[7,8] always assumes that
choice is a good and that the more options available to choose from, the better.
And since concepts such as self-determination, independence, and agency have

significant moral weight, they in turn give the rhetoric of choice much of its moral and political potency.

Current thinking about autonomy depends heavily on a particular picture of the individual autonomous agent: singular, generally disembodied, socially detached, and as far as possible "unencumbered" by affective or other ties to the surrounding world around that would restrict the freedom of personal choices. This is a *model*, in other words a caricature, and few moral philosophers would claim that real people either do or should behave as sociopathic billiard balls. Nevertheless, the model captures a persistent feature of theories of autonomy, which is an underlying belief that interpersonal connections inevitably reduce an individual's freedom, and that the fewer constraints on free choice people experience, the more likely they are to be able to exercise their autonomy.

It's a model of autonomy that has been heavily criticized from feminist, communitarian, and postmodernist moral viewpoints.[9–10] Working from more relational theories of personhood, feminist ethicists in particular argue that such an atomized model of autonomous agency is inadequate because it fails to account for the ways in which real human beings, who live deeply entangled in networks of family and community relationships, still somehow manage to act in ways that it is meaningful to describe as autonomous. The theories of *relational autonomy* developed within feminist ethics attempt to capture not only that everyday moral life is constituted by interpersonal relationships of responsibility and dependence, but also that it is precisely these relational ties that, rather than compromising it, provide the *conditions* for self-determination.[11] Social and relational ties are what make autonomy possible in material and practical terms and more subtly by enabling people to develop the capacity to reflect on their needs and desires in the first place.

From a relational viewpoint, then, autonomy is not necessarily something that is harmed by ties to other people. Instead, these constraints are an essential part of what constitutes a person, and sometimes personhood includes the voluntary relinquishment of certain kinds of choice, as discussed further in this chapter.

Control, Choice, and Autonomy: Empirical Explorations

Of course, these theories of autonomy, control, and personhood have been developed largely by professional philosophers, who are the people with the time and inclination to do so. It's only recently that bioethics has shown much interest in the practices and perspectives of the everyday moral world and the "ordinary people" making bioethical judgments.[12–13] Empirical data on moral life or opinions cannot *in themselves* be normative (other than in the descriptive sense of showing what people normally do or think), but they can extend the knowledge (the epistemic repertoire) bioethicists and others draw on when forming their normative judgments.[14] This is particularly useful given the reality that the majority of bioethicists come from a relatively homogeneous set of backgrounds and shared experiences.

Empirical and experiential information is particularly important to the bioethics of disability and to evaluating technologies like gene editing that promise to prevent or reduce it. For one thing, such knowledge brings a more accurate idea of what living with and in an anomalous body is really like. Bioethicists are often effectively required to make an evaluation of the quality of a life lived with an impairment and weigh that against the potential moral wrong of biomedical interventions that target those impairments. Yet disability is often an unfamiliar experience to bioethicists,[15] and they will need to turn to other sources of information than themselves. The issue of the quality of that information becomes important because if these sources are inadequate, biased, or just plain wrong, then the moral analysis is likely also to be flawed.

Empirical information extends our knowledge of different *experiences*. What it also does is give insight into the moral *values* that various groups and individuals find salient and the moral *rationales* they find compelling as they navigate their way through everyday bioethical choices. This kind of knowledge expansion challenges and enriches the range of what bioethics holds to be endorsable values, goals, and acts. Its significance extends beyond the work of bioethicists, though, because the relationship between what we might call professional and lay moral thinking is not a dichotomy but an interaction mediated by culture, policy, and a variety of everyday practices. The issue isn't whether professional approaches to bioethical problems are somehow better or insightful than non-professional ones, or vice versa, but about the dangers inherent in drawing on a monoculture of limited perspectives, analyses, and modes of argumentation to inform bioethical debate and policy.

So, as John H. Evans in Chapter 3 of this volume also describes, taking account of the values and evaluative processes of various publics can generate a more nuanced understanding of the concepts that lie at the heart of our bioethical deliberations. As well as a certain reluctance on the part of some bioethicists to move beyond a professional comfort zone, a second obstacle continues to be the sheer lack of adequate information on public thinking on bioethical issues. Nevertheless, the "empirical turn" within bioethics has encouraged both more openness toward the use of existing material and a greater willingness to undertake empirically oriented research.

I want now to examine some empirical material on public views about control and choice in the area of reproduction. It comes mainly from research by colleagues and me with participants from the general public in which we examined their views on the ethics of various biomedical innovations. The earliest study, Ordinary Ethics,[16] ran from 2002 to 2004 and was conducted by a team from Newcastle and Durham universities in the United Kingdom. We used the case study of prenatal sex selection for social reasons (e.g., to detect the sex of the fetus for what has been termed *family balancing*) rather than medical reasons (e.g., to detect a sex-linked condition like hemophilia A and B) to explore public opinion and the way that people form their views on an unfamiliar bioethical topic.[17,18] We held dialogue groups drawn from a variety of professional and social organizations in the northeast of England, each group with an average of six participants and ranging across age, gender, and social class, with follow-up interviews with one participant from each group to explore particular issues in more detail. In addition to this project, two separate qualitative interview studies in Switzerland between 2001 and 2006 examined people's views on genetic testing and on the disposal of surplus in vitro fertilization (IVF) embryos.[19–20] Finally, the Faithful Judgements[21] project, which ran between 2011 and 2014, focused on ethical evaluations and experiences of any form of new reproductive or genetic technology by lay people in the United Kingdom who were members of faith groups. Again, dialogue groups involving a total of around 100 people were complemented by interviews with 18 faith group members who had personal experience of fertility treatment or genetic counseling.

None of these studies was about gene editing, a technology that is not yet part of routine clinical use. Nevertheless, in practice, nearly all the groups and interviews we have held over the years included at some point a general rather than technology-specific discussion of the ethics of using reproductive and other biomedical technologies to take control and make choices. These discussions therefore provide a "thicker" insight into public thinking on the technological promise of choice and control, in particular on the limits to exercising choice over the characteristics of a future person. It's these elements that I draw on here. In addition, since the early 2000s public bodies such as the UK Human Fertilisation and Embryology Authority (HFEA) and the Medical Research Council have run public consultations on the regulation and ethics of contentious biomedical areas,[22] and the publicly available responses contain useful perspectives on issues of parental and societal choice. In the next sections, I outline the dominant themes relating to choice that emerged from these discussions and consider how they relate to bioethical thinking about choice and autonomy.

Ambivalence about Choice

These sources suggest there is a deep ambivalence about choice, especially reproductive choice. This ambivalence is intriguing because gene editing and similar biomedical reproductive interventions are positioned as universally desired because they increase the range of choice available to parents and prospective parents, and as we've just discussed, increased choice is assumed to be a good. Indeed, the claim that increasing patient choice is intrinsic to improving health-care policy has mostly gone unchallenged. For bioethics, giving central place to the *good of choice* is part of a line of reasoning that goes like this: Increasing the array of possible interventions offers more options for deciding whether, when, and increasingly what kind of children to have, which is good because more choice means greater reproductive freedom, which is good because it contributes to maximizing personal liberty and therefore also maximizes personal autonomy, which is good in itself.

In our empirical studies, by contrast, participants did make some unambiguously positive statements about the benefits of choice, but spent far more time discussing how reproductive choice might be morally problematic. They discussed whether *having* to choose might be too much of a burden for people, especially for those who feel they don't have (or perhaps that no one has) enough knowledge to predict what a choice might mean for the future "best possible" life for the child. Others argued that there is no such thing as a genuinely free choice because factors such as money, cultural assumptions, or commercial interests actively constrain the options open to people. Very often, they referred specifically to the lack of social support (material and attitudinal) for disabled people that limits parents' freedom *not* to decide against having a child with an impairment:

> If you have a disabled child, you have to battle and struggle and you are mostly unsupported. That's the context in which parents are potentially making a choice. They are not making a choice in a neutral setting. (Male social worker)

Participants were also concerned about the risk of choice becoming an end rather than a means, so that the simple offer of a range of options is treated as good in itself instead of a way of achieving a good (for them, this might be having a child without an impairment):

> To choose a sex just because you think it's good to have that choice, it's irrational. It's not based on human need. (Member of a women's group)

A further anxiety was that choice might become a morally loaded marker for some other valued quality, such as being a responsible citizen or good parent, with the result that prospective parents feel obliged to intervene[23]:

> Someone might feel that, just letting it go and leaving it up to nature, you know, it's like you're not doing the best for your baby. (Woman, mixed religious group)

Half of me's scared of all the [biomedical interventions] you can do, then a bit of me is like, oh, I'd feel guilty if we don't use it. There's so much we can do that our parents couldn't, you know, so much work [has gone into it], it doesn't seem right now to say No thanks. (Man, individual interview)

Acceptance as a Part of Parenthood

In parallel with ambivalence about the value of choice there runs a line of thought about the value of *acceptance*: that the morally right way to cope with the vagaries of chance is to accept what happens to you, at least up to a point, rather than try to change it. Based principally on the findings of the Ordinary Ethics project, we published a close analysis of our participants' discussion of the acceptance of reproductive chance around their use of the phrase "children are a gift, not a commodity."[24] This phrase, which also appears in our more recent Faithful Judgements project as well as in the public consultation material, has been dismissed by some bioethical commentators on the grounds that comparing children metaphorically to a gift only makes sense if there is some kind of religiously grounded concept of a "giver." For most people, in the context of a broadly secular society like the United Kingdom,[25] this probably isn't the case.

But to call children a gift is to use a metaphor, and metaphors are complex and overdetermined. They generally have more than one entailment (the relationship or conclusion the metaphor points toward). To describe something as a gift *could* be highlighting the existence of a giver, but it could also mean you want to invoke some other feature of gift-giving. In fact, our analysis suggested that in this context, speakers were mainly invoking ideas around acceptance rather than suggesting where the gift might come from. Western cultural rules about gift-giving and receiving mean that to say something is a gift is to say it should be accepted as it is, whether or not it's exactly what you would have chosen. In fact, for some of our participants the real value of a gift lies in those aspects of it that are unexpected and initially may even be unwanted. (When your aunt gives you an orange sweater for Christmas that fills you with dismay, you know—if you are an adult—that you must nevertheless smile and say, "How lovely! It's just what I've always wanted." It isn't done to snap, "But I wanted a blue one.") These cultural norms determine that it is not considered appropriate to want to change the features of a gift, although it would be acceptable to alter your emotional and moral response to it (and ultimately come to love your distinctive orange sweater). Our participants' use of this metaphor, therefore, suggests that for them, wanting to choose a child's characteristics means failing to treat the child as having value in him- or herself, but only in relation to the parents' desires:

> I just don't think it's right that people can actually just sit down and choose what color hair they want [for the child], what color eyes they want, because you're not loving a baby if you've got to sit down and create it like that. (Member of women's group)

At heart these are not ethical claims about the *right sort of acts*, but ontological ones about *the kind of thing* a child is and equally the kind of thing a parent is as well. It seems that using technologies like prenatal selection or gene editing to choose the characteristics of your child, at least beyond a certain point, represents parents' imposing their wishes in a way that fails to respect what the child really *is*. A few participants even went as far as to say that allowing a child to be born with an impairment, when it would have been possible to prevent their birth, showed respect for the child's uniqueness where selecting against their birth would not have done.

It's important to note that, as several other contributors discuss and as Erik Parens and Josephine Johnston note in their introduction to this volume, the sense of acceptance that is invoked here isn't of passivity or fatalism, but of conscious engagement in the enactment of a particular moral understanding of parenting. In these responses, giving up a degree of control over the characteristics of a child is regarded not as a constraint but as a *constitutive feature* of parenthood. Such an act of voluntary relinquishment becomes more significant as the number of possible interventions and opportunities for exerting control grows; there is little moral value attached to choosing not to intervene when the reality is that you can't anyway. This correlation is why reproductive control needs to be carefully and constantly (self-) limited: not because it is necessarily *wrong to treat a child like that*, but because it's *wrong for an adult to behave like that* if that adult is claiming the role of parent. Too much control risks compromising a fundamental feature of parenthood, one that parents benefit from as much as the future child:

> My mum said, "What I've learnt from you and raising you, even though you're not what I imagined initially . . . I wouldn't change you for the world." So [by exercising too much choice] you are robbing parents of that as well. (Woman, postgraduate student group)
>   I think as a parent I'm at my best when I'm not imposing my expectations on my children but rather providing them with the wherewithal to do what it is they want to do. I don't mean that . . . they can go and wreck the place if that is what they want to do, but I mean you know within social confines and

all the rest of it, to achieve what they want to achieve. . . . That doesn't mean pushing them down a particular route that actually meets *my* needs. (Older men's group)

Nuances

Few people in dialogue groups or interviews advocated unlimited parental reproductive choice, and similarly only a small number held that parental acceptance should be unlimited to the extent of accepting pretty much all inborn impairment. For the majority of the people we spoke with, a good parent exercises both some choice and some acceptance, finding a balance point that takes account of several other imperatives. Good parents *may* act to shape the features of the child of their future, but they limit their interventions to ones that further the welfare of the child and enable it to flourish, preserving its "open future"[26],[27] and thereby its future autonomy. In the Ordinary Ethics study, choosing the sex of a child for purely social reasons was not seen as a "hard case" for choice. On the contrary, because it is not about furthering the welfare of the child or enabling it to flourish better, choosing the sex was considered to be solely the expression of a parental preference and therefore not consonant with the values of parenthood. In the absence of any medical rationale for sex selection, the *child* would only benefit if being of one sex rather than another made them more acceptable to their parents—but this in itself would also prove that the parents were deficient in the constitutive parental virtue of accepting whatever comes along unless the child's welfare is thereby seriously and unavoidably threatened.

Attitudes toward disability, on the other hand, are more divided. If "whatever comes along" entails a life of insurmountable suffering or disadvantage, then intervention is generally thought to be OK, even obligatory, because the child's welfare takes priority.[28] At the same time our participants recognized that impairments are diverse, and their impact in real life—whether the genetic variation does in fact cause insurmountable disadvantage and suffering—depends a great deal on the social and material world into which a child with an impairment is born, as Rosemarie Garland-Thomson argues in Chapter 1 of this volume along with many other disability scholars and activists. Arguably, then, what becomes relevant here is the extent to which the disadvantage and suffering of genetically related impairment *is* in fact surmountable through changes in cultural attitudes to disability and provision of medical and social supports during life, so that the presumption in favor of prenatal intervention becomes rather weaker.

But the basic principle still holds: whatever is done to shape the future child's characteristics should be kept to the minimum necessary to preserve welfare and the chance of a good life. The deal with being a parent is that you don't use choice to satisfy what are solely your own personal preferences for how your future child should be. Nevertheless, the majority of our participants also acknowledged a complication to this apparently simple guideline: the lack of universal consensus on the meaning of terms like welfare, suffering, insurmountable, and so on and on how best to regulate an intervention like gene editing such that there is space for the virtue of acceptance, while also protecting the child from avoidable disadvantage and suffering.

The Good Life as Response

The desire to lead a good and flourishing life is a basic feature of being human. What constitutes the good life for humans is a more taxing question that has occupied thousands of years of philosophy and, just as importantly, of everyday human endeavor (Dan Haybron gives an overview in this volume's Chapter 2 of some historical understandings in). Whether and how the control of human and other biology contributes to the good life are the questions that preoccupy us. As a field, bioethics has a rich tradition of worrying about the exercise of control over human destiny through the manipulation of the human genome. The concerns about gene editing not only include the current uncertainty about whether it can actually deliver what it promises, but also extend to a different kind of uncertainty over whether selecting specific physical forms and functions will, in practice, achieve the overall goal of enabling people to flourish better. The public responses I've discussed here suggest that many people share an intuition that the identity and autonomy of parents are inescapably relational, which means that parents' exercise of choice is, and must be, inherently self-limited. It is not that "parents are generally regarded as having permission, and some would say obligation, to produce the best children they can."[29] Instead, they have an obligation *not* to aim for what they and others might want as the "best child" when that desire clashes with the voluntary relinquishment of choices expressing sheer personal preferences that is a constitutive feature of parenthood. The circumstances of being a parent call for a different orientation to choice, one that reflects the distinctive responsibilities, vulnerabilities, and virtues of parenthood. This orientation includes conscious self-limitation of control over the child, even in circumstances when it is possible to make life-determining decisions, like editing impairment out of the genome.

The good life is not dependent on our ability to *control* everything that happens to us, but on our ability to *respond* with appropriate adaptability, creativity, prudence, and hope to the chance and contingency of life. Choosing against the use of gene editing is not necessarily a failure to grasp the emerging opportunities for control and autonomous agency. Rather, an option for the lesser degree of control can be a positive act. The choices that people make about interventions take place within the network of relationships they have with others, and the nature of those relationships will necessarily determine the form that morally defensible autonomy can take. Here, I've explored the need to find an equilibrium between acceptance and control in parental reproductive choice. This need is a striking example of the interplay between the ethical permissibility of using whatever means become available to enable us to pursue our life goals and the constraints that moral claims and relational bonds place around the exercise of individual free agency. Part of the future project of using gene editing, and more generally of using the burgeoning repertoire of methods to control the kinds of people who populate the world, should be to explore and better understand not only how the bonds between people limit the choices they can ethically make but also how these limitations provide the contours within which the valued relationships that form a good life arise and are maintained.

Notes

1. It is generally accepted by scientists that an organism's phenotype is the product not only of its genotype, but also of other biological, environmental, and social factors. Even if genes were the only factors, the processes by which genes are made active or quiescent, produce proteins and ultimately other cellular components, and interact with each other are currently so little understood that the embodied outcome can rarely be accurately predicted just from the genetic composition.

2. The Nuffield Council on Bioethics in London published a report, "Genome Editing: An Ethical Review" in September 2016, including an accessible overview of the science to date. The full report and a summary can be downloaded from http://nuffieldbioethics.org/project/genome-editing/.

3. It's been conventional to place enhancements in a different moral category from interventions that are (or appear to be) therapeutic. Impairment and disability are seen as appropriate candidates for genomic repair or restoration because of the disadvantage and suffering that they cause, whereas nontherapeutic interventions are more open to challenge. Nevertheless, much of what I say further in the chapter is relevant to the transhumanist enhancement of human capacities as well.

4. The question of better for whom is left aside here.

5. Although it should always be kept in mind that gene editing would not affect the estimated 90 percent of impairment that is *not* genetically determined but occurs because of various common or garden life events (accidents, illness, war), and aging.

6. Keith Dowding, "Choice: Its Increase and Its Value," *British Journal of Political Science* 22 (1992): 301–314.

7. D. A. Barr, L. Fenton, and D. Blanne, "The Claim for Patient Choice and Equity," *Journal of Medical Ethics* 34 (2008): 271–274.

8. Clare Williams, Priscilla Alderson, and Bobbie Farsides, "Too Many Choices? Hospital and Community Staff Reflect on the Future of Prenatal Screening," *Social Science and Medicine* 55 (2008): 743–775.

9. Alasdair MacIntyre, *Dependent Rational Animals: Why Human Beings Need the Virtues* (Chicago: Carus, 1999).

10. Anne Donchin, "Autonomy and Interdependence: Quandaries in Genetic Decision Making," in *Relational Autonomy*, ed. C. Mackenzie and N. Stoljar (Oxford: Oxford University Press), 236–258.

11. Jackie Leach Scully, *Disability Bioethics: Moral Bodies, Moral Difference* (Lanham, MD: Rowman & Littlefield, 2008) 161.

12. Giovanni Berlinguer, *Everyday Bioethics: Reflections on Bioethical Choices in Daily Life* (New York: Routledge, 2003).

13. Hilde Lindemann, Marian Verkerk, and Margaret Urban Walker, *Toward Responsible Knowing and Practice* (Cambridge: Cambridge University Press, 2008).

14. To say this is not to counter the call by John H. Evans in Chapter 3 of this volume in favor of a "thick public debate" on gene editing and for social science research to "determine the ends held by the public that are relevant for a particular technology." But knowing what various publics think about something can't be normative in itself; what it can do is significantly shift the shape of the moral landscape on which normative conclusions rest.

15. Especially younger ones. I like to say that bioethicists tend to be rather uninterested in the realities of bodily impairment until they hit their mid fifties, and then they generally become very interested indeed.

16. The research project Ordinary Ethics: The Moral Evaluation of the New Genetics by Nonprofessionals was funded by grant 068439/Z/02/Z from the Wellcome Trust.

17. Jackie Leach Scully, Sarah Banks, and Tom W. Shakespeare, "Chance, Choice and Control: Lay Debate on Prenatal Social Sex Selection," *Social Science and Medicine* 63 (2006): 21–31.

18. Jackie Leach Scully, Tom Shakespeare, and Sarah Banks, "Gift Not Commodity? Lay People Deliberating Social Sex Selection," *Sociology of Health and Illness* 28 (2006): 749–767.

19. Jackie Leach Scully, Erica Haimes, Anika Mitzkat, Rouven Porz, and Christoph Rehmann-Sutter, "Donating Embryos to Stem Cell Research: The 'Problem' of Gratitude," *Journal of Bioethical Inquiry* 9 (2012): 1–28.

20. Jackie Leach Scully, Rouven Porz, and Christoph Rehmann-Sutter, "'You Don't Make Genetic Test Decisions from One Day to The Next': Using Time to Preserve Moral Space," *Bioethics* 21 (2007): 208–217.

21. The Faithful Judgements: The Role of Religion in Laypeople's Ethical Evaluations of New Reproductive and Genetic Technologies research was funded by grant RES-062-23-3210 from the Economic and Social Research Council.

22. The topics of these consultations have included prenatal sex selection, mitochondrial replacement technology (https://www.hfea.gov.uk/media/2618/mitochondria_replacement_consultation_-_advice_for_government.pdf), and research using human embryos (http://www.sharedpractice.org.uk/Downloads/HFEA_Report.pdf).

23. Josephine Johnston and Nicole A Vincent and Emma A. Jane make similar points in their chapters (Chapters 8 and 9, respectively): that we might "reach a point where utilizing the technology is not simply 'a choice' or 'an opportunity' for parents and prospective parents, not merely something that good parents *can* do to benefit their children, but a new responsibility of parenting, something that good parents ought to do" (Johnston).

24. Scully et al., "Gift Not Commodity?"

25. At this point, I am not entering the debate about exactly what "secular" means in twenty-first-century societies.

26. Joel Feinberg, "The Child's Right to an Open Future," in *Whose Child?* ed. William Aiken and Hugh LaFollette (Totowa, NJ: Rowman & Littlefield, 1980), 124–153.

27. Mianna Lotz, "Feinberg, Mills, and the Child's Right to an Open Future," *Journal of Social Philosophy* 37 (2006): 537–551, doi: 10.1111/j.1467-9833.2006.00356.x.

28. A sizable proportion of participants consider the welfare of other characters in the story, like the parents and other siblings, to be very relevant too.

29. Allen Buchanan, Dan W. Brock, Norman Daniels, and Daniel Wikler, *From Chance to Choice: Genetics and Justice* (Cambridge: Cambridge University Press, 2001), 156.

11

Unraveling the Human Tapestry

Diversity, Flourishing, and Genetic Modification

Robert Sparrow

Vive le difference! The idea that diversity is something we should cherish rather than regret has almost become a cliché in the multicultural and multiethnic societies of today. Technologies that allow parents to select or modify their children's genes pose a threat to diversity, at least in the longer term. If parents are choosing their children's genes, there is a chance that they will all try to have healthy, long-lived, handsome, and intelligent children. While many have advertised a world of "perfect babies" as a utopia, to some critics that loss of diversity would be a disaster. The easiest way to feel the force of this intuition is to imagine a world of clones, wherein all men had one genotype and all women had another genotype, such that there were really only two "types" of people in the world.[1] These clones might be healthy and happy. However, surely something important would be lost were we to replace the rich tapestry of human genetic diversity with one consisting of just two threads?

The discussion that follows shows that how likely it is that gene editing technologies will lead to a loss of diversity depends on the power of these technologies, the extent to which their use becomes widespread, and the sort of diversity with which we are concerned. Where gene editing poses a plausible threat to a valuable kind of diversity—and I argue that it may pose such a threat, although less often than many fear—I argue for a moderate approach. According to this approach, it is reasonable to limit the use of gene editing out of a concern for diversity, but only where conserving or securing that diversity does not require us to sacrifice the welfare of any individual too much.

Before proceeding, I should note that two related technologies—prenatal testing and preimplantation genetic diagnosis (PGD)—already offer prospective parents the chance to select against genetic disease or disability in a future child. These technologies of genetic selection pose a much larger threat to diversity than does gene editing,[2] although that may change should gene editing ever offer a realistic means to secure "human enhancement."[3] Regardless of which technology is the focus, an investigation of the value of human diversity is worthwhile for what it reveals about the ethics of the wide set of technologies and policies that could impact human diversity.

Measuring Diversity

The thought that gene editing might reduce diversity implies that we can speak of different worlds, or perhaps different communities, as having more or less diversity. Deciding which of two populations is more diverse requires taking a stand on the relative importance of different sorts of differences. Diversity might be thought to refer to the *distribution* of the differences that exist within a population, the *size* of the differences between individuals in a population, or the *number* of differences in a population. Is a small town of 1,000 people equally divided into ten slightly different "types" more or less diverse than a town of the same size with only five different types of people, but where the differences between those five types are twice as great? What about a town in which 901 of the citizens are the same "type" but the remaining 99 all differ slightly—or even radically—from one another? Each of these towns could claim to be more diverse than the others: any real society will be characterized by diversity of all three sorts, making comparisons extremely problematic.

I cannot hope to resolve here the question of how to measure diversity. For current purposes, I simply note that claims about the benefits of diversity will depend, at least in part, on both how we measure diversity *and* which sorts of diversity we value.

What Kind of Diversity Are We Talking About?

There are at least four different types of diversity that might be affected by the widespread use of human gene editing: genetic diversity, phenotypic diversity, diversity of ways of life, and diversity of life prospects. Each of these types of diversity offers different benefits, and each type of diversity could be impacted by gene editing in different ways.

As the name suggests, technologies of human genetic modification—as well as technologies of genetic selection—will first and most directly impact the extent of *genetic diversity* in the populations in which they are used. If their use is especially widespread, they will alter the relative frequency of particular genes, especially over the longer term.[4] As I will discuss further below, they might even eliminate the genes associated with certain genetic diseases or introduce particular genes into the genomes of some or all of the children born into that community.

Despite the potential impact of genetic technologies on genetic diversity, both critics[5] and advocates[6] typically agree that such technologies will not eliminate human diversity properly understood, that is, *phenotypic diversity*. They argue that, when it comes to realizing most of the purported benefits of diversity, what matters is the character of our interactions with each other, which is a function of our bodies, intellects, and personalities (our phenotypes), rather than our genes. Moreover, because phenotypes are a product of environments as well as genes, there will always be significant differences between individuals as result of their exposure to different environmental influences in the course of their different life histories. It is, for instance, hard to imagine a world in which nobody got sick or maimed or experienced significant changes in their bodily or cognitive capacities as a result of the aging process.

There is clearly some truth to the claim that environments and the impacts of those environments will continue to differ, resulting in significant phenotypic diversity. However, notice that defenders of genetic technologies do not conclude from this fact that we shouldn't be pursuing improvements in the human condition by means of genetic selection or modification. Nor do critics of genetic technologies conclude that there is no point in worrying about these technologies just because phenotypic diversity would persist. Indeed, while phenotypic diversity would not entirely disappear in a world in which genetic diversity were greatly reduced—or even eliminated—it could be reduced through the application of technologies for gene editing.[7]

There is a sense in which diversity of human phenotypes might also be considered "shallow" and, as such, insufficient to produce significant benefits simply in and of itself. Perhaps what matters is *diversity of "ways of life"*? For instance, John Stuart Mill famously argued that in order for a nation to flourish it needed to sustain a diversity of "experiments in living."[8] Think of these different ways of life as characterized by different "conceptions of the good"—different ideas about what human flourishing consists in—and also different patterns of daily activity and social relations. How much gene editing will impact diversity of ways of life will depend both on how much it impacts genetic diversity *and* on the extent to which ways of life are influenced by genetics. As Nicholas Agar has argued, it is highly unlikely that by choosing our children's genes we will ever be able to precisely control the ways of life our children grow up to endorse because the values that children grow up with—and hence the ways of life they eventually come to endorse—are extremely susceptible to historical contingency.[9]

However, even if precise control will forever elude us, some ways of life do seem to correlate roughly with the presence or absence of particular sets of genes. For instance, if—and this is a big "if"—we think of membership of a gay subculture as a way of life, then whether or not someone is same-sex attracted would seem to play a vital role in determining whether or not they adopt this way of life.

Moreover, it seems likely that genes play some role in determining whether or not an individual is same-sex attracted, with the result that any reduction in the number of people with these genes could result in fewer gay people.[10] Similarly, we know that the flourishing of "Deaf culture" depends on the existence of some critical number of deaf persons, and we know that at least some of the causes of deafness are genetic.[11] A reduction in the number of deaf persons could make it difficult for Deaf culture to continue, particularly outside high population countries or areas. These examples suggest that in societies in which gene editing is used, changes in genetic diversity will impact diversity of ways of life.[12]

The last form of diversity that I want to discuss is *diversity of life prospects*. That is to say, diversity in the opportunities available for different people to flourish. For instance, a society in which some people are born to lives of vast wealth, privilege, and freedom, while others are born into situations of poverty and social oppression with radically constrained options, is, in an important respect, a more diverse society than one in which everyone is born with equal life prospects (below, I will discuss the idea that such diversity of life prospects might itself be considered valuable). If individuals are born with different genotypes, which will eventually produce different phenotypes, it is plausible that they will, at least sometimes, have different life prospects. Some people will flourish, while others will have lives characterized by misery, hardship, and failure. The presence of some sorts of genetic diversity, then, can produce winners and losers.

There is an influential line of argument in disability studies that denies that differences in genotype or phenotype need correlate with differences in life prospects. Just as genes only produce phenotypes in conjunction with an environment, differences in phenotypes only lead to differences in life prospects in conjunction with social and institutional arrangements. Diversity of life prospects is a result of social arrangements, which are, according to this argument, consequently unjust.[13] Perhaps more important, there is good reason to be suspicious of claims about the relative extent to which different human lives go well. All too often the claim that people with particular phenotypes do not have good lives reflects either ignorance (likely due to a lack of contact with individuals living with the relevant condition) or a needlessly narrow (and frankly often bigoted) account of what human flourishing consists of. There are, after all, many ways of having a good life, as Rosemarie Garland-Thomson shows in the opening chapter to this volume. The argument concludes that rather than insisting that the lives of people with disabilities are worse than those of people without disabilities, we should understand them to be leading lives that are different but equally as good.

There is much truth in this criticism, especially when assessed against the claims of unreflective advocates of the "medical model" of disability, to which it serves as a valuable corrective. Nevertheless, the argument that we can *never* identify people as having different life prospects, or chances to flourish, is surely too strong. Some forms of cognitive or physical impairment make it exceedingly difficult, if not impossible, for the affected individuals to flourish in any realistically available environment.[14] Moreover, disability advocates typically allow that discrimination and oppression *reduce* the prospects for people born with certain sorts of bodily and intellectual capacities to flourish in our society, suggesting that they too acknowledge the possibility of diversity of life prospects. If everybody's life was equally likely to go well, we would have no grounds for resisting injustices of this nature.

What Difference Does Diversity Make?

Now that we have a better sense of the different types of diversity we can return to the larger argument about the value of diversity by addressing two further questions. First, who is diversity good for? That is to say, who benefits from diversity? And, second, why is it good? That is to say, what does it produce and how?

There are four different answers to the first of these questions, which may be distinguished in the literature. Diversity, it is argued, contributes to the flourishing of the species, the community, individuals, and "nobody" (it is an intrinsic good). For reasons of space, I do not provide an exhaustive list of all the different ways in which diversity may be of value to each of these. However, I hope that a brief survey of the most popular arguments for the value of diversity will allow us to get a sense of the potential and limits of the general argument that diversity is good.

Because species exist for multiple generations, they have properties that individuals do not, which also means they can be said to flourish or suffer independently of the flourishing of their individual members. The idea that a loss of diversity would be bad for the species is often one of the first objections to gene editing. For instance, it is argued that genetic diversity reduces the risk of humanity becoming extinct as a result of a pandemic[15] and will enable our species to adapt and evolve more quickly in response to environmental changes.[16] One form of genetic diversity, in particular, seems necessary to ensure the survival of the species: the existence of the two sexes.[17]

Arguments that diversity is good for the community are not always clearly distinguished within the literature from arguments that diversity is good for individuals. Nevertheless, several arguments that are regularly made about the benefits of diversity might reasonably be interpreted as privileging the community (e.g., its size or longevity) rather than individuals. For instance, it is often suggested that sustaining a diversity of viewpoints can help organizations flourish and respond to change.[18] And, as defenders of "neurodiversity" have emphasized, the existence of a diversity of cognitive styles (phenotypes) within a community may facilitate solving social problems.[19] Other forms of diversity may also make a contribution to this project. Mill's claim that the existence of a diversity of ways of life within a society assists in the pursuit of moral and scientific truths points to a purported benefit that accrues primarily to the community. Disability studies scholar Rosemarie Garland-Thomson has argued that, because different forms of embodiment produce different ways of knowing and valuing the world, a diversity of bodily capacities is an "epistemic resource."[20] Her argument—that disability is a "narrative resource" that can unite the human community[21]—might be interpreted as a claim about a benefit that a diversity of types of human body provides to the community rather than to individuals.

Of course, most things that benefit a community will also be good for its members. We might therefore choose to interpret each of the arguments made about the benefits of diversity to the community as really being about benefits to individuals. For example, another way that, as Garland-Thomson has suggested, bodily diversity is a narrative resource is that the encounter with "freakish" bodies can teach people without disabilities lessons about how to be more human.[22] Similarly, she has argued that disability helps us to be creative and flexible in our relation to the world by requiring us to be open to "the unbidden" and reminding us of the "inevitable growing into disability inherent in the human condition."[23] Further, the benefits to individuals of a diversity of life prospects are sometimes said to include making it possible for people to enter into certain sorts of morally valuable relationships (such as caring relationships) or to express certain attitudes or demonstrate particular virtues (such as acceptance).[24] What is perhaps the most common "folk" account of the value of diversity— that it makes life "more interesting" or "richer"—also points to a benefit that individuals might enjoy.

Notice, however, that some of the ways in which individuals may benefit from diversity look much less attractive than those I have surveyed here thus far. For example, envious preferences—preferences about the extent to which other people have their preferences satisfied—can be satisfied by the presence of diversity (e.g., when someone is made happier merely by the fact that they are better off than someone else). As I have argued at length elsewhere, making a society in which people have a uniform distribution of well-being more diverse by adding a few individuals who are extremely badly off, may, by this mechanism, lead to a significant increase in the welfare of the majority, who now feel happy that they are not badly off.[25] But it would be perverse to hold that we should therefore do this.

Finally, according to all of the accounts I have surveyed thus far, diversity is an instrumental good: it is good because of what it contributes to achieving some other good such as species survival or individual welfare. But diversity might also be an *intrinsic* good.[26] That is to say, a more diverse world might be a better world simply in and of itself, regardless of whether being more diverse contributes to the flourishing of the species, community, or individuals. Diversity might be good without being good *for* anyone.[27]

How Might Human Gene Editing Impact Diversity?

Gene editing might radically reduce diversity. The more control we can have over the genetics of our offspring, the more likely parents will be to choose their children's genes. There are good reasons, moreover, to think that parents are likely to make similar choices. Most parents will want their children to be free of genetic predispositions to cancer or heart disease and of genes that would cause them to be born without limbs or with cystic fibrosis. Parents are likely to want their children to live longer and to be more intelligent. Even if prospective parents don't initially feel strongly inclined to make these choices, the mere fact that other parents are making them may render it extremely difficult to resist. If one knows, for instance, that one's child will be growing up in a world where other children have been genetically modified to have higher IQs (pretending for a moment that this will be possible, which is most unlikely), then one may also need to enhance their IQ just to ensure that the child has a fair chance to succeed in life. This dynamic may drive parents to make the same choices whenever there are positional goods at stake, including in cases (e.g., physical appearance) where there is little reason to believe that the genes involved have any other benefits.[28] If these scenarios come to pass, genetic diversity will be reduced in societies that make use of gene editing.

Conversely, some defenders of gene editing in humans, especially transhumanists, think that the technology would actually *increase* the extent of human diversity.[29] They anticipate that different parents will want different sorts of enhancement for their children and so provide them with different genes.[30] For instance, some parents might value intelligence in a child and choose genes associated with intelligence, while others might value happiness and choose genes associated with high dopamine levels.

I am doubtful that the desires of parents with regard to the genes of their children are likely to vary that much, especially given the social forces pushing toward uniformity. Moreover, the fact that, for the foreseeable future, it will be more feasible to select against genes associated with disease conditions using PGD and prenatal testing than to produce enhancements by inserting new genes into children's genomes suggests that the application of genetic technologies to human beings is much more likely to reduce diversity by eliminating genes associated with impairments than it is to increase it by providing a wide range of human enhancements.

What, therefore, seems most likely is that genetic technologies like PGD will primarily impact the *distribution* of genotypic—and, therefore, some kinds of phenotypic—diversity within particular wealthy societies. In societies in which PGD becomes available, *most* babies will be born with a much narrower range of genetic variation than we see in children born today. However, the possibility that some people will resist PGD for moral reasons means that a small number of children in wealthy societies will still be born with the full range of human genetic variation existing today. Environmental variations, including disease and accidents, will ensure that a significant range of phenotypic variation will remain in these societies, even if most people fall within a much narrower part of that range. At a global level both of these outcomes are even more likely, given that PGD is unlikely to ever become available to the vast majority of the world's denizens, who are currently deprived of basic healthcare, public sanitation, and clean water. If gene editing eventually does prove safe and reliable enough to be used to introduce novel genes into the human genome, the size and number of genetic and phenotypic variations in wealthy societies (and therefore globally) may actually increase. These predictions—that PGD, prenatal testing, and gene editing will decrease but certainly not eliminate genotypic and phenotypic diversity—also likely characterize the impact of gene editing on the distribution of the opportunity to flourish.

The one kind of diversity that might be significantly affected by use of these technologies, at least within wealthy societies, is diversity of ways of life. Ways of life are sustained by communities, and communities must have both a minimum number of members and include a minimum percentage of the population in a particular geographic area in order to survive and to sustain a distinctive way of life.[31] Changes in the relative numbers of people born with different genotypes may threaten a community's ability to sustain those ways of life that are associated with particular genotypes. Even if some individuals remain deaf in the future, Deaf culture, for instance, will struggle to survive if sufficient numbers of parents take steps to make sure that they do not raise a deaf child.[32] For the same reasons, a small number of individuals with particular, novel, genotypes will not bring a new "way of life" into existence. Thus, while the full range of ways of life currently sustained by communities of individuals with normal genes is likely to continue to exist in the future, those associated with differences from this norm are likely to eventually disappear. New ways of life associated with novel genotypes are unlikely to replace them.[33]

Living in a Less Diverse World

If my speculations are well founded, then the threat to many of the benefits of diversity posed by human gene editing is real, but also much lower than sometimes advertised. Most goods that can be realized through the mere presence of diversity in a community are unlikely to be significantly threatened by gene editing. Should our species ever come under environmental stress, there will be sufficient genetic diversity at the global level to provide us with the genetic resources required for human evolution to continue. Neurodiversity will continue to be a feature of communities, although in wealthy societies the number of individuals with particular genetic conditions will eventually decrease. Diversity of bodily capacities will continue and will keep generating different ways of knowing and valuing the world. Writers and filmmakers will be able to draw on the experiences of people with disabilities to develop narratives that unite the human community. Those inclined to feel blessed that they are better off than others will continue to have the opportunity to do so.

The benefits of diversity that may be threatened are those that result from the presence in the community of sufficient numbers of persons with particular genetic variations. For instance, it seems plausible that some of the goods associated with diversity can only be secured if it is distributed in such a way that people regularly encounter it in their daily lives. Thus, for instance, perhaps the mere knowledge from books, films, or websites that disability exists is not sufficient for it to serve as an "ethical resource" for us. Instead, we actually need to have personal relationships, or at least encounters, with disabled persons in order to realize this benefit. This also seems likely to be true of the aesthetic benefits of diversity: diversity will only make the world more interesting or richer for us if we actually encounter it in the course of our daily lives. Finally, the loss of "ways of life" associated with particular genotypes or phenotypes may be bad for the community and its members.

When it comes to the "intrinsic" good of diversity, the implications of genetic technologies will depend on which sort of diversity is held to be an intrinsic good. It seems most plausible to hold that it is the *number* of human variations in a given setting or the *size* of the differences between them that is intrinsically valuable. If so, this value is unlikely to be jeopardized by genetic technologies. However, if we were to hold that the existence of large numbers of each and every human variation was intrinsically valuable, then genetic selection and modification is likely to impact negatively on this good.

What Price Diversity?

Although the threat to the benefits of diversity posed by gene editing is lower than might first appear, it remains true that a loss of genetic diversity could jeopardize some significant goods. Other medical technologies that shape human bodies to meet socially sanctioned ideals may pose an even greater threat to these goods than does gene editing.[34] Does the prospect of losing this genetic diversity provide grounds to resist the development and use of technologies for gene editing?

Although concern about the loss of diversity that might follow the use of gene editing and other normalizing technologies is raised by a large community of scholars and disability activists, the most explicit and extended expression of this concern has been provided by Rosemarie Garland-Thomson.[35] Garland-Thomson has argued that we should conserve disability and so resist the reduction of diversity of human genotypes that would occur if gene editing becomes widespread.[36] While I agree with some of what she says about disability and flourishing, I am worried that her argument for conservation of genetic diversity could lead us to sacrifice the welfare—and thereby the flourishing—of individuals in the name of the greater good. As I have argued at length elsewhere, promoting the flourishing of the community or the species by sacrificing the welfare of individuals treats individuals as a means to secure a benefit enjoyed by others.[37] This willingness to sacrifice the welfare of individuals for the sake of the collective was one of the hallmarks of the morally disturbing eugenics programs of the past.[38]

Conservation (or promotion) of diversity has this morally troubling character when the diversity concerned leads to diversity in the prospects of flourishing for individuals. As noted, if we held that all genotypes offer equal prospects of flourishing, then the conservation (or promotion) of genetic diversity would not result in any individual being worse off than any other. Yet, the same argument (that different sets of life options are incommensurable when it comes to their value) also makes it difficult to understand why a reduction in the amount of diversity in our environments would be problematic for either individuals or communities. The argument from incommensurability succeeds in showing that diversity is not bad for us, but at the cost of demonstrating that it isn't good for us either.

Alternatively, we could acknowledge that some genotypes offer lower prospects of flourishing. If we acknowledge this fact—as I think we must—then conservation (or promotion) of genetic diversity could in some cases result in individuals being worse off. Conservation of genotypes associated with lower flourishing will breach our obligations to future generations if we believe that we are obligated to maximize their welfare. If we instead embrace an account of our obligations to future individuals that requires us only to *satisfice* rather than maximize their welfare, conservation of genetic diversity could be acceptable as long as it doesn't require any individual to have welfare lower than this satisfactory level.[39] A plausible version of this argument might draw on the idea that because genetic selection determines which individuals come into existence rather than altering the welfare of existing individuals, we harm nobody as long as the individuals that we bring into existence have a "life worth living."[40] The argument cannot, however, be drawn on to justify imposing lower welfare on particular individuals using gene editing technologies for the sake of diversity because genetic modification of this sort will harm them. Nor can it justify refraining from surgeries or other medical procedures after conception intended to benefit children. Indeed, even when the mechanism involved is selection rather than modification, the claim that we could be justified in allowing individuals to be born with lives only barely worth living in order to conserve or increase diversity is highly implausible.

I am arguing, then, for a moderate approach to conservation or promotion of genetic diversity. On this approach, it is reasonable to limit the use of gene editing in humans out of a concern for diversity, if conserving or securing that diversity does not require us to lower the welfare of any individual too much.[41] Just how much individual welfare it would be legitimate to sacrifice for the sake of the community remains controversial and underexamined. My sense, though, is that the answer must be "not much." Despite the value of many kinds of diversity, we should cherish and perhaps conserve—or even promote—it only where doing so avoids lowering the welfare of any individuals by more than a trivial amount.[42]

Notes

1. *Types* here refers to *geno*types. As the example of identical twins proves, genetic identity does not mean phenotypic identity, so a society of clones might nevertheless include a great deal of diversity; I discuss the relation between genetic and other types of diversity further in the text.

2. In the vast majority of circumstances, couples desiring to avoid the birth of a child at risk of genetic disease will be able to use PGD to achieve the birth of an unaffected child. Only where a couple is unable to produce an unaffected embryo would gene editing offer a therapeutic benefit that PGD could not. Even in this rare circumstance, couples could secure the birth of a healthy child if they were willing to use donor gametes. For this reason, "therapeutic" genome editing is more properly thought of as a technology to allow couples to realize their desire to be a genetic parent rather than a technology to allow them to raise a healthy child.

3. For an overview of the potential of this technology to be used for this purpose, see Antonio Regalado, "Engineering the Perfect Baby," *MIT Technology Review* 118, no. 3 (2015): 27–33.

4. Chris Gyngell, "Enhancing the Species: Genetic Engineering Technologies and Human Persistence," *Philosophy & Technology* 25, no. 4 (2012): 495–512; Russell Powell, "The Evolutionary Biological Implications of Human Genetic Engineering," *Journal of Medicine and Philosophy* 37, no. 3 (2012): 204–225.

5. Rosemarie Garland-Thomson, "The Case for Conserving Disability," *Journal of Bioethical Inquiry* 9, no. 3 (2012): 339–355.

6. James Hughes, *Citizen Cyborg: Why Democratic Societies Must Respond to the Redesigned Human of the Future* (Cambridge, MA: Westview Press, 2004).

7. Modern medical technologies have already impacted the distribution of human diversity in wealthy nations. Public health initiatives such as providing clean drinking water or clearing land mines have had an even greater impact. We should not allow the valid observation that these initiatives have not entirely eliminated phenotypic diversity among human beings to distract us from this obvious truth.

8. John Stuart Mill, *On Liberty*, ed. David Spitz (New York: Norton, 1975).

9. Nicholas Agar, *Liberal Eugenics: In Defence of Human Enhancement* (Oxford, England: Blackwell, 2004), 124–126.

10. Niklas Långström, Qazi Rahman, Eva Carlström, and Paul Lichtenstein, "Genetic and Environmental Effects on Same-Sex Sexual Behavior: A Population Study of Twins in Sweden," *Archives of Sexual Behavior* 39, no. 1 (2010): 75–80. For a useful discussion of the significance of this and similar literature, see Olivier Lemeire and Andreas De Block, "Philosophy and the Biology of Male Homosexuality," *Philosophy Compass* 10, no. 7 (2015): 479–488.

11. Robert Sparrow, "Implants and Ethnocide: Learning from the Cochlear Implant Controversy," *Disability and Society* 25, no. 4 (2010): 455–466.

12. Robert Sparrow, "Liberalism and Eugenics," *Australasian Journal of Philosophy* 89, no. 3 (2010): 499–517.

13. Michael Oliver, *Understanding Disability: From Theory to Practice* (Basingstoke, England: Macmillan, 1996).

14. Linda Barclay, "Justice and Disability: What Kind of Theorizing Is Needed?" *Journal of Social Philosophy* 42, no. 3 (2011): 273–287; Jackie Leach Scully, *Disability Bioethics: Moral Bodies, Moral Difference* (Lanham, MD: Rowman & Littlefield, 2008); Tom Shakespeare, *Disability Rights and Wrongs* (New York: Routledge, 2006); Susan Wendell, *The Rejected Body* (New York: Routledge, 1996).

15. Françoise Baylis and Jason S. Robert, "The Inevitability of Genetic Enhancement Technologies," *Bioethics* 18, no. 1 (2004): 1–26; Gyngell, "Enhancing the Species"; David T. Suzuki and Peter Knudtson, *Genethics: The Clash between the New Genetics and Human Values* (Cambridge, MA: Harvard University Press, 1989).

16. Gyngell, "Enhancing the Species"; Powell, "Evolutionary Biological Implications."

17. Paula Casal, "Sexual Dimorphism and Human Enhancement," *Journal of Medical Ethics* 39, no. 12 (2013): 722–728; John Harris, "Sparrows, Hedgehogs and

Castrati: Reflections on Gender and Enhancement," *Journal of Medical Ethics* 37, no. 5 (2011): 262–266.

18. Scott Page, *The Difference: How the Power of Diversity Creates Better Groups, Firms, Schools, and Societies* (Princeton, NJ: Princeton University Press; 2008); James Surowiecki, *The Wisdom of Crowds: Why the Many Are Smarter than the Few and How Collective Wisdom Shapes Business, Economies, Societies, and Nations* (New York: Doubleday, 2004).

19. Thomas Armstrong, *Neurodiversity: Discovering the Extraordinary Gifts of Autism, ADHD, Dyslexia, and Other Brain Differences* (Cambridge, MA: DaCapo Lifelong/ Perseus, 2010); Chris Gyngell and Thomas Douglas, "Stocking the Genetic Supermarket: Reproductive Genetic Technologies and Collective Action Problems," *Bioethics* 29, no. 4 (2015): 241–250.

20. Garland-Thomson, "Conserving Disability," 346–347.

21. Garland-Thomson, "Conserving Disability," 344–345.

22. Garland-Thomson, "Conserving Disability," 344–345

23. Garland-Thomson, "Conserving Disability," 348–349.

24. Erik Parens, "The Goodness of Fragility: On the Prospect of Genetic Technologies Aimed at the Enhancement of Human Capabilities," *Kennedy Institute of Ethics Journal* 5, no. 2 (1995): 141–153.

25. Robert Sparrow, "Imposing Genetic Diversity," *American Journal of Bioethics* 15, no. 6 (2015): 2–10.

26. Timothy F. Murphy, "The Genome Project and the Meaning of Difference," in *Justice and the Human Genome Project*, ed. Timothy F. Murphy and M. A. Lappé (Berkeley: University of California Press, 1994) 1–13; Parens, "Goodness of Fragility."

27. An obvious problem with the argument that diversity is an intrinsic good is that it would seem to require us to maximize the level of the relevant sort of diversity. In order to avoid this implication, it might be suggested that some particular amount or level of diversity was an intrinsic good. Quite how this level should be determined remains an open question.

28. Gregory S. Kavka, "Upside Risks: Social Consequences of Beneficial Biotechnology," in *Are Genes Us? The Social Consequences of the New Genetics*, ed. Carl Cranor (New Brunswick, NJ: Rutgers University Press, 1994), 155–179; Jonathan Glover, *Choosing Children: Genes, Disability, and Design* (Oxford: Oxford University Press, 2006).

29. Nick Bostrom, *The Transhumanist FAQ: A General Introduction*, Version 2.1 (Oxford, England: World Transhumanist Association, 2003); Powell, "Evolutionary Biological Implications," 214.

30. Another mechanism by which diversity might increase is the implications of ine-quality of access to technologies for human gene editing. If wealthy people are able to purchase enhancements that poor people are not, this would increase the range of ge-netic diversity within the species. Some writers have even speculated about the pos-sibility of "species splitting." See, for instance, Lee M. Silver, *Remaking Eden: Cloning, Genetic Engineering and the Future of Human Kind* (London: Phoenix, 1999), 4–8.

31. The Internet, which allows some aspects of ways of life to be sustained online, complicates but does not fundamentally challenge this claim.

32. Joseph J. Murray, "Genetics: A Future Peril Facing the Global Deaf Community," in *The Deaf Way II Reader*, ed. Harvey Goodstein (Washington, DC: Gallaudet University Press, 2006), 351–356; Sparrow, "Implants and Ethnocide"; Harlan Lane and Benjamin Bahan, "Ethics of Cochlear Implantation in Young Children: A Review and Reply from a Deaf-World Perspective," *Otolaryngology—Head and Neck Surgery* 119, no. 4 (1998): 297–313.

33. Insofar as the ways of life associated with particular genetic or phenotypic conditions tend to differ significantly from those adopted by persons with "normal" phenotypes, it is reasonable to anticipate, then, that the widespread adoption of gene editing might lead to a to a significant reduction in the size of the variation between different ways of life in each society. It seems unlikely, though, that there are that many ways of life that originate in genetic differences. The most plausible candidates are the various Deaf cultures around the world and—more controversially—a "homosexual way of life." More controversially still, it's possible that particular ways of life that are contingently associated with various phenotypic markers of racial or ethnic difference might also be threatened. Beyond these, however, I struggle to identify ways of life that might be threatened by genetic editing. I therefore suspect that the impact of gene editing on the number of different ways of life in each society is likely to be small. That being said, because each way of life may contain within it valuable insights about the many good ways to lead a human life, the loss of even a small number of different ways of life may represent a moral tragedy.

34. Erik Parens, ed., *Surgically Shaping Children: Technology, Ethics, and the Pursuit of Normality* (Baltimore: Johns Hopkins University Press, 2006).

35. Rachel Hurst, "Are Disabled People Human?" in *Unnatural Selection: The Challenges of Engineering Tomorrow's People*, ed. Peter Healey and Steve Rayner (London: Earthscan, 2009) 60–66; David S. King, "Eugenic Tendencies in Modern Genetics," in *Redesigning Life? The Worldwide Challenge to Genetic Engineering*, ed. Brian Tokar (Montréal: McGill-Queen's University Press, 2001) 171–181; Wendell, *The Rejected Body*, 82–83.

36. Garland-Thomson, "Conserving Disability."

37. Sparrow, "Imposing Genetic Diversity."

38. Of course, the *most* disturbing feature of the historical policies justified by eugenic concerns was their endorsement of the murder or forced sterilization of people judged to represent a danger to the genetic "health" of the community. None of the advocates of a concern for population-level genetics in the contemporary philosophical debate embrace such policies. Whether the willingness of esteemed philosophers to contemplate genetic modification of future individuals for the sake of the community or nation might lead other people to embrace such policies is a further question. For discussion, see Robert Sparrow, "Ethics, Eugenics, and Politics," in *The Future of Bioethics: International Dialogues*, ed. Akira Akayabashi (Oxford: Oxford University Press, 2014), 139–153.

39. Satisficing involves making sure that a good is secured to at least some minimum value.

40. Derek Parfit, *Reasons and Persons* (Oxford, England: Clarendon Press, 1984).

41. For instance, I think the willingness of most discussants in debates about new reproductive technologies to restrict access to these technologies where they are likely to produce large shifts in sex ratios at birth reflects the belief that the difference between the life prospects of men and women in realistically available social circumstances is small.

42. Thanks are due to Nick Agar, Rosemarie Garland-Thomson, James Hughes, and Josephine Johnson for comments and discussion over the course of the drafting of this chapter.

12

Creaturehood and Deification as Anchors for an Ethics of Gene Editing

Michael Burdett

New gene editing technologies are inciting scientists and the public to ask difficult questions about the technologies' safety and efficacy. But safety and efficacy are not our only concerns; we are also asking what those technologies might mean for human lives and for our understandings of the nature of a good—or flourishing—life. In an article in the *Washington Post*, "Pondering 'What It Means to be Human' on the Frontier of Gene Editing,"[1] Jennifer Doudna, the Berkeley scientist who is one of the inventors of CRISPR-cas9, reflected on the many possible uses of the technology that she helped to create. Doudna not only recognized the importance of assessing the technology's safety and efficacy in humans, but also noted the far-ranging and ethical questions raised by these new technologies. To illustrate the potential significance of altering a person's genes, Doudna recounted a powerful interaction she had with the mother of a child with Down syndrome. The mother explained to Doudna that she would never seek to change her child with the gene editing technology that Doudna invented: "I love my child and wouldn't change him. There's something about him that's so special. He's so loving in a way that's unique to him. I wouldn't change it." The scientist teared up retelling the story, saying to the reporter, "It makes you think hard about what it means to be human, doesn't it?"

In this chapter, I consider what it means to be human in an era of gene editing technologies, using ideas from philosophical and religious scholarship. I call these ideas "visions of the human being." These visions are central to understanding the relationship between gene editing and human flourishing because they are "at work" in our definition of human flourishing, and they will shape people's responses to the technologies. We can't formulate an ethics of gene editing without reference to the plurality of visions of the human being that undergird human flourishing. What's more, because gene editing might enable changes to human nature, these visions will play a significant role in helping people determine which uses of the technology will be acceptable and which unacceptable. People will use these visions of the human being as a guide, asking,

Do the changes these technologies might make to human beings align with my overall vision of the human being and what makes us flourish?

My particular contribution draws on my faith and relies on a Christian vision of the human being, which I think can provide a helpful heuristic for charting— and guiding—responses to new gene editing technologies. This Christian vision sees human flourishing in the context of gene editing as the successful navigation between two elements of human existence: "creaturehood" and "deification." Both elements are important for developing a robust conception of human flourishing and for allowing us to respond well to the uses of gene editing applications.

Human beings are at an important stage in their evolutionary history. Advances in genetics, robotics, informatics, and nanotechnology over the last several decades have sparked great speculation about the possible personal, moral, and special ramifications of applying them to the human body. That speculation is especially acute where the technology could alter capacities that shape personhood directly. Memory, behavior, and sociality are just some of the things that might be affected by future genetic engineering. This possibility invites us to ask, Toward what end ought we employ these new techniques? What vision of the human being do we seek? These are questions not only for those individuals who will use the technologies, but also for us all.

Changes to the nature of persons don't merely affect isolated individuals; they raise important considerations for the public and policymakers. Seeing decisions about whether and how to use these technologies solely as private decisions does a disservice to our shared responsibility to the future and ignores the possible negative social ramifications of allowing "market forces" and "power relations" to dictate our progeny's lot. Hans Jonas's questions, posed decades ago, have never been so timely: "Who will be the image-makers, by what standards, and on the basis of what knowledge?"[2] Scientists and the public recognize the imperative of these questions. It is time that policymakers, public intellectuals, and scholars face them head on.

To Understand Human Flourishing We Need to Understand Our Visions of the Human

To develop an ethics of gene editing, we need some delineation of what it means for a human being to thrive or flourish. Understandings of human flourishing vary, but they all incorporate or rely on specific visions of the human being. Alternative or competing versions of human flourishing can presuppose very different visions of the human being. For example, hedonistic conceptions imagine the human being as primarily a pleasure center and view increasing pleasure as the aim of human life. Consequently, if we are trying to develop some kind of publicly acceptable conception of "human flourishing," even if that conception is pluralistic, tentative, and piecemeal, we must clearly identify the visions of the human being that undergird it.[3]

Traditionally, we get visions of the human being from religion, philosophy, or other worldviews. By worldview, I mean a system of beliefs that underlies a person's actions, goals, and motivations. Worldviews can be explicitly acknowledged by the person holding the view, or they can be entirely unconscious. They are the epistemological prism—the way of seeing—that colors our world, provides and expresses "ultimate concerns," and influences our dispositions and affections. They are intimate to the individual. For many, they are the systems in which we live and find meaning in the world. Hence, they bear a great resemblance to traditional religions in terms of their role in people's lives.[4]

Before turning to consider the visions of the human being at work in religion, philosophy, other worldviews, I first want to address some possible objections to the inclusion of religious perspectives in public debates about emerging technologies.[5] There is a long tradition of calling on religious ideas in ethical, specifically bioethical, reflection. Many leaders in the field, particularly at its origin in the 1960s, were motivated by religious concerns.[6] More recently, however, the use of religious perspectives has declined, perhaps due to concern that consulting religion is fraught with partisan bias and complicates public discourse. Hence, much of contemporary discourse relies on pure philosophical analysis. While I believe that philosophical sources are imperative to the discussion, religious voices also belong in public debate for several reasons.

First, there are no "views from nowhere": no purely objective positions or worldviews. As Lisa Sowle Cahill has argued, in response to criticism about utilizing religious sources on bioethics issues, "the 'secular' sphere is not neutral, since all participants inevitably come from communities of identity, and continually participate in many such communities."[7] Second, it is in the nature of public discourse today to have a plurality of positions and belief systems that will give rise to distinct ethical applications. Further, discounting some voices just because they are religious seriously misunderstands and undermines the contemporary move to transform secular public discourse into a postsecular landscape. Following the work of Charles Taylor, Hans George Gadamer, and other theorists, instead of truncating dialogue in the public sphere so that everyone must abide by the rules set in place by the liberal humanist position, we should seek to move into a postsecular sphere dominated by dialogue. We should seek common exchange and possible agreement with others outside our own worldview while utilizing the "home" resources, beliefs, and language available within our specific worldview.[8] Finally, despite mid-twentieth century proclamations that religion is on the decline in modern societies, religion is playing a much larger role in politics and individual lives than these sociologists predicted.[9] This is particularly the case with bioethical matters. Research showed that the religious public relies on religious discourse to help them make their own individual bioethical decisions.[10] Since a pervasive strategy has been to allow individuals, within reason, to employ biotechnological techniques toward their own defined aims and in harmony with their beliefs, we won't be able to understand the future social impact of these decisions without reference to religious reasoning and deliberation.

Three "Visions of the Human" at Work in the Gene Editing Debate

The specific possibility of using gene editing technologies for human enhancement highlights just how much overall belief structures and visions of the human can bring to bioethical discourse. Here, I review three sources of these visions: transhumanism, liberal humanism, and Christianity. Of course, many other ideas that supply people with a vision of the human being could be represented here; indeed they have been in this volume.

Transhumanism explicitly depicts and defines a vision of the human being in the context of gene editing. That vision understands the human being to be (1) primarily an entity defined by intellect and rationality, (2) made up most primordially of information, and (3) directed by pure will and freedom.[11] As extreme technophiles, transhumanists advocate for the near-unfettered use of technologies, including genetic technologies, to transcend current human capacities. What these transhumanists get right is that they think long term when considering the repercussions of gene editing: they recognize the impacts it might have on our future societies, species, and selves.

Liberal humanism shares with transhumanism many common core values and convictions. Both are committed to human progress and rational thinking and treat the flourishing of the human species as an end in itself. But whereas transhumanism seeks to move beyond current biological limitations through the deployment of radical transformative technologies, liberal humanism takes a more cautious approach and advises its adherents to tarry on the value of our present life and the virtues that arise in its current form. Instead of relying on enhancement technologies to improve the human condition, liberal humanism focuses on improving the human, largely through relational, cultural, and educational approaches. For example, Alain de Botton counseled his fellow humanists to approach art galleries as one might the psychologist's couch: as a form of therapy.[12] Art engages the basic existential and meaning-rich questions that help to orient one's life and can act as a guide to transformation and a better life. In addition, human transformation can be obtained through relation. Philosophically dense approaches like that of Emmanuel Levinas[13] rest on the simple claim that transformation and transcendence is reached through interpersonal relationships. Childbearing, in particular, is given a privileged role by these humanists. Passing not only our biological material to the next generation but also our habits and personalities is a source of tremendous hope.

Two central ideas are at work in Christian approaches to gene editing. The first is the vision of humans as creatures made by God. The second is the vision of humans as "children of God" (deification) who express and participate in some of God's characteristics, particularly their creativity as a source of transcendence in the world. Both ideas are in a fertile tension, a tension that is explored by sociologist John H. Evans, whose work is absolutely central to understanding public views of genetic engineering. Evans unpacks the religious public's attitudes and their reasons for accepting or rejecting particular biotechnological applications. He noted that while many religious people are wary of using bioengineering for enhancement purposes, these religious bioconservatives do not believe that any change to the human genome is sacrilegious. They do not think that human beings should be left as they are. Rather, their religious faith teaches them that human beings are seriously flawed creatures in need of transformation. Their religious reasoning compels them to try to discern "which human changes God would like." In other words, as Evans argued citing Christian bioethicist Paul Ramsey, Christians are seeking to "play God as God plays God."[14]

Christians share this sentiment with transhumanists: human transformation is required. The difference between them lies in their diverging visions of the human being.[15] For the transhumanist, the plan for human transcendence comes not from God but from individual human desire, technical acumen, or social consensus. For the religious, God holds the final plan for nature/creation and humanity, as revealed by their extensive reference to "nature," "God," and "humanity" in the context of bioengineering. In this way, they are utterly reliant on their religious faith as a compass and moral guide.[16]

Creaturehood and Deification: Emphasizing Both Aspects of the Christian Vision of the Human

As a person of faith, I think that the Christian claim that human beings are "creatures" bound for deification can provide a rudimentary framework for assessing gene editing. This framework does justice to the perspective of those in the faith while providing important translational value and resonance outside the Christian faith. Allow me to explain.

Initial Christian discourse on human biotechnology has appealed to the important tension between creaturehood and deification as discrete anchor points in the debate. Christians leaning toward creaturehood stress that human beings are created with limits. For example, we are created with limited mental and physical capacities, and we will die someday. Moving beyond those delineated boundaries means transgressing God's ordained order in creation, of which human beings are one part. Infraction of the created and moral order comes at a cost to humanity by stunting our well-being, growth, and virtue. What's more, as discussed in the next paragraph, many theological scholars argue that only when our limits are affirmed can we truly flourish: greater happiness and virtue are achieved by acknowledging that humans are creatures and by living within ordained limits rather than seeking to exceed them through human biotechnological change.

Scholars like Celia Deane-Drummond, Brent Waters, Gerald McKenny, Jeanine Thweatt-Bates, and myself have all appealed in some way to creaturehood as an important rejoinder to the prospect of using gene editing for human enhancement, such as might be advocated for by transhumanists. Deane-Drummond has consistently argued against radical human enhancement projects because their goals often neglect the inherent good in creaturely life, instead representing the distinctive features of creaturehood as problems or limitations to be overcome.[17] Advocates of human enhancement take an entirely functional view of the body, failing to see how current embodied life is the locus of human experience and relation with others and the world, and that it is therefore central to human flourishing. Jeanine Thweatt-Bates made the same argument in a more radical way: she argued for the inherent good in the plurality of human embodied experiences, such as might be found in the disability community.[18] And I have argued that important Christian virtues (mercy, grace, humility, and love) arise in the context of a community that acknowledges its plurality, limitation, and weakness because the members all have to rely on one another for the common good of all.[19] Brent Waters and Gerald McKenny also emphasized the role that limitation, an important marker for creaturehood, has for genuine human flourishing. For Waters, birth and mortality are distinctive features of creaturehood that ought to be maintained.[20] Indeed, he claimed that the goods that come from our contingency—our dependence and mortality—far outweigh the vapid benefits of the extended life promulgated by transhumanists. Similarly, McKenny argued that final human goods cannot be obtained through technological transformation of natural capacity, but only through divine grace.[21]

Other Christian scholars in the gene editing debates emphasized the other pole in this dialectic, which I call deification. They argue that humans have been given a unique role in creation: we are to cultivate the world around us and bring it to fruition. Indeed, one of the most prominent interpretations of the image of God in the biblical text is that it requires human beings, as God's proxy, to make the world better; this role is the very thing that is meant by saying that human beings are made in God's image.[22] Some take this role to extend beyond our surrounding environment to include ourselves. They argue that we have been tasked with transcending our limitations through our own creative endeavors. Where spiritual disciplines and other indirect cultural techniques were the engines of this transformation in the past, they see science and technology simply as the latest tools to be used on ourselves to realize this vision.

Appeals to deification in the context of gene editing human enhancement are much less common in contemporary Christian literature than are appeals to creaturehood. Nevertheless, there is a clear thread of Christian thinkers who advocate for something like human transformation by technological and scientific means, and they generally rely on their belief in deification.[23] For example, the nineteenth-century Russian Christian philosopher N. F. Fedorov held that utilizing science and technology to overcome death was necessitated by Christ's example in the resurrection. If we are to be like Christ, like God, we have some role to play in overcoming this limitation as Christ did. The Jesuit theologian Pierre Teilhard de Chardin advocated for something similar by suggesting that the road toward final deification at the Omega Point (i.e., the culminating end of history and creation), while largely instituted and enacted by Christ, is paved with human evolution and human initiation.

Contemporary theologians Ted Peters and Ronald Cole-Turner are much more positive about the contribution technological human enhancement might make to the "glorified human" than are their colleagues. While Peters is quick to claim that no human ingenuity, enhancements included, will ever solve the basic problem at the heart of human nature—sin—he does think that we could use science and technology to make cosmetic alterations to human nature that have genuine theological implications. He said: "If through drug or genetic intervention we could enhance our disposition to love and expand our capacity for effecting that love in our relationship to others, then we might find this kind of science and technology knocking on the door of the *imago dei*. But, this certainly is not the case among the champions of enhancement we see today."[24] So, even though he remains agnostic about whether current science and technology can contribute to the kind of transformation of the human being spoken of by Christian theology, he is open to the possibility that future enhancements could contribute to spiritual matters and, yes, to theology. Cole-Turner is even more open than Peters here: he speculated that drugs like psilocybin (found in some mushrooms) might have genuine theological import and critiqued Christian scholars for failing to appreciate deification as a motivating principle in the human enhancement debates.[25] Similarly, another theologian, Todd Daly, warned Christian scholars against overspiritualizing deification that, in turn, does not do justice to its clear physical and bodily dimension, which he said is at the heart of the Christian tradition and which could then be impacted by techno-logical human transformation.[26]

What is overlooked in these prototypical Christian responses and in many non-Christian arguments of the same nature, and what conceptually drives my proposal, is that both deification and creaturehood are required for an adequate theological understanding of the nature of human beings. Simply focusing on one element without acknowledgment of the other's claim to the issue dims the vision of the human being at the heart of the Christian message. We are what some Christians call "created creators"—we have been created and, hence, de-pend on our creaturely life to sustain us—and we are "children of God" who transcend our present existence by actively cultivating and shaping our world in creative ways akin to God. Acknowledging the interplay and tension between creaturehood and deification is a good starting point for a robust vision of the human, one that could guide us to genuine human flourishing in the context of the gene editing debates.[27]

A Secular Counterpart: Accepting Human Limits and Creativity

In closing, I'd like to suggest that this theological template of the human being has value outside the Christian faith and in public discourse on human flour-ishing and gene editing. The argument I make is very similar to the via media between two well-worn responses to enhancement that Erik Parens seeks both in the introduction to this volume and in a previous text, Shaping Ourselves,[28] al-though he utilizes less explicit theological language than I am proposing.[29] In his book, Parens described one response to enhancement as defined by "gratitude"—similar to my rendering of "creaturehood." This response invokes "the human capacity to recognize that we have been thrown into being by forces we don't yet understand and that we didn't create," and that this fact about our existence "feels worthy of celebration."[30] I agree with Parens that this stance toward our present condition views human life as a gift worthy of our respect, celebration, and de-light. Whereas Parens does not acknowledge any gift-giver, the religious believer is moved to worship God for this divine blessing and giftedness.[31] The dispo-sition, however, is similar, and the terms creaturehood in Christian circles and gratitude outside it invoke similar lauded virtues like humility, vulnerability, fra-gility, relationality, and solidarity. The second response to enhancement Parens identified is "creativity," and it pairs with what I have been calling deification. This response emphasizes that human beings are by their very nature creators, a capacity that is virtuous and to be celebrated. Associated virtues in the deifica-tion/creativity strand include ingenuity, freedom, and growth. Most important, just as I have argued here that both elements of the Christian understanding of humans are needed to respond well to contemporary gene editing technologies, so, too, does Parens argue, if from a distinctly nonreligious perspective, that both are needed in the enhancement debate.

Parens isn't the only advocate here. Other contributions in this volume have also sought a "thicker account of the human." I affirm with Garland-Thomson (Chapter 1), Jennings (Chapter 17), and Roberts (Chapter 14) that we need to expand human flourishing to include a greater plurality of human embodiment relations, which will likely mean creating greater social and environmental room for those we might deem wrongly to be in need of genetic alteration. This expansion in thinking certainly "thickens" our account of human flourishing and the underlying visions of the human they presuppose. I have sought to indicate here that a thicker account of the human being will mean delving deeper into the often-religious/ideological moorings of our discussions, even recognizing how present nonsecular approaches for a thicker anthropology often depend on their historical reception of religious categories and sources.[32] What is more, if, as Gaymon Bennett indicates in Chapter 16, dignity plays a tremendous role in our ethical imaginary today, then religious visions are indispensable to our public discourse on gene editing because they can provide both constructive and critical voices to others at the table.

But even when I acknowledge the value of other, nonreligious, thick accounts of the human being, I do not think that human flourishing can be reduced to or equated entirely with these other accounts, however thick they might be. A public, dialogical rendering of Christian theological anthropology is not the complete vision to which Christians subscribe. For one thing, a Christian vision of the human being can affirm from whence human dignity is derived, rather than asserting the existence of human dignity by fiat or deriving it from some structural or relational component of human nature, or from human life alone. (Among other things, these strategies for grounding human dignity are vulnerable to challenges about why certain features are selected or what to do when they are missing in particular individuals.) For the Christian, human dignity is based on the infinite worth ascribed to it by a loving creator in all the plurality of human embodiments and relations we find. In this way, a Christian approach to human flourishing can be both constructive to the dialogue and critical of it.

The understanding of the nature of human beings that I have proposed here— one that relies on both our creaturehood and our deification—has theological moorings and is rooted in religious convictions. Nonetheless, it has substantial value as a heuristic outside religious contexts. The challenge now is to undertake a thorough study, within both religious and nonreligious communities, of how to strike this balance between creaturehood or gratitude and deification or creativity both in our individual private communities and in public discourse. The future of gene editing—and of human flourishing—depends on it.

Notes

1. Joel Achenbach, "Pondering 'What It Means to Be Human' on the Frontier of Gene Editing," *The Washington Post*, May 3, 2016.
2. Hans Jonas, *The Imperative of Responsibility: In Search of an Ethics for the Technological Age* (Chicago: University of Chicago Press, 1984), 21.
3. This needs to be plural and broad to include factors generally left out, which is why studying race, gender, and disability is so important for this venture. But we should not mistake a broadening of definition for having no definition at all; clearly some boundary work is necessary in order to distinguish between human flourishing and, say, beetle flourishing.
4. See Paul Tillich, *What Is Religion?* (New York: Harper & Row, 1969); Terry Eagleton, *Ideology: An Introduction* (London: Verso, 1991).
5. Much of this argumentation is derived from Ronald Cole-Turner, "Religion and the Question of Human Germline Modification," in *Design and Destiny: Jewish and Christian Perspectives on Human Germline Modification*, ed. Ronald Cole-Turner (Cambridge, MA: MIT Press, 2008) 1–28.
6. For example Richard McCormick, Joseph Fletcher, and Paul Ramsey might be considered figureheads of bioethics, and all three address bioethics with clear religious motivations and unapologetically religious intentions. See Albert R. Jonsen, "A History of Religion and Bioethics," in *Handbook of Bioethics and Religion*, ed. David E. Guinn (Oxford: Oxford University Press, 2006) 23–36; John H. Evans, *The History and Future of Bioethics: A Sociological View* (Oxford: Oxford University Press, 2012).
7. Lisa Sowle Cahill, "Theology's Role in Public Bioethics," in Guinn, *Handbook of Bioethics and Religion*, 37–60. Outside of bioethics many others have argued against reducing public discourse to mere liberalism. See, for example, Alasdair C. MacIntyre, *Whose Justice? Which Rationality?* (Notre Dame, IN: University of Notre Dame Press, 1988).
8. Gadamer spoke of the "fusion of horizons" as a way to begin that discourse with others outside a shared worldview. Fruitful dialogue is possible when we recognize our shared history and the common future that underlies our basis for understanding each other. See Hans-Georg Gadamer, *Truth and Method* (London: Continuum, 2004). Also see Charles Taylor, "Comparison, History, Truth," in *Myth and Philosophy*, ed. Frank E. Reynolds and David Tracy (New York: SUNY Press, 1990) 37–56.
9. Excellent challenges to the "secularization thesis" can be sought in Craig J. Calhoun, Mark Juergensmeyer, and Jonathan VanAntwerpen, eds., *Rethinking Secularism* (Oxford: Oxford University Press, 2011); Charles Taylor, *A Secular Age* (Cambridge, MA: Belknap Press of Harvard University Press, 2007).

10. See John H. Evans, *Contested Reproduction: Genetic Technologies, Religion, and Public Debate* (Chicago: University of Chicago Press, 2010).

11. See Michael Burdett, *Technology and the Rise of Transhumanism: Beyond Genetic Engineering* (Cambridge: Grove Books, 2014).

12. Alain De Botton and John Armstrong, *Art as Therapy* (London: Phaidon Press, 2013).

13. See Emmanuel Levinas, *Alterity and Transcendence* (New York: Columbia University Press, 1999); Emmanuel Levinas, *Totality and Infinity: An Essay on Exteriority*, trans. Alphonso Lingis (Pittsburgh: Duquesne University Press, 1969).

14. John H. Evans, *Playing God? Human Genetic Engineering and the Rationalization of Public Bioethical Debate* (Chicago: University of Chicago Press, 2002), 130.

15. John H. Evans, "Future Vision in Transhumanist Writings and the Religious Public," in *Perfecting Human Futures: Transhuman Visions and Technological Imaginations*, ed. J. Benjamin Hurlbut and Hava Tirosh-Samuelson (Wiesbaden, Germany: Springer, 2015) 291–306.

16. Evans, *Contested Reproduction*.

17. For example, Celia Deane-Drummond, "Taking Leave of the Animal? The Theological and Ethical Implications of Transhuman Projects," in *Transhumanism and Transcendence: Christian Hope in an Age of Technological Enhancement*, ed. Ronald Cole-Turner (Washington, DC: Georgetown University Press, 2011) 115–130; Celia Deane-Drummond, "Remaking Human Nature: Transhumanism, Theology, and Creatureliness in Bioethical Controversies," in *Religion and Transhumanism: The Unknown Future of Human Enhancement*, ed. Calvin Mercer and Tracy Trothen (Santa Barbara, CA: Praeger, 2015) 245–254. Also see Celia Deane-Drummond, *Genetics and Christian Ethics* (Cambridge: Cambridge University Press, 2006).

18. Jeanine Thweatt-Bates, *Cyborg Selves: A Theological Anthropology of the Posthuman* (Farnham, England: Ashgate, 2012).

19. Michael Burdett, *Eschatology and the Technological Future* (London: Routledge, 2015).

20. Brent Waters, "Whose Salvation? Which Eschatology? Transhumanism and Christianity as Contending Salvific Religions," in Cole-Turner, *Transhumanism and Transcendence* 163–176; Brent Waters, "Flesh Made Data: The Posthuman Project in Light of the Incarnation" in Mercer and Trothen, *Religion and Transhumanism*, 291–302.

21. Gerald McKenny, "Transcendence, Technological Enhancement, and Christian Theology," in Cole-Turner, *Transhumanism and Transcendence*, 177–192.

22. For an exhaustive treatment of this view, see J. Richard Middleton, *The Liberating Image: The Imago Dei in Genesis 1* (Grand Rapids, MI: Brazos Press, 2005).

23. Michael Burdett, "Contextualizing a Christian Perspective on Transcendence and Human Enhancement: Francis Bacon, N. F. Fedorov, and Pierre Teilhard De Chardin," in Cole-Turner, *Transhumanism and Transcendence*, 19–36.

24. Ted Peters, "Can We Enhance the Imago Dei?" in *Human Identity at the Intersection of Science, Technology and Religion*, ed. Nancey C. Murphy and Christopher C. Knight (Farnham, England: Ashgate, 2010), 215–238.

25. Ronald Cole-Turner, "Going Beyond the Human: Christians and Other Transhumanists," *Theology and Science* 13, no. 2 (2015) 150–161; Ronald Cole-Turner,

"Spiritual Enhancement," in Mercer and Trothen, *Religion and Transhumanism*, 369–384.

26. Todd T. W. Daly, "Chasing Methuselah: Transhumanism and Christian Theosis in Critical Perspective," in Cole-Turner, *Transhumanism and Transcendence*, 131–144.

27. I have intentionally tried to avoid using oft-cited terms like *co-creation* or *subcreation* so I do not prematurely define how God's creativity relates to human creativity. Space does not permit me to unpack the nuance of affirming both creaturehood and deification in our present biotechnological age or how terms like cocreation or subcreation might or might not be useful in this context. Rather, at this early stage, my sole aim is to suggest creaturehood and deification cannot be separated without undue damage to a robust and ecumenical theological anthropology that is needed to provide a more robust vision of the human in the context of gene editing.

28. Erik Parens, *Shaping Our Selves: On Technology, Flourishing, and a Habit of Thinking* (Oxford: Oxford University Press, 2014).

29. He even noted how important the religious roots of his contention were to his proposal. See Parens, *Shaping Our Selves*.

30. Parens, *Shaping Our Selves*, 61.

31. There is an entire "secular" tradition that seeks to localize this sense of gratitude in the gift of Being itself. Heidegger and other post-Heideggerians (e.g., Jacques Derrida) make much of this when invoking the inherent ambiguity of the German "to be," *es gibt*, which is literally translated as "it gives". See George Pattison, *Routledge Philosophy Guidebook to the Later Heidegger* (London: Routledge, 2000); Martin Heidegger, *What Is Called Thinking?*, trans. J. Glenn Gray (New York: Harper & Row, 1968); John D. Caputo and Michael J. Scanlon, eds., *God, the Gift, and Postmodernism* (Bloomington: Indiana University Press, 1999).

32. See Gaymon Bennett. *Technicians of Human Dignity: Bodies, Souls, and the Making of Intrinsic Worth* (New York: Fordham University Press, 2016); Hans Joas, *The Sacredness of the Person: A New Genealogy of Human Rights* (Washington, DC: Georgetown University Press, 2013).

13

Recovering Practical Wisdom as a Guide for Human Flourishing

Navigating the CRISPR Challenge

Celia Deane-Drummond

Why might scientists be interested in thinking about the implications of their work through the lens of ancient religious texts that were written hundreds of years ago? Geneticists in particular are likely to be among those who are least likely to take such thinkers seriously, even if they might concede that scientists may adhere to strongly held values, including religious ones. The training of a scientist is to bring distance between personal views and their scientific work, though the sociology of different scientific practices shows that cultural and other values do inevitably play a part in the way scientific hypotheses are born, developed, and even tested.[1]

Michael Burdett argues in Chapter 12 of this volume that religious perspectives need to be taken seriously in public debates as they bring to the ethical discussion perspectives that may otherwise be overlooked. His stress on the twin theological concepts of creaturehood and deification as "anchors" portrays the theological framework or scale in which Christian theological ethics can be worked out, though the precise way that is worked out will also depend on which particular theological traditions are being stressed. One of my aims in this chapter is to argue, like Burdett, that specific classic resources in the Christian traditions—and Catholic traditions in particular—*do* have something important to contribute to scholarly debates about the new genetics, including what look like innovative "solutions" to genetic disorders, such as those being developed through CRISPR-Cas9 and related technologies. The dialectic of creaturehood and deification in Burdett's analysis resonates to some extent with my own perspective, which seeks to find a balance between the material, earthly reality while being cognizant of what Christian faith attributes as the ultimate goal of deification, or as I stress in the analysis that follows, the beatific vision. Classic traditions also challenge unexamined and narrowly individualistic notions of the good by showing how different conceptions of human flourishing at different scales or levels serve to inform each other.

As someone who trained originally in the natural and life sciences, I have a reasonable sense of the drive behind scientific discovery. Where that drive is directed toward ends that, to a scientist at least, look like clever techniques to prevent the worst kinds of individual suffering, or even extend natural human capability, the possibility that there might be any objections to that technology seems Luddite and perhaps even incomprehensible, especially in a North American context where individual freedom is an assumed good.

To help understand more clearly where such objections arise and possible ways forward in that discussion, I lay out as clearly as I can both the substantive objections arising from a particular religious standpoint and those tools that are at the disposal of Christian theologians in making their arguments about how particular processes are perceived from that religious starting point. Those substantive objections arise from a distinct understanding of each and every human being: as made in God's image, in a relationship of love with God as maker of all that is, and patterned after Christ as exemplar in the beatific vision (which I elaborate further in the chapter). The majority of people in the world practice some form of religion, with Roman Catholicism having the highest number of adherents. Ethical discourse that ignores religious belief entirely may be missing the mark in terms of both resources available and likely impact.

Theology habitually draws on a mixture of scripture, philosophy, tradition, and experience. Roman Catholic theology in general puts much greater weight on tradition compared with Protestants, who generally give priority to scripture, but the basic combination is common across different denominational traditions. Theologians who are ethicists tend to be rather more inclined to stress philosophy, though heated debates on method rage among moral theologians just as much as in any area of theology or any area of science. CRISPR-Cas9 and other new technologies would fall broadly under the category of what theologians term *experience* insofar as the questions these technologies raise are about how to navigate our human experiences with the world. While scripture might have something in a very broad sense to contribute about the created world as such and the place of humanity in that world, there are few if any specific biblical instructions about how to act in relation to new technologies. What theological traditions do stress, however, are particular habits of mind or dispositions called virtues. These virtues are developed from the basic biblical golden rule to love God and neighbor as oneself as the means toward the hoped-for future. In this future, human flourishing is envisaged as being fully embedded in this world, but it is a world transformed, rather than a world that is first annihilated through an apocalyptic natural or God-sent disaster. In this transformed world, ethical frameworks about right action and the particular way in which human flourishing is portrayed are both significant theologically.

Rather than engage in biblical exegesis, for this chapter I turn to the work of a theologian who not only has shaped Catholic Christian thought, but also has exerted a strong influence on many Protestant writers, namely, the medieval theologian and scholar Thomas Aquinas. Aquinas inspired a religious community begun by Saint Dominic in the twelfth century and still active in the present. The Dominicans are one of the most philosophically and intellectually sophisticated Roman Catholic religious orders. Their vision of what it means to flourish in a given community provides a case study of the practical implications of that theological tradition. In other words, Thomistic thought is not confined only to dusty book stacks; it also has a lived expression in specific community life. Gaining some insight into the primary texts of Thomas Aquinas opens a window into not only how theologians perceive the world, but also what it means to flourish in a Christian way in a Christian community, insights that are relevant to understanding what it means for any person to flourish in any community.

Because Aquinas drew heavily on Aristotle, he provided an interesting example of how classic theologians are able to navigate both theological territory, which he gained largely from that other highly influential figure, Augustine of Hippo, and secular philosophical traditions. The Aristotelian tradition is still influential in philosophy today, giving Aquinas's work the ability to resonate with and challenge current philosophical debates. For this chapter, I then ask, Can human flourishing according to this vision ever be compatible with the use of new techniques like CRISPR-Cas9? Focusing on the virtue of practical wisdom or prudence, I address some of the controversial ethical issues at stake theologically and seek clues to ethical conduct and human flourishing in contested public debates about genetic engineering.

While the portrait of what the future world looks like in theological terms will sound strange to ears that are not tuned to such concepts, for religious believers, at least those with a classical bent, this portrait is not only meaningful but also awe inspiring. The strange worlds painted by science fiction writers are no less strange; it is just that they are products of pure fictive imagination. Theologians, on the other hand, believe that their accounts of the future come not only from an overactive imagination, but also from contact with the ground of all reality, namely, God. In as much as theological accounts of the future are rooted in respected traditions and scriptures, they are understood as inspired by the work of the Holy Spirit. In this sense, rather like in Plato's vision of the cave, the world around us can seem like shadows in comparison to the ideal world that is presented in the theological vision of the future. That future vision, also known as the beatific vision, can impinge on the present and help interpret future hope, summarized in the more general theological term *eschatology*. I urge patience, therefore, among readers who are not familiar with this language in the very short section that follows in order to begin to understand the depth of meaning that such visions present to the human mind.

Human Flourishing through the Beatific Vision

The ultimate end for human beings—an end that is only possible in the world to come, according to the thought of Thomas Aquinas—is to be fully immersed in the beatific vision. In this world, all that can be hoped for is to glimpse and live in accordance with that beatific vision. To some extent this vision compares with Zhuangzi's understanding of the "heavenly perspective" referred to by Richard Kim in Chapter 5 of this volume, in that it takes the believer away from too much preoccupation with their own desires, but there are important differences as well. While detachment is an important movement in Christian understanding of the perfection of virtues, the Christian goal is not so much an emptying, but a filling up with knowledge of God, understood through the example of Christ. Beatific knowledge, or the vision of God, is therefore the final goal or *telos* of the human life as made in the image of God, *imago Dei*.[2] It is one way of representing the end point in the process of deification (becoming like God) described by Michael Burdett in Chapter 12 of this volume.

The effort to become like Christ is perfected through suffering. True human flourishing is, therefore, the good that is known and experienced by imitating Christ and even believing that one *becomes* Christ's body on Earth through communal participation in the Eucharist. According to Aquinas, Jesus Christ was, unlike those who are merely imitating Christ, uniquely capable of enjoying both uncreated and created beatitude. Created beatitude, accessible to all humanity, is received by God's grace working in the human person; it never arises through our own efforts in the manner of, for example, acquired virtues, but is infused or given by God's grace.

Uncreated beatitude is given uniquely to the Son of God and is related to a different understanding of the nature of the person; Christ is the perfected image of God in the way that relates to a unique filial relationship between God the Father and God the Son. Human beings, on the other hand, are in the image of God, but only by being images of the perfected divine image that is the Christ. For Aquinas there was a hierarchy in knowing: first through the senses of our bodies, second through intellectual understanding that allows for a universal knowledge, and then through is knowledge that is given through divine grace.[3]

For Aquinas, the beatific vision was a sublime elevation in the power of understanding and the mind: It is received by grace, and it is through that light that the human creature becomes even more God-like.[4] This kind of knowing by grace is oriented toward pure goodness alone, while knowledge gained through the senses and intellectual understanding is a mixture of good and bad.[5] Revelation that is received by grace "does not tell us what God is," but it "helps us to know him better."[6] This kind of knowing is more than simple faith or assent to particular beliefs since it is a personal knowledge of God.[7]

This pattern of knowing in Christianity is related to the structure of character development through the virtues, in that the *acquired* virtues are developed through learning and instruction, while the *infused* virtues are given by God's grace through the power of the Holy Spirit. The gifts of the Holy Spirit are distinct again and are received rather than earned. The idea of receptivity also has some common ground with Daoism, but again, receptivity and letting be are not sufficient for there is a positive content to what is received. There are, of course, implicit dangers in this pattern of thinking insofar as it seems to put an emphasis on distinctions between this world and the next. It also suggests an idealization of a future glorified in God, where knowledge of God seems to be mediated through the grace-filled elevation of the human mind. At the same time, such a vision helps to qualify and relativize the manner *and* content of any individual good sought in this life since the ultimate good is to become like Christ and attain the same beatific vision of God. Hence, Christian perfection is always perfection *in the virtues* that are expressed in communal contexts and true flourishing or happiness is found in God alone.

This vision sets up the collective goal of human life in a way that is distinct from secular interpretations of human flourishing, even though there may be some overlap between them. In Christian thought, the test of true human flourishing, then, is filtered through and measured in the light of the complete good found in beatitude. According to this vision we are *not necessarily obliged* to follow the goals set or even the kind of flourishing that is portrayed as a good in secular terms. A secular vision of flourishing will assume that all kinds of impairments need to be fixed, the goal being to remove physical forms of suffering simply as a matter of course. The goal of the beatific vision is not perfected bodies, but perfection in relationship with each other and with the God of love whose understanding of perfection relates to human qualities of virtue, rather than perfection in physical characteristics alone. That does not mean that suffering is simply accepted since the virtue of justice protests against inequity of all kinds, including racism, sexism, colonialism, and so on. Indeed, secular and theological perspectives can overlap in setting as a priority the flourishing of the most impoverished, marginalized members of human societies.

The CRISPR Challenge

How might the beatific vision of the good inform our understanding of those goods sought through new genetic engineering technologies? I am not going to dwell on the scientific or technical aspects of this new technology except to say that, as a biologist, the scientific evidence suggests that the CRISPR technique is more precise than older, cruder techniques of genetic engineering. Most scientific discussions about CRISPR are likely to lean toward specific medical applications, especially its seeming promise to address currently incurable human diseases and its use as a tool in the knowledge of human genetics.

The broader public debate has narrowed its focus to worries about the slippage toward human enhancement and issues of justice concerning access. And many of the specific ethical questions that arise in advisory bodies are the same ones that are already familiar to those who have worked in the ethics of human genetics, namely questions of safety, scope of use, and means of achieving the ends sought. Such bodies are most comfortable dealing with issues like safety, a focus that amounts to, as John Evans argues in Chapter 3 in this volume, a thin version of ethics that misses thicker ethical concerns.

What I offer here is not a claim around which consensus might be built, but rather an approach or way of thinking that can help to rescue our ability to talk about more than safety and efficacy. This approach, which I have developed in the past, retrieves the virtue of practical wisdom, a tool that is *even more* relevant now that speculation about the possibility of accurate human gene editing is closer to becoming a reality.

Infused Theological Virtues

Aquinas believed that the theological virtues of faith, hope, and charity could not be learned or acquired but were given by the grace of God. Charity, defined as love of God, spills over into love of all that God has made, especially other human beings made in the image of God. Hence, virtues that are *infused* into a person by a direct act of God can be experienced in this life and not just the life to come. The capability of humans to show compassion over the long term is one of the distinctive characteristics of human beings that reaches deep into evolutionary history.[8] While there has been a heated and long-standing debate in philosophical and psychological literature about the place of empathy and compassion in moral life, the significance of charity from a theological perspective is undisputed. Further, just as empathy is a prerequisite for compassion, so compassion is a prerequisite for *mercy*, a virtue that can be both acquired and infused by divine grace. Mercy and compassion are modeled on divine mercy and compassion, which are considered to be limitless.

Experiences of divine grace can impact a person's ability to care for others, including those who are severely disabled. Psychological research conducted by Michael Spezio and his colleagues at selected L'Arche communities, which house those with severe disabilities, have shown that the carers closely identify with members of the community in a way that is distinct from how people interact in the normal population. These caregivers see their actions as possible because of a religious experience of God's grace.[9] How compassion needs to be expressed in particular circumstances is also judged through the lens of practical wisdom: practical wisdom adjudicates what it means to show compassion. Yet if new genetic technologies move too quickly to try to fix or eliminate a specific need or disability, they may actually undercut more substantive virtues and human abilities, like compassion, which are at the heart of human community life and which make us human.

A Recovery of Practical Wisdom

When Aquinas envisaged his account of the beatific vision achieved by God's grace he was speaking in terms of "infused" virtues, which are given by God. But there were, he believed, smaller steps that ordinary people could take to acquire virtues, even those people who did not necessarily have any particular religious faith. Crucial to those small steps is the exercise of practical wisdom. Practical wisdom, then, is a source of insight and is a virtuous disposition that is particularly useful in the conduct of ordinary human affairs. As it is aimed at the common good (which I discuss further in this chapter), it can be applied in specific circumstances in different ways. Hence, a particular decision that follows the exercise of practical wisdom takes into account multiple factors in making that decision, even while keeping an open eye on whether that decision serves to achieve the goal of the common good. But for the religious believer, true practical wisdom will also be informed by the beatific vision when considering how to promote the ultimate goal of human flourishing.

While the moral virtues, such as justice and courage, on their own will incline their possessors toward right action, this inclination is not sufficient, which is why practical wisdom is so important. As Aquinas wrote: "The bent of moral virtue towards the mean is instinctive. Yet because the mean as such is not found after the same manner in every situation, the bent of nature which works uniformly is not enough, and requires to be complemented by the reasoning of [practical wisdom]."[10] Hence, practical wisdom helps to recognize those subtle differences that lead to a different course of action in given circumstances. Part of the challenge for CRISPR-Cas9, as with other new and potentially influential technologies, is that ethical decision-making should consider not only the implications for one individual or family, but also the wider social and political implications. Truly moral decisions aren't based on autonomy alone.

Practical wisdom, for Aquinas, has eight qualities, all of which are important in making a good decision. These qualities are memory, teachableness, acumen, insight, reasoned judgment, foresight, circumspection, and caution.[11] Memory (*memoria*) must be "true to being," which means that it must "contain in itself real things and events as they really are and were."[12] And it does not take long to realize that historical reflection forces a closer look at the long shadow of eugenics in the application of genetic science, a manipulation of human reproduction and discrimination against those with disabilities for ultimately political ends.[13]

Teachableness (*docilitas*), or open-mindedness, is a quality that many scientists will respect since without open mindedness discovery is much more difficult. But it is also a reminder that decisions are always embedded in complex networks of human needs and interests. Acumen (*solertia*) includes the ability to act clearly and well in the face of the unexpected. What if, for example, the CRISPR technology was approved for use in a fatal single-gene disease such as Tay-Sachs and wholly unexpected results followed? For example, there is hostility toward Jewish populations because funding is being channeled to ends perceived to be for the good of a specific ethnic group. Would the momentum of research be such that it would be hard to speak out? Acumen makes it possible to act correctly even when the time to make a decision is compressed. *Insight* and *reasoned judgment* are also on the list of intellectual virtues that practical wisdom requires. Yes, some readers will ask questions regarding, for example, *whose* insight and *which* reasoned judgments are assumed in such an account, but these questions do not undermine the effort to discern what should be done. What seems reasonable to one may not be to another, but insofar as prudential reasoning includes deliberation, it takes into account different points of view.

Which additional elements need to be in place for practical wisdom to be possible? The first element here is *foresight*, which is the human corollary of divine providence since divine providence always aims at the ultimate good, while foresight seeks to imitate that orientation. Foresight is the ability to know if certain actions will lead to a desired goal. The judgments of practical wisdom are not fixed or certain in ways that might be the case for a simple application of rules or principles. Rather, "because the subject matter of [practical wisdom] is composed of contingent individual incidents, which form the setting for human acts, the certitude of [practical wisdom] is not such as to remove entirely all uneasiness of mind."[14] This component is crucial for judgments about gene editing, especially in view of the fact that many of the so-called predictive beneficial effects have not come to pass in genetic medicine. Is this new and, due to its specificity, seemingly very promising technology an exception to that trend, or is interest in CRISPR yet another example of overenthusiasm in the wake of a new and exciting discovery? Are the uncertainties sufficiently strong to be tolerated or not? And who will be the major beneficiaries?

Aquinas also included *circumspection* and *caution* in the list of the components of practical wisdom. Circumspection is the ability to understand the nature of events as they are now, while foresight is the ability to understand events as they might be in the future. The difficulties with CRISPR include that it is very hard for a nonspecialist to fully understand what is in fact certain knowledge or what is less secure. Caution has to do with imprudent acts that are too hasty and avoiding obstacles that might get in the way of sound judgments, though caution that leads to inaction is not really what Aquinas had in mind either. In this sense, freezing all action due to an overinflated sense of caution may not be appropriate, but caution does keep in mind the overall trajectory of scientific research in this field. Caution here refers not only to safety issues, but also to wider, more substantial questions about the kind of human community that is envisaged—in other words, what human flourishing actually means. In addition, Aquinas also recognized the place of *gnome*, that is, the wit to judge when departure from principles is called for in given situations.

Practical wisdom as setting the mean of the moral virtues not only is primarily concerned with individual prudential decisions, but also should inform political governance. While Aquinas's discussion of practical wisdom bears some relationship to that in Aristotle, in this respect it is different, for Aristotle confined his attention to individuals. For Aquinas, political practical wisdom "bears the same relation to legal justice that ordinary [practical wisdom] does to moral virtue."[15] The common good is that which is related to the good of all and the good of each, and in Aquinas's time, that included the state.[16] While the rule of nation-states is more complicated now with international laws and transnational companies whose power exceeds that of some states, the overall intention of political practical wisdom toward the common good still applies.

Part of the debate over gene editing relates to what that good means and for whom. In other words, what does it mean for a community to flourish? Compared with the individualism that prevails today, Aquinas was more communitarian. So where individual practical wisdom clashes with economic or state practical wisdom, the former has to give way to the latter. Hence, "the good of the individual is subordinate to the good of the people. . . . The virtue engaged with the furthest end is the superior and commands the other virtues."[17] Distributive justice and political practical wisdom work together for the same end, though they can be distinguished in their role.[18] While the rhetoric of the "common good" was once used to promote eugenic practices, in the current context of deliberations over the use of gene editing technologies—especially when filtered through the light of Christ and the beatific vision of true human flourishing—use by a powerful elite of such technologies to promote racial purity would be necessarily excluded. Hence, rather than opposing eugenic practices by avoiding any collective sense of what the good might require and resorting to individual autonomy as the way forward, a more promising approach is to insist on greater scrutiny of what social, political, and collective goods require using the tools of distributive justice and political practical wisdom.

Just as individual practical wisdom sets the mean for the moral virtues, so political practical wisdom sets the mean for distributive justice. Distributive justice is concerned with the relationship between the community and individuals, but what this distributive justice might require is not self-evident in all cases and needs to be supplemented by political practical wisdom, in much the same way as correct decision-making for the moral virtues must be supplemented by individual practical wisdom.

Political practical wisdom is one way of helping to heal the rift between public and private morality, the false divide between a "subjective" virtue ethic that is concerned with individuals and principled "objective" approaches that are more often concerned with wider social contexts. It is particularly useful for adjudicating heated public contestations regarding gene editing technologies since much of the discussion seems, as it is with many controversial issues, to rest on key exemplars, which in turn provide the basis for lobbying either in favor of or against this technology.

Take, for example, the case made by Erika Check Hayden based on the example of Ruthie Weiss, who has albinism and has appeared in media reporting on CRISPR.[19] Check Hayden reported that when you ask patients like Ruthie, or her parents, whether they would have used CRISPR to prevent albinism, the answer is a resounding, No. Why? Because what makes Ruthie Ruthie is the challenge she has faced and the particular determination to live in spite of these disadvantages. This is a poignant story about the virtue of perseverance in the face of hardship, yet it leaves me unconvinced. After all, Ruthie would have been a very different child if engineering had been permitted, making it impossible to project back into the past and ask whether some of those unique characteristics could be compromised.

Emotive arguments like this are also too anecdotal. Yes the voices of those who have been excluded from discussion need to be taken into account and even given priority, but that process must be fair. Equally poignant anecdotal stories could have been told about how a particular affected individual has suffered and continues to suffer unbearably due to a genetic condition. While many parents of children with Down syndrome also say that they do not wish to change their child's chromosomes, others disagree. It is easy to find and use anecdotal evidence on both sides of the debate in a way that parallels heated discussions about stem cell and regenerative medicine. Analysis based on isolated anecdotal cases will not work.

What difference might the adoption of practical wisdom make to current policy decision-making on the application of new genetic technologies to particular cases, in particular those cases related to gene editing and related technologies? Current scientific narratives about how to make such policy decisions concentrate on issues of "efficacy, safety and specificity."[20] These are all short-lived issues of process; the assumption is that as long as these obstacles are overcome, gene editing and allied genetic technologies can be applied to whatever situation presents itself as amenable to genetic manipulation under the banner of particular "therapeutic" desires. Practical wisdom is therefore not simply about individuals making decisions about whether to use this technology in specific cases—situations that often fall under the medical-bioethical rhetoric of respect for autonomy—with the individual patient left to decide. Rather, the important point to make is that practical wisdom applies to different levels: the level of the individual, yes, but also the level of the family, the community, and the state or system of governance.

Such an approach, which stresses a movement away from isolating the individual and toward complex multivalent levels in envisaging the good, applies whether or not a specific Christian and Thomistic understanding of that good is sought. Individual goods in the approach I am arguing for are not denied. But such goods are sought within a much broader context of what that good might mean as embedded in specific social contexts operating at different levels. Within each of these levels, practical wisdom necessarily takes account of efficacy, safety, and specificity since these are all ingredients relevant to that element of practical wisdom or prudence known as circumspection. Circumspection, of course, is just *one aspect* needed for a prudential decision–policy-making that is prudential and is not content to limit its parameters to issues of practical safety and efficiency.

Bigger questions relate to that part of practical wisdom called *foresight*, which involves taking account of broader consequences, such as whether the technology is desirable at all for the common good, who is really going to benefit from the use of the technology, what implications are relevant for a given community, what impact such applications might have on the use of resources, and so on. Further, which population groups will be used in clinical trials that will inevitably be set up to test efficacy, such as gene technologies that work to "correct" AIDS or other immune deficiency diseases such as severe combined immune deficiency (SCID)? Single-gene diseases such as Tay-Sachs may seem obvious as a first step in the application of CRISPR and may even be preferable for conservatives since the manipulation will be on sex cells rather than the embryo, but a prudential decision in a given community will also place such seeming advantages in a wider social and political context.

Practical wisdom also helps to judge what the virtue of justice requires in given circumstances insofar as it is oriented toward the common good. It seems highly likely that the most vulnerable will be the target of clinical trials in the lead up to large-scale therapeutic applications. Are all such treatments necessarily desirable as ends to promote overall human flourishing? A similar point is made by Jackie Leach Scully in Chapter 10 in this volume where she argues that removal of disease through gene editing, which seems to some an unambiguous good, may on closer examination not be so. For Scully, the balance between control and acceptance is important. However, in the Thomistic tradition practical wisdom provides the means, at least, to attempt to take account of a multiplicity of factors in decision-making, including what such "balance' might look like in practice, for example, by giving moral priority to the weak, but not *just* those who are suffering various diseases.

Concluding Remarks

Roman Catholics who are concerned about human dignity tend to focus exclusively on the status of the embryo, as if that is the *only* ethical quandary raised by debates about human genetics research. This no-embryo filter leads to an unfortunate shrinking in the scope of what is at stake in such debates. There is also often a bland acceptance of technologies such as adult stem cell research that do not involve use of human embryos, perhaps due to nervousness about being perceived as antiscience. Such a stance is clear but is not necessarily fully responsible since techniques that appear innocuous—somatic gene therapy being another prime example—when looking through the "no human embryo" filter are in fact not necessarily free of moral quandaries.

In the first place and more substantially, should such technologies necessarily be developed at all? Certainly, the beatific vision questions an overreliance on technology to "fix" perceived problems of individual suffering, especially when those fixes risk undercutting substantive perspectives on what it means to flourish in a virtuous human community. Other quandaries are interrogated in the light of practical wisdom, which takes *both* principles and consequences into account in a holistic deliberative judgment while recognizing that absolute certainty in making those judgements is never possible. Relevant questions include, Which diseases should be targeted? Who is going to benefit most? Which population groups will be asked to participate in clinical trials? How might such technologies impact wider issues of racial, sexual, or cultural discrimination?

Practical wisdom, insofar as it sets the mean of the moral virtues, will enable clear insight into what justice and compassion require in given contexts.

The beatific vision is a reminder that the goal of the Christian life and the ultimate form of human flourishing is that envisaged as hidden in God, yet disclosed in part through contemplation on the life of Christ. That vision reins in the aspiration toward perfect human bodies implicit in much genetic engineering agendas and challenges the too easy adoption of the any-means-to-an-end approach to either bodily perfection or extended life span that is characteristic of much transhumanist rhetoric. There are ambiguous cases to navigate here in that the lines between "enhancement" and "treatment" are often blurred; what counts as a condition worthy of such treatment and for whose benefit?

The quick fix solution of what some have called "moral enhancement" is also alien to the slow and patient development of virtues useful for the moral life and may even undermine human freedom.[21] Are vaccines and genetic interventions aimed at the *prevention* of disease properly thought of as treatment or enhancement?[22] Practical wisdom does not offer a clear response in advance, but it does put priority on taking account of the views of the most marginalized and excluded in society. In this sense, what is perceived as a good by secular governments is unlikely to align with the kind of flourishing society envisaged through a Christian lens informed by practical wisdom and in the light of the beatific vision of human perfection of virtues. A Christian understanding of the pursuit of human flourishing does not deny aid toward those individuals who suffer, but it does encourage greater acceptance of those whose bodies or whose genes are not considered "ideal" in terms of physical function.

Practical wisdom, by insisting on an examination of the different aspects of what makes a good decision and different levels of decision-making, forces onto the agenda the full complexity of a problem, seeking understanding of all levels, not just the circumspective one, while providing at least some tools for that decision-making. Practical wisdom is not a panacea, but it may be an important alternative to the idea that all we need to do is apply fixed principles such as respect for individual autonomy to ethical problems that are, at root, the same.

Christians also have hope in another means to arrive at good decisions, namely by means of an infused virtue that is given directly by God. Talk of such "infused" virtue may make secularists blanch, as it might seem to provide religious justification for all kinds of acts. But infused virtue has the same source as charity, love of God, and love of neighbor. Aquinas wrote that "the [practical wisdom] of grace, however, is caused by God's imparting."[23] And Aquinas was ready to admit that practical wisdom can be spoiled in all kinds of ways, and where truths are forgotten, practical wisdom no longer flowers into action and becomes "blocked."[24]

Hence, the virtue of charity in one sense even trumps that of practical wisdom, for without charity prudential decision-making becomes disconnected from its source as rooted in the love of God and neighbor. While charity is more commonly associated with wisdom, understood as right relationship with both God and neighbor; practical wisdom is associated with making right judgments. Practical wisdom also encompasses the ability to learn from others, or teachableness (docilitas).[25] Charity is the "mother and root" of all virtues.[26] Isolated acts of charity are insufficient guides for decision-making, as are isolated cases of what justice requires. The Catholic conception of the common good aligns with secular understanding of human flourishing, but here again there are difficult issues to decipher on whose good is being promoted and for what ends. Practical wisdom may provide a useful companion tool to charity and justice since charity is more than simply the emotive elements in empathy, but involves compassionate judgments about what is right in given circumstances.[27] This, then, is a broad framework for decision-making through a prudential lens, a guide that is less about absolute rules of right or wrong, yet is taking appropriate responsibility for human flourishing according to specific virtues of the human community, namely those virtues of practical wisdom, charity, compassion, and mercy.

Notes

1. Philosophy and sociology of science studies engage in heated debates about the meaning of scientific objectivity. Andrew Pickering has proposed an interesting model of the production of scientific knowledge as a complex "mangle" of practices, theories, machines, and social relations. Andrew Pickering, *The Mangle of Practice— Time, Agency and Science* (Chicago: University of Chicago Press, 1995).
2. Thomas Aquinas, *Summa Theologiae, The Grace of Christ, Vol. 49, 3a, 7–15,* trans. Liam G. Walsh (London: Blackfriars, 1974), 3a, Qu. 9.2.
3. Thomas Aquinas, *Summa Theologiae, Knowing and Naming God, Vol. 3,* 1a, 12–13, trans. Herbert McCabe (London: Blackfriars, 1964), 1a Qu. 12.4.
4. Aquinas, *Knowing,* Qu. 1a 12.4; 12.5.
5. Aquinas, *Knowing,* Qu. 1a 12.12.
6. Aquinas, *Knowing,* Qu. 1a 12.13.
7. Aquinas, *Knowing,* Qu. 1a 12.13.
8. Celia Deane-Drummond, "Empathy and the Evolution of Compassion: From Deep History to Infused Virtue," *Zygon,* 52, no. 1 (2017): 258–278.
9. Michael Spezio, "Forming Identities of Grace and Cognitive Models of Self for Others in L'Arche Communities" (public lecture, Center for Theology, Science and Human Flourishing, University of Notre Dame, Notre Dame, IN, September 2, 2016), https:// www.youtube.com/channel/UCyObd-6TG0q4SLA7NAVUohw.

10. Thomas Aquinas, *Summa Theologiae, Prudence, Vol. 36*, 2a2ae, 47–56, trans. Thomas Gilby (London: Blackfriars, 1973), 2a2ae, Qu. 47.7.
11. Aquinas, *Prudence*, 2a2ae, Qu. 49.
12. Josef Pieper, *Prudence*, trans. R. and C. Winston (London: Faber and Faber, 1970), 26.
13. As documented in, for example, the work of Jon Marks, *Tales of the Ex Apes: How We Think About Human Evolution* (San Francisco: University of California Press, 2015).
14. Aquinas, *Prudence*, 2a2ae, Qu. 47.9.
15. Aquinas, *Prudence*, 2a2ae, Qu. 47.10.
16. Aquinas, *Prudence*, 2a2ae, Qu. 47.11.
17. Aquinas, *Prudence*, 2a2a, Qu. 47.11.
18. Porter treats distributive justice and political prudence as two sides of the same coin, though this is a confusing articulation since it implies they are identical, which may not be her intention. Jean Porter, *The Recovery of Virtue* (London: SPCK, 1994), 104.
19. Erika Check Hayden, "Should You Edit Your Children's Genes?" *Nature* 530, no. 7591 (2016): 402–405, http://www.nature.com/news/should-you-edit-your-children-s-genes-1.19432.
20. David Cox, Randall Platt, and Feng Zhang, "Therapeutic Gene Editing: Prospects and Challenges," *Nature (Medicine)* 21, no. 2 (2015): 121–131.
21. Celia Deane-Drummond, "The Myth of Moral Bio-Enhancement: An Evolutionary Anthropology and Theological Critique," in *Religion and Human Enhancement: Death, Values and Morality*, ed. Tracy Trothen and Calvin Mercer (New York: Springer, 2017), 175–189.
22. For discussion, see Cox et al., "Therapeutic Gene Editing."
23. Aquinas, *Prudence*, 2a2ae, Qu. 47.14.
24. Aquinas, *Prudence*, 2a2ae, Qu. 47.16.
25. For further discussion of the relationship between prudence and the gift of counsel, see Celia Deane-Drummond, *The Ethics of Nature* (Malden, MA: Blackwell, 2004), 13.
26. Thomas Aquinas, *Summa Theologiae, Virtue, Volume 23, 1a2ae, 55-67*, trans. W. D. Hughes (London: Blackfriars, 1968), 1a2ae Qu. 62. 4.
27. Celia Deane-Drummond, "Empathy."

PART V
FLOURISHING TOGETHER

14

Whose Conception of
Human Flourishing?

Dorothy Roberts

Advocates of human inheritable (germline) genetic modification argue that selection of human traits—eliminating undesirable ones and amplifying those that
are desirable—can benefit human societies. This argument, that having certain
genetic traits and not having others (whether as an individual or as a species)
increases well-being, assumes an understanding of what it means for humans to
live well—to flourish. Yet the meaning of human flourishing embraced by these
advocates is neither objective nor universally accepted. Rather, the concept of
human flourishing that undergirds their claims tends to import socially biased
assumptions about what human flourishing means. In particular, it promotes
the traits of socially advantaged groups and focuses on individual enhancement rather than social change. By assuming a concept of human flourishing
that privileges these interests, arguments in favor of gene editing can reinforce
socially unjust hierarchies. Moreover, the idea that gene editing can improve
human flourishing distracts us from what we know are flourishing's most powerful predictors. For individuals to flourish, they must be situated in societies
that promote their flourishing. Those who are enthusiastic about gene editing
either assume that those social conditions are already in place, leading them to
fixate on what remains to be improved (their genomes), or have great faith in
the power of changing the biology of individual human beings, but little faith in
changing the unjust structure of the societies in which human beings live.

A full and just deliberation of the ethics of human genetic modification must
include a more robust consideration of the meaning of human flourishing. How
do we ensure that this deliberation will entail the needed scrutiny of underlying
and biased assumptions? One important way is to include the perspectives of
groups that are disadvantaged most by social inequalities. Yet, public discussion thus far has narrowly included scientists, bioethicists, and patient advocacy
groups (what have been called "professional elites"). Their arguments in favor of
genome modification, based on false assumptions of scientific objectivity and
a universal concept of flourishing, not only neglect other perspectives but also
affirmatively exclude them from view. To better advance ethical uses of genomic

modification, we need a more diverse conversation. People with disabilities, poor people, queer people, people of color (especially women of color), and others at various intersections of these social positions must be centered on defining the meaning of human flourishing and articulating the role that gene editing technologies might play in promoting flourishing for all.

The Assumed Conception of Human Flourishing

The prominent ethical debates about human genetic modification have focused on the safety and misuse of gene editing technologies. An influential 2015 article in *Science* by key scientists and bioethicists in this field, including David Baltimore, Jennifer Doudna, and George Church, called for research to "manage the risks arising from the use of the CRISPR-Cas9 technology," which they identified as "the possibility of off-target alterations, as well as on-target events that have unintended consequences."[1] In their view, managing these risks centers on weighing the potential safety and efficacy of gene editing against its potential benefits: "Higher risks can be tolerated when the reward of success is high, but such risks also demand higher confidence in their likely efficacy." This understanding of success places human biology at the very center of the analysis.

In summarizing ethical issues raised at the 2015 International Summit on Human Gene Editing, Tracy Hampton noted similar concerns "regarding errors and other unintended effects with unknown consequences."[2] The issues raised by the International Summit statement by the organizing committee also included "the risks of inaccurate editing" and "the difficulty of predicting harmful effects," as well as "the possibility that permanent genetic 'enhancements' to subsets of the population could exacerbate social inequities or be used coercively."[3] All of these ethical concerns center on the risks of using gene editing technologies in the wrong way. While the inclusion of justice concerns is notable, the committee's framing accepts that genomic modification will make human beings better off as long as no one is physically harmed and the technology is available to everyone. It fails to question the claim that human flourishing will be furthered if the procedures achieve what they are designed to do and are distributed widely. According to this view, as the technologies improve and the risk of "undesirable side effects" or "off-target alterations" diminishes, gene editing can ethically proceed because it will improve the quality of human lives. The nature of human flourishing is left out of the debate focused on safety, efficacy, and access, not because it is ignored but because it is assumed.

As John Evans argues in Chapter 3 of this volume, a thin debate about the ethics of gene editing assumes a limited set of ends (e.g., autonomy and relief of human suffering) and questions only whether the means (e.g., CRISPR-Cas9) are efficacious to achieve these limited ends. A thick debate about the ethics of gene editing asks, as Evans put it, "*about* the ends or goals that we should or should not pursue," including the more controversial goal of human flourishing. Without a thick debate about the ends of gene editing, our ethics become guided by the technologies when in fact the technologies ought to be governed by our ethics. But even a thick debate about human genome modification risks reinforcing social injustices if it does not attend to social assumptions underlying conceptions of human flourishing. The only way to have a truly thick debate that unearths and contests these social assumptions is to include socially disadvantaged groups, whose traits are devalued and who have a greater stake in social change.

How Mainstream Concepts Import Unjust Social Assumptions

Some bioethicists predict that gene editing will create new standards of normalcy or a new social hierarchy of genetic haves and have-nots.[4] I am concerned with how gene editing incorporates the devaluation of certain group traits and with how it distracts attention from ways of increasing human well-being that address *current* unjust social hierarchies and ideologies. It is not an accident that the assumed understanding of human flourishing has been determined by what improves the well-being of those who are the most privileged in society and in a way that legitimizes their privileged position. In particular, it has elided structural inequalities that advantage them and disadvantage others. Thus, the most socially privileged people have a vested interest in supporting a definition and means of increasing human well-being that focus on individual enhancement rather than on social change, and that blame lack of well-being on individual deficits rather than on unjust social structures. The argument that scientists can edit genes objectively without social bias ignores the biased view of human flourishing that underlies the promotion of gene editing in the first place. Moreover, it is not enough to argue that gene editing can take place alongside efforts to end societal inequities when those advocating for gene editing obscure the need for social change to achieve human flourishing.

There are two main reasons why socially privileged people have a vested interest in a view of human flourishing that supports development and use of gene editing. First, the practice of genetic selection has long been characterized by confusing unjust social hierarchies with inherited traits. This was a principal aspect of the pre–World War II eugenics movement in the United States and Europe.[5] Eugenicist thinking was promoted by not only government agents but also mainstream scientists and remains very alive in genomic research and policy discussions today.[6] Francis Galton, the father of eugenics, confused inherited social privilege with inherited intelligence when he wrongly assumed that the British elite achieved their stature because of their innate "genius."[7] Galton's fundamental flaw persists in contemporary concepts of human flourishing, which tie flourishing to the innate capacities of individuals. The problem with the thin version of the ethical debate is not only that its list of ends is too narrow—enhancing autonomy and reducing human suffering—but that these ends are viewed as products of individual traits, such as disabilities, rather than as products of social structure.

Second, the dominant perspective devalues the traits that socially disadvantaged groups possess as if these traits diminish a universally accepted understanding of human flourishing. Conversely, it values the traits of socially advantaged groups as if they objectively enhance human flourishing. As Dan Haybron points out in Chapter 2 of this volume, a common concept of human flourishing is its Aristotelian definition as the fulfilling of our natures. But what constitutes human nature? For Aristotle, the answer centered on the capacity for reason. Others have focused on physical perfection or intellectual ability. It is important to note that these and other answers have been profoundly shaped by the deeply embedded history of dividing human beings into races and sexes that are seen as evolving separately, having inherently distinguishable traits, and naturally belonging to different human communities.[8] In much the same way, a history of discrimination against people with disabilities has fueled the idea that disabilities are departures from ideal human nature.[9]

Today, popular images of genetic perfection in advertising, news media, and movies routinely exclude people with disabilities and people of color. The phrase "the perfect baby" associated with assisted reproductive technologies is typically accompanied by a photo of a white baby, usually with blond hair and blue eyes, as if to highlight his or her racial purity. This imagery reflects and reinforces the racial inequities in reproductive laws and policies. At a time when wealthy white people have disproportionate access to technologies designed to produce genetically screened babies in the type and number they desire, a host of laws and policies discourage poor women of color from having babies at all.[10] The multibillion-dollar market devoted to technologically facilitating affluent peoples' procreative predilections stands in glaring contrast to appalling racial disparities in infant and maternal mortality rates.[11]

The argument that gene editing promotes human flourishing is based on an understanding of human flourishing that is unexamined and systematically biased. This understanding is shaped by the views of the most privileged people and is biased in favor of the traits that they happen to possess. The privileged have a vested interest in the belief that the suffering of socially disadvantaged people stems from their inherent traits rather than from unjust social hierarchies. While it is dominant, the view of human flourishing held by the most privileged people is only partial.

Editing Genes Can't Change Structural Inequities

Having seen that arguments in favor of human genetic modification incorporate an assumed but partial concept of human flourishing, we can turn to the inadequacies of that concept. A significant flaw in the dominant view of human flourishing is that it points us toward genetic modification by distracting us from the most significant predictors of well-being. This view of human flourishing imagines that it depends on individual modification rather than social change. Gene editing involves altering the traits of individual human beings in order to improve their well-being and that of future generations. It relies on the alteration of human traits, rather than changes to the social structures that render those traits advantages or hindrances.

Disability rights scholars and activists have long criticized the medical model of disability because it focuses on the disadvantages created by the bodily defects of people with disabilities rather than on the barriers that people with disabilities face because of discrimination against them.[12] The idea that genetic modification to eliminate certain disabilities is required to enhance human flourishing makes the same kind of mistake. It assumes that the reason people with disabilities are not flourishing already stems from their own physical limitations and not from limitations imposed by social structures. Yet, we know that improving social structures can vastly improve the lives of people with disabilities. For example, children with Down syndrome live longer and have more fulfilling lives today than they did thirty years ago because of the adoption of policies that include them in typical social and educational settings, provide them with better healthcare, prohibit discrimination against them, and support their families.[13] These changes did not require the children to no longer have Down syndrome.

The claim that intelligence can be improved by genetic modification suffers from a similar flaw. The very notion that intelligence is inherited genetically and can be identified at the genetic level ignores the social construction of intelligence and the social purpose of measuring it.[14] Most IQ tests measure a narrow range of intellectual skills (e.g., memory and general knowledge) or limited forms of thinking (mainly linguistic and mathematical) and focus on past learning, which reflects educational opportunities.[15] Because intelligence is complex and includes many equally important kinds of intelligences (which the tests ignore), we should not expect geneticists to identify a gene or genes that predict it. Moreover, scientists have used the concept of inherited intelligence to legitimate unjust social hierarchies by claiming that social inequality results from group differences in intelligence.[16] Because the very meaning of intelligence is disputed and some groups of people perform poorly on widely accepted tests for social reasons, intelligence tests privilege dominant social groups. Yet research has shown that mental test performances of groups improve along with the groups' social mobility.[17]

By attributing children's intellectual deficiencies to genes, researchers divert attention from the social impediments to children's intellectual flourishing. Indeed, opponents of equal education have exploited genetic theories of intelligence to claim that groups who score lower on IQ tests are incapable of benefitting from social interventions.[18] Other researchers studying the genetics of intelligence have argued that genetic testing can help determine which children need educational interventions the most. Yet we already know that intellectual enhancement programs are more likely to address social disadvantages if they nurture children's intellectual capacities by more equally distributing educational resources without relying on genetic testing.

Why, then, do scientists continue to focus on gene editing and other biological interventions as ways of improving well-being? This is because socially privileged people have relatively more to gain from genetic modification than from social change. People in socially advantaged positions are not as affected by the structural impediments to human flourishing, so they have less of a stake in eliminating them than they do in amplifying the genetic traits that they prefer. People who are socially disadvantaged, however, will continue to be at greater risk of illness and disability because of structural inequities, regardless of the potential for genetic modification.[19] Eliminating the genes associated with cystic fibrosis, for example, will do nothing to eliminate breathing problems caused by living in neighborhoods located near toxic waste sites, working in hazardous jobs, and experiencing stress from racial discrimination. The fantasy that genetic engineering will allow parents to determine "how healthy [their] children are actually going to be" ignores the structural causes that make many children sick and disabled.[20] This is a fantasy only the most privileged people in our society can maintain.

Increasing Access to Gene Editing Won't Solve the Problem

Concerns about social inequality are often framed as a matter of distribution of gene editing technologies. According to this view, human genetic modification would only be unjust if it were not equally available across society.[21] Granting access to these technologies only to people who are already socially privileged will enhance their privileged status, exacerbating existing inequalities by adding to them the gap between genetic haves and have-nots. Framed this way, the problem of social injustice can be solved simply by increasing access to gene editing, perhaps by making it universally accessible.

The focus on increasing access to technologies, however, incorporates the dominant assumptions about human flourishing rather than questioning them. If it is assumed that gene editing, done correctly, will promote human flourishing, then it follows that it is a good thing to increase access to the technology. But if that assumption is wrong, then it cannot be assumed that greater access to gene editing will increase human flourishing. Further, making genetic modification more widely available does not resolve the more fundamental question of what human flourishing is or how best to promote it.

A related ethical concern has to do with the coercive use of gene editing. In response, it is commonly assumed that giving individuals the freedom to choose whether to modify the genes of their children, as well as which traits to prefer, avoids the problem of forcing people to accept a particular concept of human flourishing.[22] According to this view, increasing access to gene editing inevitably enhances human flourishing because it allows parents to choose their children's traits. Yet this response underestimates the persuasive power of social norms. As Siddhartha Mukherjee wrote, "If the history of the last century taught us the dangers of empowering governments to determine genetic 'fitness,' then the question that confronts our current era is what happens when the power devolves to the individual."[23]

Putting genetic modification in the hands of individuals doesn't solve the problem of socially biased concepts of human flourishing. Even though prenatal genetic testing is not mandated by the government, pregnant women are made to feel that they have primary responsibility for making the "right" genetic decisions.[24] It is increasingly routine for pregnant women to get prenatal diagnoses for certain genetic conditions, such as Down syndrome and trisomy 18. They are typically expected to opt for abortion to select against any disabling traits identified by genetic testing.[25] Many obstetricians provide these tests without much, if any, explanation or deliberation because they consider such screenings to be a normal part of treating pregnant patients. Women who decide not to use genetic testing and have a baby with disfavored traits report being admonished and shamed by their doctors.[26] The existing expectation that women will use genetic testing to select their children's traits will only be exacerbated by the expansion of access to gene editing technologies. Gene editing is likely to become more of a duty than a choice.

As genetic screening becomes an expected part of pregnancy, we are seeing its wider incorporation into healthcare systems.[27] Unlike coercive programs of the past, these screening programs rely on the sense of obligation individuals feel to control their children's traits at the genetic level, shifting the spotlight away from state responsibility for ensuring healthy living conditions and ending discrimination against people with disabilities. While transferring the power to determine genetic fitness from the state to individual parents put an end to dehumanizing state policies like mass sterilization of people deemed genetically unfit, it has generated significant social pressure on women to ensure their children's genetic fitness. It is likely that pressure from government policies and medical practices will intensify as gene editing is considered a parental duty and cost-saving measure.[28]

The justice problem raised by gene editing isn't just that some people will lack access to genome modification owing to an inability to pay for it or to other structural barriers. The problem is that we are operating with a concept of human flourishing that devalues certain groups of people and diverts attention from the structural impediments to human flourishing. Gene editing can promote this inadequate conception of human flourishing even if individual parents rather than government agents are expected to enhance the genetic makeup of children. Increasing access to modification technologies without questioning the concept of human flourishing that supports them can intensify, not diminish, social inequality.

Including Groups Disadvantaged by Unjust Social Hierarchies

The National Academies of Science, Engineering, and Medicine recognized that ongoing deliberations over human genetic modification should "engage a wide range of perspectives and expertise—including from biomedical scientists, social scientists, ethicists, health care providers, patients and their families, people with disabilities, policymakers, regulators, research funders, faith leaders, public interest advocates, industry representatives, and members of the general public."[29]

This list must include groups that are disadvantaged by the current social hierarchy, whose traits are devalued, and who have a greater stake in social change.[30] In addition to people with disabilities, this means people of color, women, low-income and cash-poor people, queer people, and especially people at intersections of these social positions. Although patient advocates are not uniform, they tend to be concerned with questions of safety, efficacy, and access and can't be a substitute for members of these groups.[31]

The framing of the questions will also be important. Abstract arguments about the potential future affected by genome modification allow scientists and bioethicists to ignore already existing social inequities and the role technologies play in perpetuating or contesting them. By failing to acknowledge—let alone deal with—current unjust social structures, debates about human modification contribute to ways of thinking that help to maintain those same injustices. Deliberating the ethics of human genetic modification in a pretend world without structural inequality validates the false view that human well-being depends on genes alone and not primarily on social structure.

A thicker deliberation of human flourishing requires a commitment to creating a world without race, sex, class, and other social hierarchies. To move toward a human future that is liberated from these unjust hierarchies, we would not ignore but squarely face them. The only way to have this kind of thick debate about human flourishing is to include socially disadvantaged groups in ethical discussions and decision-making about human genetic modification.

Notes

1. David Baltimore, Paul Berg, Michael Botchan, Dana Carroll, R. Alta Charo, George Church, Jacob E. Corn, et al., "A Prudent Path Forward for Genomic Engineering and Germline Gene Modification," *Science* 348, no. 6230 (2015): 36–38.
2. Tracy Hampton, "Ethical and Social Questions Look Large as Gene Editing Moves Closer to the Clinic," *JAMA* 315, no. 6 (2016): 546–548.
3. Steven Olson, Committee on Science, Technology, and Law; Policy and Global Affairs, *International Summit on Human Gene Editing: A Global Discussion* (Washington, DC: National Academies of Sciences, Engineering, and Medicine, 2016).
4. Francis Fukuyama, *Our Posthuman Future: Consequences of the Biotechnology Revolution* (New York: Farrar, Straus & Giroux, 2000); Pete Shanks, *Human Genetic Engineering: A Guide for Activists, Skeptics, and the Very Perplexed* (New York: Nation Books, 2005).
5. Alexandra Minna Stern, *Eugenic Nation: Faults and Frontiers of Better Breeding in America* (Berkeley: University of California Press, 2015).
6. Dorothy Roberts, *Killing the Black Body: Race, Reproduction and the Meaning of Liberty* (New York: Vintage, 20th anniversary ed., 2017); Dorothy Roberts, *Fatal Invention: How Science, Politics, and Big Business Re-create Race in the Twenty-first Century* (New York: New Press, 2012).
7. Francis Galton, *Hereditary Genius: An Inquiry into Its Law and Consequences* (repr., 2012; London: Forgotten Books, 2012).
8. Roberts, *Fatal Invention*.
9. Erik Parens and Adrienne Asch, eds., *Prenatal Testing and Disability Rights* (Washington, DC: Georgetown University Press, 2000).
10. Roberts, *Killing the Black Body*.
11. Amnesty International, *Deadly Delivery: The Maternal Health Care Crisis in the USA* (London: Amnesty International Secretariat, 2010); Marian F. MacDorman, Eugene Declercq, Howard Cabral, and Christine Morton, "Recent Increases in the US Maternal Mortality Rate: Disentangling Trends from Measurement Issues," *Obstetrics & Gynecology* 128, no. 3(2016): 447–455.

12. Parens and Asch, *Prenatal Testing*.
13. Jennifer Jacob and Mardra Sikora, *The Parent's Guide to Down Syndrome: Advice, Information, Inspiration, and Support for Raising Your Child from Diagnosis Through Adulthood* (Avon, MA: Adams Media, 2016); Nancy J. Roizen and David Patterson, "Down's Syndrome," *The Lancet* 361, no. 9365 (2003): 1281–1289.
14. Dorothy Roberts, "Can Research on the Genetics of Intelligence Be 'Socially Neutral'?" *The Hastings Center Report* 45, no. S1 (2015): S50–S53.
15. Stephen J. Gould, *The Mismeasure of Man* (New York: Norton, 1981).
16. Tukufu Zuberi, *Thicker Than Blood: How Racial Statistics Lie* (Minneapolis: University of Minnesota Press, 2001).
17. Richard E. Nisbett, Joshua Aronson, Clancy Blair, William Dickens, James Flynn, Diane F. Halpern, and Eric Turkheimer, "Intelligence: New Findings and Theoretical Developments," *American Psychologist* 67, no. 2 (2012): 130–159.
18. Arthur R. Jenson, *Educability and Group Differences* (New York: Harper & Row, 1973).
19. Roberts, "Embodying Race," in *Fatal Invention*, 123–146; Gilbert C. Gee and Chandra L. Ford, "Structural Racism and Health Inequities," *DuBois Review* 8, no. 1 (2011): 115–132.
20. Antonio Regalado, "Engineering the Perfect Baby," *Technology Review*, March 5, 2015, quoting Harvard geneticist David Sinclair.
21. Olson et al., *International Summit*.
22. Nikolas Rose, *The Politics of Life Itself: Biomedicine, Power, and Subjectivity in the Twenty-First Century* (Princeton, NJ: Princeton University Press, 2007).
23. Siddhartha Mukherjee, *The Gene: An Intimate History* (New York: Scribner, 2016).
24. Dorothy Roberts, "Race, Gender, and Genetic Technologies: A New Reproductive Dystopia?" *Signs* 34, no. (2009): 783–804.
25. Cynthia M. Powell, "The Current State of Prenatal Genetic Testing in the United States," in Parens and Ash, *Prenatal Testing*, 44–53; Marsha Saxton, "Why Members of the Disability Community Oppose Prenatal Diagnosis and Selective Abortion," in Parens and Ash, *Prenatal Testing*, 147; Amy Harmon, "Genetic Testing + Abortion = ???" *New York Times*, May 13, 2007, http://www.nytimes.com/2007/05/13/weekinreview/13harm.html?mcubz=0
26. Brian Skotko, "Mothers of Children with Down Syndrome Reflect on Their Postnatal Support," *Pediatrics* 115, no 1 (2005): 64.
27. Wolfgang Van den Daele, "The Spectre of Coercion: Is Public Health Genetics the Route to Policies of Enforced Disease Prevention?" *Community Genetics* 9, no. 2 (2006): 40–49; Kristin Bumiller, "The Geneticization of Autism: From New Reproductive Technologies to the Conception of Genetic Normalcy," *Signs: Journal of Women in Culture and Society* 34, no. 4 (2009): 875–899.
28. Robert Sparrow, "Ethics, Eugenics, and Politics," in *The Future of Bioethics: International Dialogues*, ed. Akira Akayabashi (Oxford: Oxford University Press, 2014).

29. Olson et al., *International Summit*.
30. Ruha Benjamin, *People's Science: Bodies and Rights on the Stem Cell Frontier* (Stanford, CA: Stanford University Press, 2013).
31. E.g., Sharon Shaw Reeder, "The Patient Perspective," *Gene Watch* 27, no. 3 (2014): 10–12.

15

Reprogenetic Technologies Between Private Choice and Public Good

Maartje Schermer

No man is an island.

—John Donne

If resistance waits till life is reduced nearly to one uniform type, all deviations from that type will come to be considered impious, immoral, even monstrous and contrary to nature. Mankind speedily become unable to conceive diversity, when they have been for some time unaccustomed to see it.

—John Stuart Mill

Much of the bioethical debate on reprogenetic technologies has focused on the potential risks and benefits for individuals. Reprogenetic technologies include not only familiar technologies such as prenatal screening and preimplantation genetic diagnosis (PGD), but also emerging ones such as prenatal whole-genome sequencing and germline gene editing. It is argued that these technologies are beneficial because they prevent children being born with severe disabilities or suffering from terrible diseases. It has also been claimed that in the future they may enable the selection or creation of children with specific positive traits or enhanced capacities and hence an even better chance of leading flourishing lives.[1] For prospective parents, these technologies already enable and enlarge reproductive choice and will perhaps increase the range of those opportunities in the future. However, it is also argued that these technologies carry unknown risks to the health of children thus conceived, limit their "right to an open future," and are often burdensome and sometimes risky for the prospective mother. Moreover, it is argued that the increase in the number of possible choices may give prospective parents more responsibility than they can bear (see Iyengar and Kuman, Chapter 7, this volume, for a sophisticated version of this argument).

Although these are all valid considerations, in this chapter I shift the focus of attention away from this individualistic level toward a societal perspective.

Instead of looking at risks and benefits and the meaning of these technologies for the flourishing and self-understanding of individual humans—as many of the chapters in this volume do—I want to explore how emerging reprogenetic technologies can both undermine and promote the flourishing of communities and societies. Individual human flourishing is inextricably bound up with the structure, functioning, and values of the communities and society in which people live, as Dorothy Roberts and Bruce Jennings also stress in Chapters 14 and 17, respectively, in this volume. Communities determine the preconditions for flourishing and influence individuals' choices and options. Conversely, individual choices to use certain technologies often have effects beyond one's individual life and may, directly or indirectly, affect other individuals as well as society at large. Individual choices can have effects at the collective level, and these effects may be favorable or unfavorable. Reprogenetic technologies thus shape who we are and how we flourish not only as individuals but also as a collective. Although some will find this self- evident, in most of the bioethical discourse, the individualistic perspective reigns.

In this chapter I argue that in order to understand what these technologies mean for us, and for human flourishing, we need to take the collective level into account and ask what these technologies mean for society as a whole. I thus focus on the public or common good, rather than on the individual good. First, I explore what the public good *is* and how reprogenetic technologies can affect it, for better or worse. Next, I ask which forms of governance we might deploy with regard to reprogenetic technologies so that they can contribute to the public good—or at least not thwart it. What kind of regulations, institutional checks and balances, practice guidelines and criteria, public awareness campaigns, and so on should we consider and what kind of limitations should we perhaps impose either on the development of such technologies or on individual choice for the sake of the public good? The general claim I want to argue for is that reprogenetic technologies can contribute to the public good, but only when certain social conditions and side constraints are in place, and that this can sometimes entail influencing or even limiting individual choice.

Why We Should Consider the Public Good

Instead of focusing too narrowly on individual choice and well-being, the bioethical debate about reprogenetic technologies should start paying more attention to the collective and public dimensions. There are a number of reasons for this.

First, as science and technology studies have taught us, new (bio)technologies often affect everyone in some way and not just the people who choose to use them.[2] Individual choices regarding the use of technologies may lead to aggregate effects—also called "externalities"—that also have an impact on those who do not use the technology themselves. Some harms and benefits of technologies present themselves at a collective level, and it is often impossible for individuals to opt out of these. Consider, for example, the risks of climate change and global warming caused by the sum of many individual choices to use cars, airplanes, and energy-consuming equipment. These risks also affect people in developing countries who may not even have access to these polluting technologies. Another example would be the benefits and drawbacks of altering the germline. Using germline gene editing for one's offspring is never a strictly individual choice because it will affect future generations. More important, germline engineering could alter the human gene pool, which may have unforeseen collective effects. Many single genes or genetic variants have effects on many different aspects of the human phenotype, a phenomenon that geneticists call *pleiotropy*. Hence, eradicating for example a gene for one specific disease might at the same time lead to decreased resistance among the population against another disease,[3] while adding new genetic material, like resistance for certain diseases, might also have unforeseen collective effects. Likewise, it has been argued that if parents would start selecting, for example, specific cognitive traits for their children, which might give them a positional advantage as individuals, this choice might come at the expense of diversity in cognitive styles, which would arguably be a loss for society.[4]

Another way in which individual choices to use technologies can have a collective impact is by influencing how we perceive the world, how we conceive of ourselves, and how we relate to each other. An everyday example is the use of braces and teeth whiteners, which has changed the norms for appearance. At one time, crooked, brownish, or even rotten teeth were considered "normal"; nowadays only a perfectly straight and shiny white smile is. This change in norms and expectations affects all of us, not least those who have crooked teeth but no desire or no money to correct them. Likewise, when we start using reproductive and genetic technologies to select and perhaps even enhance our offspring, one aggregate effect of this might be that norms of normality and health will shift and that "imperfections" come to be less accepted and differences less tolerated (for more on the shifting norms of parenting, see Nicole Vincent and Emma Jane's Chapter 9 in this volume). Although it is often hard to say whether such changes are, overall, for better or for worse, the point is that they affect everyone, whether they use the technology, or approve of it, or not. Hence, reprogenetic choices not only are "self-regarding," but also have a public impact.

Finally, biotechnologies that have benefits for individuals may at the same time have a negative impact on social justice and equality. Technologies that help shape future children may reinforce existing inequalities, especially when they are expensive or access to them is otherwise limited. Already, disadvantaged people live shorter and unhealthier lives than wealthy ones and have fewer opportunities. If some can benefit from new reprogenetic technologies while others cannot, the existing socioeconomic divide with regard to health and well-being may grow. If we consider justice to be an important component of the public good, as I think we should, then we should look beyond the individual benefits and risks of technologies.

The Tension between Individual Choice and Public Good

Again, what is good when regarded from the individual perspective may not always be so from a collective point of view. This maxim also works the other way around: what is good from a collective perspective may be harmful for individuals or may infringe on their rights. To complicate matters further, there are good reasons to be apprehensive about invoking the public good in discussions about reproductive and genetic technologies. The historical misdeeds inspired by the eugenic movement, which were ostensibly carried out in the name of the public good, still hang over the debate like a dark cloud. It is, for this reason, completely understandable that bioethicists shy away from speaking about collective interest or the public good in relation to reprogenetic technologies. The concern is that invoking population-based arguments will lead to an inhumane or unjust sacrificing of individual interests, rights, and well-being for the greater good of the community, and that some dominant idea of the common good will effectively exclude certain groups of people who hold different views. The notion of human dignity is often invoked to counter these tendencies (see Gaymon Bennett's Chapter 16 in this volume for a detailed analysis of the evolution of this concept). In bioethics, proponents of biotechnological enhancement advocate "liberal eugenics" and stress the fundamental differences with the old eugenics, which was state driven, coercive, and "negative" (aimed at eliminating persons deemed inferior). In contrast, liberal eugenics is positive (aimed at increasing health and enhancing capacities) and driven by the free choice of individual prospective parents.[5]

Freedom of choice is one of the most important ethical principles within a liberal ethical framework, only limited by the classical harm principle formulated by John Stuart Mill.[6] This principle is not very well suited, however, for dealing with the collective effects of individual actions described in the previous section. It assumes a direct one-on-one relationship between actor and potential victim, not the complex web of relationships and interdependences that characterizes today's technological and globalized world. I would argue, therefore, that a current interpretation of the harm principle needs to take a more critical look at so-called self-regarding actions (actions that only directly affect individuals themselves). Such an interpretation should take indirect collective harmful effects of technologies into account. However important individual freedom of choice is, we must acknowledge that many of our choices and actions are not strictly self-regarding because we are intertwined with other individuals and because we live together in relationships and communities; hence most of what we do has some impact on others.

All this does *not* mean I want to claim that well-being should be sacrificed for the public good, or that individual choice should be made completely subservient to collective interests. But I do think that some restrictions on individual freedom, or some inconveniences, can be justified with an appeal to the common good. In fact, we already have regulations in place that limit individual freedom for the sake of the collective. We are all obliged to pay taxes, for example; some countries have compulsory military service or jury duty; and in case of serious epidemics of infectious diseases, people can be put in quarantine. In making policy about new technologies we may sometimes need to balance individual interests, including freedom of choice, against the public good. Individual rights and interests may weigh heaviest in many if not most cases, but we can only properly weigh them if we have a clear picture of the collective interests at stake. We therefore need to explore what the potential benefits and drawbacks of reprogenetic technologies are when considered from a public good perspective.

Reprogenetic Technologies and the Public Good

One way to define the public good is by simply identifying it with the aggregate of individual goods. However, I think this definition is too thin. The public good is more than the mere sum of individual goods or individual well-being. It also entails the fair distribution of individual well-being and individual opportunities for flourishing among members of society. In other words, the public good entails social justice. Moreover, it includes the social and environmental conditions that affect the well-being of individuals and that can only be created and maintained collectively.[7] This entails institutions, social structures, and basic values (i.e., freedom, equality, solidarity, and tolerance) that enable members of a society to live together peacefully and to flourish according to their own conception of the good life. The public good can thus be understood as a collection of elements that together make up a flourishing society: a society that offers all its members sufficient genuine opportunities to flourish and to live together peacefully. Although this conception of the public good needs further

theoretical elaboration and justification, I for now take it as my working definition. What does such an understanding of the public good imply in the context of
reprogenetic technologies? And how could reprogenetic technologies affect the
public good thus conceived?

Potential Contributions to the Public Good

Reprogenetic technologies might contribute to the public good in a number of
ways. Most obviously they may prevent suffering by children who would have
been born with serious congenital disease or disability, and their families; this
could result in a decrease in the net amount of suffering in society. Whether this
potential benefit will materialize depends, among other factors, on the amount
of suffering that these diseases and disabilities actually cause, which for some
conditions is contested. Scholarship in disability studies has questioned the self-
evident way in which disabilities are often conceived of as "bad" for people and as
the cause of unnecessary suffering, as Rosemarie Garland-Thomson explains in
Chapter 1 of this volume. This and other insights of disability studies ought to be
taken into account when assessing the potential benefits of disability-preventing
technologies.

Second, reprogenetic technologies might also increase the health and well-
being of future people, or at least increase their chances of leading healthy and
happy lives, by selecting or engineering certain positive traits and capacities in
children-to-be. In his book *Beyond Humanity*, Allen Buchanan discussed four
properties that he believes are the most likely candidates for biomedical enhancement in the near future, as well as most likely to increase productivity
and hence human development and well-being in society as a whole: cognitive
capacities, longevity, health (compressed morbidity), and immunity. Although
Buchanan defined *productivity* rather broadly as "how good we are at using existing resources to create things we value," the further examples he used have
strong economic overtones.[8] It appears as if the main public good that he believes
biomedical enhancement could help attain is a healthy workforce and increased
gross national product. There lies a serious danger in defining the public good
in such a narrow way as it implies that individual contributions to the common
good are to be evaluated in terms of economic value. In fact, the public good
should be interpreted much more broadly, to include valued practices like
arts and science and immaterial goods such as solidarity, justice, and peace.
Increasing or improving these elements of the public good may require enhancement of different traits and capacities than would be required to increase economic productivity.[9]

Next, an important consideration when thinking about the use of reprogenetic technologies for the public good is that promoting certain individual traits or capacities can have positive aggregate effects. In other words, the collective benefits of some selected-for or enhanced traits can be more than the sum of individual benefits. Herd immunity is a perfect example of this; when a sufficient number of individuals in a community are immune to a disease, the ones who are not immune are nevertheless protected because the disease-causing virus or germ cannot get a foothold in that community. So, vaccination of a sufficiently large percentage of individuals can also protect those who are not vaccinated. Herd immunity is a public good, and there are examples of regulations where mandatory vaccination programs are in place (for example, under legislation passed in California in 2016) to ensure these benefits for the community. It has been suggested that gene editing technology could be used to engineer immunity to certain diseases into the germline. Like vaccinations, this use of gene editing could create herd immunity to certain communicable diseases in future populations, which would also protect those who were not immune themselves.

Likewise, small gains in health, or other capacities, that may appear insignificant from an individual perspective may be important when viewed from a collective perspective. Buchanan and others have argued, for example, that from the perspective of the public good, a small gain in the cognitive abilities of all members of a population might be more valuable than significant increases in abilities for some individuals.[10] In a similar vein it could be argued that selecting or editing genes that contribute to—or are known to be protective against—common diseases such as diabetes, cancer, cardiovascular disease, or dementia might significantly contribute to population health by decreasing the prevalence of these diseases, even though on an individual level it would not always be clear how much benefit this conferred. Suppose, hypothetically, that a simple vaccine could change a specific gene variation that conferred a 20% higher risk of getting a specific disease into a healthier variation. This would not guarantee that those who were vaccinated would not get the disease in question, and if they did not, they would never know if it was due to the gene editing or for other (e.g., environmental) reasons. Their risk of getting the disease would decrease, however, and the prevalence of the disease in the population would drop. This would even be worthwhile if the contribution of these genetic variants to the disease in question is relatively small because on a population level a small decrease in the prevalence of a major disease like diabetes would be very significant. The benefits of gene editing thus need not be clear or substantial for individuals in order to confer an important benefit for society.

Potential Threats to the Public Good

A first concern about the impact of further expansion of reprogenetic technologies on the public good is that it will cause increased inequalities and injustice in society, especially when such technologies would be used for selecting or enhancing competitive traits or capacities. Social justice is an integral part of the public good as I conceive it; the public good is not merely the sum total of individual well-being, but requires that well-being is distributed justly. A just society offers sufficient genuine opportunities for flourishing to all its members and ensures fair distribution of the benefits and burdens of collective enterprises. This idea of social justice builds on Amartya Sen and Martha Nussbaum's capability approach, which argues that genuine opportunity to do and be what one has reason to value (i.e., to effectively be able to live the kind of life one considers "good") involves more than the formal availability of options or the fair distribution of primary goods.[11] In their *Social Justice*, Madison Powers and Ruth Faden[12] deployed a similar notion of opportunity and argued that justice requires sufficient minimal levels of well-being for all (see also Bruce Jennings's Chapter 17 in this volume).

Reprogenetic technologies might increase inequality and injustice by primarily benefiting those who are already well off. For example, if such technologies are prohibitively expensive for some people, access to them is effectively unequal. The burdens of genetic disease may thus fall harder on those who do not have the means to use these technologies to prevent them. Wealthier and better educated people might at the same time start using biotechnological opportunities to ensure further advantages for their offspring, creating an ever-more-unequal society.

Another important component of the public good concerns the social and environmental conditions that affect the flourishing of members of society and that can only be produced and maintained collectively. These include important public goods like sanitation or infrastructure and well-functioning social institutions, but I want to focus here on sociocultural factors, like "the shared norms and behavior that create and maintain substantive social values such as solidarity and trust."[13] These are all goods that are created as a result of conscious or unconscious collective action and are not easy to change or ignore individually. As I discussed previously, technologies can play a part in shaping and changing shared expectations and norms even among those who do not use the technologies themselves.

Maintaining basic social values such as freedom, solidarity, equality, and tolerance should all be considered part of the public good, at least in liberal pluralistic societies such as the United States and Europe. Individual freedom is necessary for individuals to pursue their own views of the good life, while the values of equality and tolerance demand respect for others' views, and the value of solidarity implies a willingness to mutually support one another in their pursuit for flourishing. These values enable societies to flourish by creating the "space" necessary for various modes of individual flourishing to exist alongside each other. As Mill argued, diversity among people in views and in ways of life is an essential element of well-being, both individual and societal.[14] As also argued by Rosemarie Garland-Thomson and Robert Sparrow (Chapters 1 and 11, respectively), diversity is important because it challenges our own views and because people with different views, dispositions, lifestyles, and abilities can make complementary contributions to society. A narrow collection of clones from a handful of "originals" could never make up a flourishing society.

One concern about the social impact of reprogenetic technologies is that diversity among people and tolerance regarding differences may come under pressure. The use of these technologies may indeed diminish some diversity among people, for example, by preventing the birth of people with certain diseases or disabilities, but it has rightly been argued that not all diversity is worth preserving. I fully agree with Sparrow when he argues in Chapter 11 that preserving disability for the sake of diversity, while disregarding the well-being of the individual would not be justifiable. However, the impact of some diseases and disabilities on the well-being of individuals remains contested. For example, the Dutch government program that offers prenatal screening is criticized by some because it is said to send the message that Down syndrome is an undesirable condition, a disability that should be prevented. Not everyone agrees with this evaluation of Down syndrome. While proponents of the prenatal screening program argue that the offer of screening enhances the opportunities for reproductive choice and is not meant to send any normative message about Down syndrome, critics continue to worry that it will adversely influence the acceptance of people with Down syndrome. For a flourishing society, both the acceptance and inclusion of people who are physically or mentally different, as well as tolerance toward people who make different reproductive choices than one would make for oneself, are necessary.

Reprogenetic technologies that shape future generations will also co-shape our cultural norms and perceptions concerning normality, (dis)ability, performance, and individual responsibility for health. They may reinforce a cultural belief in our ability to control and direct health, happiness, and success in life. That belief might have a negative impact on both well-being and solidarity. A strong cultural emphasis on personal responsibility for and a belief in the malleability of health can lead to feelings of personal failure and worthlessness in those who do not "succeed" (e.g., people who do not perform at the highest levels, who become ill, or who have a disabled child). It can also lead to blaming the victim: others may start holding them personally responsible. This may in turn lead to a loss of solidarity, as has also been pointed out by Michael Sandel.[15] Since solidarity with others is at least partly based on the recognition that some people are simply luckier than others, and that we do not always earn or deserve our fate, the idea of solidarity loses ground when the notion of luck is replaced by a belief in total control and personal responsibility.

What Kind of Governance Might the Public Good Require?

The potential contributions of reprogenetics to the public good, as well as potential drawbacks, do not solely depend on the technology itself. They are also, perhaps primarily, dependent on the ways in which these technologies will be regulated and the societal context in which they are embedded. The differences between the United States and the Netherlands may be instructive here, and I refer to some Dutch examples when discussing possible policy measures that take the public good into account. It is not my intention to deliver a blueprint of policy recommendations, but rather to provoke further thought about possible directions.

Already in 2003 a report of the Dutch Health Council noted that enhancement technologies might threaten "some intangible public goods" and argued "it is one of the tasks of the State to investigate threats to the public good, and if necessary to consider what policy measures can be adopted to protect it."[16] One policy option would be to leave everyone to choose freely whether to use these technologies and for which purposes as long as they can afford to pay for them. This is the "genetic supermarket" option. From the perspective of the public good as I have sketched it, this would not be the most desirable option, mainly for reasons of justice. It might also frustrate the creation of positive aggregate effects if individuals merely pursued their own interests without regard for collective consequences—a so-called collective action problem—and it could thus have indirect negative effects on social values.

Another regulatory option would be to enforce or prohibit the use of certain reprogenetic applications. Prenatal or preconception genetic screening programs could be made mandatory, as is the case for premarital beta-thalassemia carrier screening in Cyprus. Conversely, the use of preimplantation genetic selection for non–health-related purposes, such as enhancements or sex selection, could be prohibited, as is currently the case in the Netherlands. Or prenatal screening and abortion for conditions such as Down syndrome could be prohibited, the latter being the case in North Dakota. All these policy options clearly limit personal freedom and individual choice and hence stand in need of justification. In some specific instances the public good might provide such a justification, although in many cases individual freedom will be found more important; this depends on a careful weighing of the importance of free choice versus the public good at stake in any specific case.[17]

A third policy option, which avoids limiting personal freedom without leaving things up to the market, is to install government programs to promote certain applications of the technology while discouraging others. Using incentives or disincentives, such as subsidies, limiting availability of technologies to certified centers, or campaigns raising awareness of potential positive and negative collective effects, would not infringe on individuals' free choice (or at least do so to a lesser degree than mandating or prohibiting certain choices). Still, conscious attempts to influence individual choice, especially by the government, stand in need of some justification; an appeal to the public good can provide this. In the next section I illustrate how policy regarding reproductive technologies in the Netherlands aims at defending the public goods of justice and solidarity while also defending the public good that is freedom of choice.

The public good of social justice, which entails that sufficient genuine opportunities to flourish are open to all, requires that reproductive choice and hence access to reprogenetic technologies should be available for everyone equally. Reproductive choices are such significant life-shaping choices and have such high impact on the ability to flourish—both for the prospective parents and the child-to-be—that the capability to make such choices should be guaranteed. In the Netherlands, most forms of prenatal testing[18] as well as PGD on medical indication are covered in the basic package of the mandatory health insurance; premiums for this insurance are partly income dependent. Abortion services are also available to all and covered by national insurance.[19] At the same time, the cost of caring for children who are born with any disorder or disease are also carried collectively either through the mandatory insurance scheme or through national budgets for long-term care. Supporting both the option of avoiding and welcoming the birth of a child with a disability means that prospective parents are truly free to choose whether to use prenatal testing, or other reprogenetic technologies, without being constrained by financial concerns.

The Health Council of the Netherlands, which advises the government on these issues, has always emphasized that a responsible implementation of prenatal screening and PGD requires certain societal preconditions: "In order to make individual choice possible, social solidarity is needed with those who are confronted with these choices. The right to self-determination requires solidarity and vice versa. Personal decisions regarding these important matters must be respected by society."[20] This position requires that "facilities and conditions for care, support, and integration of people with disabilities must be guaranteed. It is an important task of the government to promote and monitor this." Without such societal conditions in place, it is argued, reproductive choice is not really free and self-determination is limited.[21] Moreover, I would add that without such conditions, values like tolerance, inclusion, and solidarity come under threat. If we take the public good into account, policy on health-related reprogenetic technologies should include measures to ensure equal access and truly free individual choice—that is, choice that is not dominated by financial considerations or social pressures.

While justice requires equal access to technologies that can alleviate or prevent serious health problems, it does not require access to every conceivable biotechnological option. In the Netherlands, for example, PGD is only allowed for a strict set of serious medical conditions (such as Huntington's disease or Duchenne muscular dystrophy). It is not permissible to perform PGD for conditions that are classified (by a special indication committee) as nonserious or nonmedical (such as sex or eye color), regardless of whether people would be willing to pay out of pocket.[22] Many other countries also prohibit sex selection in order to protect gender diversity and counter discrimination. Especially in countries like India, where women are disvalued, allowing prospective parents to select the sex of their child runs the real risk of creating a gender imbalance in society, which is not in the public interest. Restricting individual choice of prospective parents can, in this context, be justified.

Concerns regarding an increase in inequalities related to the possible use of reprogenetic technologies for enhancement purposes can seem rather far-fetched given the current state of the technology. However, we could imagine tackling this potential long-term problem through a general prohibition on using gene editing techniques for enhancing "normal" traits or by limiting it to enhancements that stay within a certain "normal range." From the public good perspective it would also be an option to promote (e.g., subsidize) the type of enhancements that will be beneficial for all, like increased immunity, decreased susceptibility to certain diseases, or small increases in cognitive or communicative abilities in the general population. Although this is still speculative (especially the bit about cognitive and communicative enhancements), it is not too early to start discussing, as societies, how reprogenetic technologies may affect the public good, for better or for worse, and to what extent this justifies some limitations on individual choice.

In the meantime, it is important to understand that if we truly want to contribute to the public good, it will in many cases be more effective to try to change social structures and institutions than to try to change the biology of individuals. Dorothy Roberts, in Chapter 14 in this volume, is right, I believe, in her worry that discussions around gene editing may distract from nonbiotechnological ways of tackling existing injustices. A good public education system that enables everyone to live up to their potential, regardless of social background, would most likely be a more effective and safer way to achieve overall gains in cognitive performance than editing the genome. Cognitive enhancement by biomedical or reprogenetic means would not even be very effective in the absence of such structures and institutions since even smarter children will not learn much without proper schooling. Justice is better served by improving access to care and to education systems in which attention and assistance are based on need rather than ability to pay. Justice also requires legislation to ensure equal rights for people with disabilities and measures to effectively create equal opportunities in the real world, not just in name. In the enhancement debate, such nonbiomedical means for improvement sometimes tend to get lost from sight. Proponents of enhancement appear to put all their cards on achieving a better world through biomedical means and tend to forget the importance of social structures and social institutions.

Conclusion

In contemplating reprogenetic technologies in relation to human flourishing, we should ask not only what this means at an individual level but also what it means for a society to flourish. Individuals in pluralistic democratic societies have different—even widely diverging—views of what individual flourishing entails; hence, such societies should accommodate a variety of ways to "live a good life." Individual freedom of choice regarding how to live one's life is therefore very important. However, reproductive and genetic technologies that may shape future generations have an impact at the societal level, and choices regarding the use of such technologies not only are self-regarding but also affect others. Taking the public good as a lens to look at these technologies enables us to see the possible tensions between individual choice and collective interests more clearly. As Erik Parens might phrase it, for an in-depth understanding of what is at stake, it is important to be able to oscillate between comprehending persons "as individuals" and "as members of societies."[23]

In this chapter I have explored the kind of governance that we might consider and the kind of limitations that we should perhaps impose on the development and use of reprogenetic technologies for the sake of the public good. I have also argued that reprogenetic technologies can contribute to the public good only when certain social conditions are in place. Social institutions and arrangements that protect justice and promote values like tolerance, inclusion, and solidarity are indispensable to embed new technologies in society in such a way that they can contribute to, rather than thwart, flourishing—both individually and collectively.

Notes

1. The dividing line between prevention of disease or disability and the improvement or enhancement of physical and mental traits is not always very clear. One may merge imperceptibly into the other, as with enhanced immunity, and certain traits that are considered disability by some are seen as unproblematic or even desirable by others (e.g., deafness). I therefore do not make a very strict distinction here between treatment, prevention, and enhancement but rather consider them as on a continuum. The common denominator is between technologies that enable us to influence—and to a certain extent control—what kind of people there will be.

2. Edward Hackett, Olga Amsterdamska, Michael E. Lynch, and Judy Wajcman, eds., *The Handbook of Science and Technology Studies* (Cambridge, MA: MIT Press, 2008) and Peter-Paul Verbeek, *What Things Do: Philosophical Reflections on Technology, Agency, and Design* (University Park: Penn State University Press, 2005). For specific examples in the field of reproductive technologies, see Maartje Schermer and Jozef Keulartz, "How Pragmatic Is Bioethics? The Case of In Vitro Fertilization," in *Pragmatist Ethics for a Technological Culture*, ed. Jozef Keulartz, Michael Lorthals, Maartje Schermer, and Tsjalling Swoerstra (Dordrecht, the Netherlands: Kluwer Academic Press, 2002), 41–68, and Dirk Stemerding, Tsjalling Swierstra, and Marianne Boenink, "Exploring the Interaction between Technology and Morality in the Field of Genetic Susceptibility Testing: A Scenario Study," *Futures* 42, no. 10 (2010): 1133–1145.

3. One well-known example is sickle cell disease. Individuals who are homozygous for the sickle cell gene (i.e., have two copies) have the disease, but those who are heterozygous (have only one copy of the gene) do not become ill and have, moreover, better resistance against malaria.

4. Chris Gyngell, "Valuable and Valueless Diversity," *American Journal of Bioethics* 15, no. 6 (2015): 38–39; Chris Gyngell and Tom Douglas, "Stocking the Genetic Supermarket: Reproductive Genetic Technologies and Collective Action Problems," *Bioethics* 29, no. 4 (2015): 241–250.

5. See, for example, Nicholas Agar, *Liberal Eugenics: In Defence of Human Enhancement* (Malden, MA: Blackwell, 2004); Allan Buchanan, *Beyond Humanity* (Oxford: Oxford University Press, 2011).

6. John Stuart Mill, *On Liberty* (London: Parker, 1859).

7. This conception of the public good is inspired by the notion of public health as understood in public health ethics. See especially Marcel Verweij and Angus Dawson, "The Meaning of 'Public' in 'Public Health,'" in *Ethics, Prevention and Public Health*, ed. Macel Verweij and Angus Dawson (Oxford: Oxford University Press, 2007) 13–29. See also Angus Dawson, "Resetting the Parameters: Public Health as the Foundation for Public Health Ethics" in *Public Health Ethics*, ed. Angus Dawson (Cambridge: Cambridge University Press, 2011) 1–19.

8. Buchanan, *Beyond Humanity*, 44.

9. One way in which it has been suggested that enhancement of certain traits or capacities in the population could be conducive to the public good is by so-called

moral enhancement. Arguably, increasing capacities for empathy or cooperation, for example, would be in the public interest as it might help to create more peaceful and cooperative societies. There is a lot more to be said about the pros and cons of such an approach than there is room for in this present chapter, but see Jona Specker, Farah Focquaert, Kasper Raus, Sigrid Sterckx, and Maartje Schermer, "The Ethical Desirability of Moral Bioenhancement: A Review of Reasons," *BMC Medical Ethics* 15, no. 1 (2014): 67.

10. Buchanan, *Beyond Humanity*; Anders Sandberg and Julian Savulescu, "The Social and Economic Impacts of Cognitive Enhancement," in *Enhancing Human Capacities,* ed. Julian Savulescu, Ruud ter Meulen, and Guy Kahane (Chichester, England: Wiley-Blackwell, 2011) 92–112; Nick Bostrom and Rebecca Roache, "Smart Policy: Cognitive Enhancement and the Public Interest," in Savulecu, ter Meulen, and Kahane, *Enhancing Human Capacities*, 138–149. Some of these authors have also argued that significant cognitive enhancement for a few individuals could result in great social benefit (e.g., when supersmart researchers would find a cure for cancer).

11. Ingrid Robeyns, "The Capability Approach," *Stanford Encyclopedia of Philosophy,* last modified 2011, https://plato.stanford.edu/entries/capability-approach/.

12. Madison Powers and Ruth Faden, *Social Justice: The Moral Foundations of Public Health and Health Policy* (Oxford: Oxford University Press, 2006).

13. Dawson, "Resetting the Parameters," 16.

14. Mill, *On Liberty.*

15. Michael Sandel, "The Case Against Perfection," *Atlantic Monthly*, April 2004, https://www.theatlantic.com/magazine/archive/2004/04/the-case-against-perfection/302927/.

16. Health Council of the Netherlands, *Human Enhancement* (The Hague: Health Council, 2003), 16.

17. Other justifications might come from protecting the interests of the persons themselves (paternalism), from harm to others (harm principle), or from more contested moral values such as the status of the embryo. As said previously, it is not my purpose here to perform this weighing. My main point is to show which public interests are at stake.

18. Ultrasound at 20 weeks is covered for all. A risk-estimating combination test (ultrasound and blood) for Down syndrome and trisomy 13 and 18 is covered for women with increased risk. Others have to pay for this test out of pocket. Discussion about covering prenatal screening for all, to guarantee equal access, is ongoing. Invasive follow-up testing (amniocentesis) after an initial positive combination test is covered for all. As of April 1, 2017, women can also choose to use the Non Invasive Prenatal test instead of the combination test as part of a nationwide implementation study.

19. Termination of pregnancy is allowed until 24 weeks' gestation if the woman finds herself to be in an "emergency situation" due to her pregnancy. In practice this means that the evaluation of the women herself is decisive. The woman should be informed of alternative solutions, like adoption. There is a five-day legally required "reflection period" between the first request of the woman and the actual termination. The

termination may only be performed by a physician in an abortion center or hospital with a special license from the Health Department.

20. Health Council of the Netherlands, *Genetic Screening* (The Hague: Health Council, 1994), 18.

21. Health Council, Genetic Screening, and Health Council of the Netherlands, *Prenatal Screening: Down's Syndrome, Neural Tube Defects, Routine-Ultrasonography* (The Hague: Health Council of the Netherlands, 2001).

22. The current rationale for this is a rather paternalistic concern for the burdens to the prospective parents, especially the women; concerns about the moral value of the embryos that are discarded in the process; and the wish to maintain a distinction between medical and nonmedical (i.e., enhancement) uses. However, concerns about discrimination, equality, and diversity might become more prominent if the technological possibilities would evolve.

23. See Erik Parens, *Shaping Ourselves: On Technology, Flourishing, and a Habit of Thinking* (Oxford: Oxford University Press 2015).

16

The Politics of Intrinsic Worth

Why Bioethics Needs Human Dignity

Gaymon Bennett

Talk of "protecting human dignity" has become a fixture of modern counterpolitics.[1] Indeed, as an anchor point of human rights discourse, humanitarianism, and religious ethics, it has become one of the most prominent modes of political critique to appear in the past half-century.[2] "Dignitarian politics" has become so widespread that advocates now find themselves in the unexpected position of having to contend with the consequences of their own success: everyone, it seems, can lay claim to human dignity, raising the worry that the term has come to mean too little by being made to do too much.[3]

The perceived overuse of dignity talk, and the sense that overuse leads to "thin" conversations, has led some people to give up on the term. Indeed, it has, over the past decade, slowly been marginalized in bioethical discourse, leaving it in the hands of religious bioethicists—a perceived artifact of theology left to the theologians.

That marginalization is a loss. As I explain in this chapter, the power of talk of human dignity in twentieth-century politics and ethics lies not so much in its precise definitions; indeed even in those places where dignity has been most vigorously asserted, the philosophical meanings of the term have sometimes been left up for grabs. The power of talk of dignity lies, rather, in its diagnostic force: it has allowed modernity's critics to call into question and thus put to the test the worst excesses and critical limitations of that most quintessentially modern form of power, biopolitics.

Biopolitics, as I explain in what follows and as others suggest in this volume, is centrally concerned with normal and normalizing constructions of human life and the potential of science and technology to renormalize human life through technical and political intervention. The trouble with biopower is that it is, on its own terms, neither inclusive nor constrained: it is concerned only with increasing the norms (usually selected by those in power) of a particular population (often those already on the leading edge). As a result, biopolitics often amplifies the worst excesses of modern life, reproducing its blind spots.

The power of dignitarian politics is that it put into play a figure of human value that could be weighed against the biopolitical, reframing human life as an object of intrinsic worth. With gene editing technologies, the dreams of modernity are very much still with us. It is therefore worth revisiting and rethinking the place of dignitarian politics in and for bioethics, asking how they might yet help us make sense of and, where necessary and possible, free ourselves from those dreams.

Proceeding in the spirit of the challenge that John Evans lays out in Chapter 3 of this volume (i.e., the challenge of equipping ourselves with concepts and arguments sufficient to the bioethical demands of the day), I offer here one way of rethinking the value of human dignity. First, I introduce readers to the recent history of "human dignity," tracing key shifts in its meanings and uses, especially as they pertain to counterpolitics. Second, I argue that those meanings and uses remain crucial to understanding and critically engaging with the legacy of biopolitics. Third, I argue that engaging the legacy of biopolitics remains centrally important to the project of bioethics, especially as it confronts the aspirations of gene editing. In this way, I take stock of how human dignity has become a vital part of who we are today as citizens of a world governed in no small part by biotechnology. I conclude that we cannot give up that part of ourselves without seriously compromising our collective ability to make sense of and resist the governance of biotechnology. To quote the scholar Sheila Jasanoff, "In all of its guises, actual or aspirational, technology functions as an instrument of governance . . . [shaping] not only the physical world but also the ethical, legal and social environments in which we live and act."[4] Talk of human dignity remains vital to facilitating a conversation about what is at stake in a world of biopolitics: how it functions and whether and how we can move beyond its limitations.

Biopower and Human Dignity as Counterpolitics

Despite the diverse uses to which the term *human dignity* gets put, several features of the term tend to remain constant. Most important, dignity is almost always evoked as an intrinsic and inviolable, albeit vulnerable aspect of human life.[5] That aspect, in turn, gets talked about as if were timeless and self-evident— as if in the face of human outrage nothing could be more natural than protecting dignity. The reality, however, lies elsewhere. The idea that human dignity is intrinsic (and thereby self-evident) is, in fact, a relatively recent innovation in moral reasoning. It was crafted through institutional transformations that took place over the last half century. Human dignity as it is used today can thus be thought of as a contemporary term, even though the phrase has been around for centuries.

It matters that human dignity is contemporary and that its seeming self-evidence is actually an innovation. It matters because it means the idea of human dignity was crafted for our times: it is a central, if troubled, fixture of modern counterpolitics. Dignity was born in response to the perceived excesses and deficiencies of modern forms of power. Specifically, it was born as a critical response to what has been called "biopolitics" or sometimes "biopower."[6] This means that dignity and biopolitics are linked, and to understand the former one must also understand the latter.

Like human dignity, the term *biopolitics* is used in various ways in various contexts. In this chapter, I use it to designate a specific way power is exercised, that is, a specific manner of government. This "manner of government" is one that seeks to increase the vitality (i.e., the health, productivity, and security) of targeted human populations. It does this by connecting the exercise of power to the knowledge and technology produced by modern science, especially those sciences that bear on the shape of human life: from agriculture to public health, economics to bioengineering.

Biopolitics is sometimes talked about as if it is always nefarious. But the value (and thus strength) of biopolitics is that it has, on average, increased longevity and decreased morbidity for many in the world's wealthiest populations.[7] European nations, where biopower was born, have been free from plague and famine for well over a century. The limit of biopolitics, however, is that it increases the vitality of some at the expense of others: it "makes live, and let's die," as the historian Michel Foucault famously put it.[8] This limit means that biopolitics can sometimes intensify the forms of exploitation, domination, and marginalization that are otherwise latent in the societies that seek to "make live." Moreover, because biopolitics has no internal principal of self-limitation, it functions as an inexhaustible demand. As Bruce Jennings persuasively demonstrates in his reflections on "entangled humanism" in Chapter 17 of this volume, biopolitical regimes sometimes cannot be squared with the cultivation of other kinds of goods—goods that lie beyond the indefinite improvement of human vitality.

This is where human dignity enters. Over the last half-century, human dignity, conceived as intrinsic and inviolable, has been asserted precisely as a safeguard against the deficiencies and excesses of biopolitics.[9] And because so much of biotechnology today—including the gene editing technologies that have inspired this volume—continues to be imagined and pursued in a broadly biopolitical manner, it is not surprising that talk of human dignity has made its way into bioethics. What is surprising, however, is that the turn to human dignity in bioethics has often functioned differently than in other domains of counterpolitics. The reasons for this difference are varied, but they rest in large part on the difficulty of specifying just what it is about the "dignified human" as a biological being that needs to be secured against biopolitics. Because of this seemingly unresolvable difficulty, some bioethicists have proposed giving up on the term *human dignity* altogether.[10] That, I argue, is a mistake.

The History of Biopower and Human Dignity

In the second half of the twentieth century, the term *human dignity* became a commonplace of counterpolitics.[11] Talk of protecting human dignity became such a normal part of political culture that such talk could be taken for granted; for many, it became intuitive. And in counterpolitics, the goal of protecting human dignity became an intuitive way of resisting the dominant norms and forms of modern power.

Before the 1940s, human dignity had been a relatively marginal term. It had circulated in the halls of medieval theology, and it made an appearance in nineteenth century labor politics. "Dignity" (usually used without the qualifier "human") had originally been a status term.[12] To be a person of dignity was a state to aspire to, achieve, and inhabit. As such, dignity was rarely connected to universal or intrinsic notions of humanity or human nature. It is true that from the Renaissance forward dignity was often talked about as a potential latent in all humans. But it was a potential realized only by the few. It might be realized through the cultivation of higher capacities (e.g., the rule of reason over the passions) or through association with certain institutions (e.g., a sovereign became dignified when crowned or a laborer could experience dignity in work).[13] But it was neither intrinsic nor self-evident, as it came to be in the postwar era. Put differently, in the prewar era, there had been plenty of talk about the distinctive worth of the human and plenty of talk about dignity. But the two weren't usually paired.

The seeming counterexample was the philosophy of Immanuel Kant, for whom dignity (the concept if not always the word) was, in fact, basic to what it meant to be human.[14] Yet for Kant, and for many of the forms of "liberal humanism" that were impacted by his thought, dignity was derivative of the fact of being a human *person*, with personhood being defined by specific qualities, such as being able to govern oneself—being autonomous. For Kant, dignity was not— as it would be for the later framers of "dignitarian politics"—simply a self-evident fact of "human-ness," a fact that could be recognized and declaimed but never "proven." For many in this tradition of liberal humanism, the stakes of dignity turned entirely on the fate of the individual. Yet as Bruce Jennings exemplifies in his reflections on "ecological humanism," for dignitarian politics, the value of human life is more capaciously interwoven into social and even cosmic realities. Indeed, for twentieth-century dignitarians, it was crucial that human dignity *not* be identified with a particular feature of the individual human for fear that anyone seen as possessing that feature in insufficient measure would be robbed of dignity. Dignity needed to be treated as self-referential and self-justifying, that is, declared as the ground of human value and not derivative of some other trait, capacity, status, or relation.

This idea that human dignity is intrinsic and self-referential first began to take shape in the late nineteenth century. At that time, a growing number of concerned actors—notably in international law, social reform, and religious ethics—undertook sustained efforts to confront what they saw as the failings of modern forms of power.[15] They frequently did this in the name of intrinsic human worth, eventually framing their efforts in terms of dignity. For these actors, modern power was "modern" precisely in as far as it was built on the belief that the world can (and will) be progressively improved through "technocratic" projects, that is, through projects designed to reorder human affairs on the basis of modern notions of rationality, hygiene, and productivity.[16] These projects included such things as public health campaigns, government-organized agriculture research, and redesign of urban infrastructures. What these projects had in common is that they "rationalized" and "secularized" human well-being. These projects were, in other words, "biopolitical." They sought to directly link the exercise of power to scientific knowledge about human life. "Power" not only included politics in the strict sense, but also included the cultural influence of institutions as diverse as corporations, hospitals, schools, and churches.

Although the term *biopolitics* is sometimes used loosely by cultural critics, several specific features are crucial for understanding the subsequent emergence of dignitarian politics. Above all, biopolitics "sees," and thus intervenes on, the vital dimensions of human populations. It does this by way of statistical modes of reasoning, seeking to "normalize" these vital dimensions.[17] That is to say, it seeks to (1) determine the statistical "norm" of a population relative to a particular vital dimension, (2) decide whether and how those norms might be improved, and (3) create mechanisms (from policy and law, to public clinics and health campaigns) aimed at changing those norms. Biopower seeks to shift the overall norms of a population relative to a particular dimension, such as birth rates, death rates, disease prevalence, wealth, or the price and availability of food.[18] But it might also focus, more controversially, on dimensions like race, productivity, age, gender, sexuality, and intelligence.

Biopower is indifferent to the condition of any particular individual or group within that population, so long as the overall norms improve. It trades on the expectation that the health of populations can be increased indefinitely: vital statistics can always be improved. In this, biopolitics has no intrinsic principle of self-limitation or equality: improvement is always relative. At first blush, this way of calibrating power can appear value free. After all, biopolitics can never tell you which norms to valorize or whose lives to improve. It just tells you how to improve them. The twist is that once the vitality of populations takes hold as a defining goal of the exercise of power—whether political, economic, scientific, or religious power—then biopolitics becomes not only a "normalizing" force in the statistical sense, but also a "normative" force in the sense of creating a binding moral obligation. Biopolitics at that point is no longer only about improving norms, but also about the idea that norms *must* be improved. The political culture is thereby committed to the open-ended improvement of health, wealth, and security.

The open-ended logic of "make live and let die" has become a defining feature of modern life. It can be seen, for example, in the way nation-states presume an unlimited reach of sovereignty within their own territories as the flip side of an unlimited responsibility for the welfare of their people. It can likewise be seen on economic fronts in the "naturalization" of markets. Markets have come to be imagined as semiautonomous environments within which the lives of everyday people can be indefinitely incorporated and made productive. Above all, these dynamics can be seen in the manner and extent to which science and technology have been made engines of the biopolitical project. Modern science and technology have been funded on the expectation that human vitality, with its related economic value, can be indefinitely increased so long as it is grasped in sufficiently scientific terms.

For all its success in shifting statistical norms, biopolitics has been marked by an evident ethical wrinkle. The indefinite normalization of populations has inevitably translated into growth for some and withering for others. And in its most pathological moments, this "growth for some" has led to the direct and purposeful elimination of others—the "racial hygiene" campaigns of the Third Reich being only the most notorious example. Biopolitical regimes have tended to reproduce and even amplify the most pernicious aspects of existing social relations. So, although by the late nineteenth century Western Europe had broken centuries-old cycles of famine and plague, these successes frequently entailed a corollary intensification of domination and exploitation, from the crippling number of working poor required for the rise of industrialization to the medicalization of childhood, gender, and sexuality as part of the rationalizing of social relations and to the widespread degradation of environmental integrity entailed in the scale-up of industrial farming.

Equally troubling, but less evident, biopolitics has also restricted the goals that can be taken seriously by modern regimes of power. Only those aspects of human life commensurate with normalization (things whose value is relative) get to count. In this light it is retrospectively unsurprising that, by the early twentieth century, counterpolitical actors—from activists, to diplomats, priests, and radicals—had begun talking about human worth as intrinsic and definitive, self-evident, and so self-evidently vulnerable that it needed to be made a central concern of institutional life. Human worth, in their view, was not derivative of a quality like productivity, citizenship, or reason or of the expression of a private value like the Christian belief that humans are dignified because they are made in the image of God. These dignitarians instead began to talk about human worth as a point of absolute limitation against which the biopolitical claims of national sovereignty, economic rationalization, or technoscientific improvement could be put to the test.

The upshot is that by midcentury, political discourse became attuned to an ethics of intrinsic human worth. By the 1950s talk of human dignity was on its way to becoming commonplace in counterpolitics. And by the late 1960s, human rights activists (to pick one prominent example) could demand the protection of human dignity as a key component of international development. Human dignity was set against the biopolitics of normalization.

The Institutional Rise of Human Dignity

The founding of the United Nations in the 1940s was decisive in transforming an emergent politics of intrinsic worth into an institutional commitment to human dignity. Equally important were internal developments in the Roman Catholic Church in the 1950s and 1960s concerning its role in the modern world. The 1970s, in turn, saw the global proliferation of human rights, making human dignity the predicate of a vast apparatus of nongovernmental organization. Given the limits of this chapter, I provide a brief sketch of the transformations that took place at the United Nations and the Vatican. This sketch sets the stage for understanding how human dignity was subsequently received by, and partially transformed through, bioethics.

The United Nations provided the institutional setting within which human dignity would be given its "founding function" for modern politics.[19] Its function was founding in that the conception of dignity put forward at the United Nations subsequently became definitive for dignitarian politics. It was also founding in that human dignity was put forward as a seemingly self-evident foundation for human rights.

The centerpiece of the UN efforts in this regard was the work of the UN Commission on Human Rights (CHR) and their drafting of the Universal Declaration on Human Rights.[20] Broadly speaking, the CHR was given the task of formulating the terms for an international moral order rooted in the language of dignity and human rights. These terms and this imagined order might then be used to moderate an international political order rooted in national sovereignty, one whose troubles had been on vivid display in World War II. The CHR's mandate was inspired, in part, by the legacy of the League of Nations.[21]

The League of Nations had sought to establish itself as a clearinghouse for the claims of displaced and persecuted peoples who needed political protection but who couldn't count on the rights of citizenship enshrined in the modern state. Given the number of such people in Europe and elsewhere after World War II, this legacy remained apposite, and the language of human dignity and human rights seemed appropriate to the task. The "human" as a bearer of fundamental rights, after all, could be said to be more basic than the "citizen" as a subject of national sovereignty.

To that end, the Universal Declaration included five references to dignity. Nowhere, however, did the document actually define the term. It simply asserted dignity as the predicate of fundamental political goods. The declaration puts it this way: The "recognition of the inherent dignity and of the equal and inalienable rights of all members of the human family is the foundation of freedom, justice and peace in the world."[22] It goes on to offer a list of rights, the protection of which is taken to be the manner in which dignity is recognized. Protect rights, and you recognize dignity; recognize dignity, and you secure a foundation for political goods.

What this use of dignity seems to mean—as multiple critics have pointed out—is that what was really at stake postwar was not so much an explanation of dignity (its meaning or sources) but a fight over who gets to define which rights get treated as fundamental. The trouble is, while it's true that the declaration gives more space to listing rights than defining dignity, the *manner* in which this came to be the case has been largely ignored. This lack of attention makes it seem as if the framers of dignitarian politics at the CHR were deliberately "thin" on philosophical grounds, that is, that they simply used the term as a prop for rights and didn't worry too much about its definition and sources.[23] Yet they did, in fact, think intensively about what dignity means and where it comes from. The remarkable thing about human dignity at the United Nations (and at the Vatican in its own way) is not so much that the term was made to be philosophically *thin*, but that it was made to seem politically *self-evident*.

Early in deliberations, the CHR sought to find language that would adequately express a grounding rationale for dignitarian politics. Yet almost as soon as those efforts began, it became clear that the members of the commission were not going to be able to agree on terms.[24] Commission members put forward a range of candidate formulations, but other members criticized those formulations as carrying too much cultural or political baggage. For example, language was put forward that connected "human dignity" to the idea of the "human person"— dignity as respect for persons. But this language was rejected as too Kantian and therefore too European and too secular. Others put forward language that connected dignity to the idea of being "created equally." This language was rejected for implying that dignity is rooted in the idea of being a creature of a creating god.

In the end, Eleanor Roosevelt, the CHR chair, made the pragmatic decision to end discussion and declare the recognition of dignity without extensive language on dignity's source, ground, or even meaning (though the declaration ultimately included one reference to the dignity of persons and one to the equal dignity of all men and women).[25] Dignity was simply declaimed as the basis of rights and thereby the foundation of political goods like peace, freedom, and justice. The decision was pragmatic. By asserting dignity, members could disagree on where it comes from, while agreeing on what it demands. But this pragmatic solution tacitly brought with it an understanding of human dignity that is its own point of reference. Dignity, in other words, was effectively defined as a political reality inherent in being human, one that needs to be declared, recognized, and protected, but not explained by reference to something else. Roosevelt's political pragmatism thus had the effect of shaping the United Nation's "political ontology," its assumptions about the underlying nature of political reality and its relation to that reality. Dignity was established as a reality whose source is identical to itself.

This recasting of dignity's political ontology, if circumstantial in origin, was suited to the task of countering biopolitics. Over the preceding two centuries, biopolitical reasoning had transformed the central question of power in Europe and other parts of the world from a moral one concerning legitimacy (i.e., who has the right to govern?) into an empirical and operative one concerning political methods (i.e., how to govern in a manner consistent with the "scientific" nature of the "vital" object being governed)[26] This didn't mean that political ideologies, or other questions of value or legitimacy, completely disappeared. It meant that the everyday life of power increasingly relied on empirical engagement with the life of populations.

Where biopolitics had displaced a moral question with an empirical one, the assertion of human dignity in the Universal Declaration brought the two back together, but in a new way. The language of human dignity was clearly a moral language (i.e., a language bearing on questions of legitimacy). But it was also a reality claim about the nature of political life, that is, that political goods such as justice, peace, and freedom derived from the recognition of dignity. Dignity, in short, was put forward as the nature of the object to be governed, a nature that reveals itself when it is recognized or neglected.

The figure of human dignity as self-grounding and the source of political goods was not, strictly speaking, new. The humanistic politics of the nineteenth century, especially those connected to the labor movement, had drawn deeply on the language of dignity.[27] And these politics had, at times, asserted dignity as if self-evident. But those assertions tended to focus on dignity as an experience—the worker's experience of indignity under conditions of industrialization—and not a defining quality of being human per se. One prominent exception was Roman Catholic social theory.[28] In the late nineteenth century, the Catholic Church began to elaborate a political theology of work and dignity, treating dignity as a defining quality of the worker him- or herself, qua human, one that needed protection in order to come to full actuality. The indignity experienced by the working class was taken to be a sign that the essential being of the worker was being violated.[29]

Because human dignity was said to be rooted in a divinely created soul, the anthropology underlying Catholic social theory initially kept the Church on the outside of other institutional transformations connected to the politics of intrinsic worth. Yet by the middle of the twentieth century a number of Catholic theologians, working alongside secular colleagues in anthropology and political science, began to suggest that if dignity is an intrinsic feature of human life, and not just a derivative quality, then the protection of dignity ought to establish a point of common political, ethical, and cultural interest between the Church and institutions of secular modernity.

The problem was how to conceive of dignity as fundamentally human while continuing to affirm the classical theological idea that human worth is a function of humanity's relation to God—the idea that the worth of the human is found in the play of "creaturehood" and "deification" that Michael Burdett elucidates in Chapter 12 of this volume.[30] Drawing on a legacy of medieval thought, these theologians argued that humans are, in their very nature (creaturehood), oriented toward "supernatural" ends, that is, oriented, by nature, to participation in "supernature" (deification). More controversial—for both the Church and secular moderns—was the theologians' insistence that a relation between nature and the supernatural is intrinsic to the makeup of a human being itself. Moreover, the theologians took this to be a claim about material reality itself and not only an assertion of faith. Material reality, they argued, has been called into being by the divine. Moreover, that "call into being"—that participation of the supernatural in nature—is identical to what it means to have dignity. The point is not just that humans are endowed with dignity by God.[31] The point, rather, is that humans are called into existence by and for a supernatural end, and that fact of being called is part of their very nature. This argument seemed to shift the terms of the Church's pastoral obligations. If the goal of a moral life is to live in a manner consistent with dignity as the defining aspect of human nature, then the Church had an obligation to help people do this, whether those people are part of the Church or not.

These lines of theological reasoning ultimately proved institutionally transformative. In 1962, Pope John XXIII, who had been part of these theological discussions, used his power as pontiff to convene a council of all the leaders of the Roman Church.[32] The Second Vatican Council, or Vatican II, took up precisely this question of dignity and the Church's pastoral relation to the modern world. In his opening address, John asked, What is the nature of the Church, such that it should have a pastoral relation to the modern world? And what is the modern world, such that it should be open to a pastoral relation to the Church? His answer to both turned ultimately on dignity as an intrinsic quality of being human in the world.

In October 1965, two months before the end of Vatican II, Pope Paul VI, who had succeeded John, addressed the UN General Assembly. Paul proposed that the mission of the Church, alongside the United Nations, was to care for human dignity. The timing of his address was strategic: Paul was hoping to push through a vote on the last document of the Second Vatican Council, "The Pastoral Constitution on the Church in the Modern World." Although its underlying reasons were different, the Pastoral Constitution shared with the UN Declaration a sense that dignity is so intrinsic to what it means to be human that it can simply be asserted and recognized. Critics of the Pastoral Constitution worried that its take on human dignity effectively "naturalized" the "supernatural" by making an otherwise-divine quality inherent to human life. Supporters saw it the other way around, that dignity pointed beyond itself to the divine. Either way, Vatican II advanced a figure of human dignity that resonated with the legacy of the UN Declaration.

The Vatican and the United Nations both offered what has been called an "archonic" view of human dignity because it is simultaneously primordial and normative. *Archonic* is a word that scholars invented to name something that is essential and fundamental about human life and therefore sets the terms for how humans ought to be treated. The term combines two Greek words: *arche*, meaning "primordial," and *archon*, meaning "to judge." Archonic human dignity was asserted against the circumstantial and relativistic logic of biopower.

Human Dignity and Bioethics

The ontological status of archonic dignity—how it exists both within and beyond the circumstances of history—was elusive from the outset. But this elusive quality was part of its strength. Human dignity was made to function as a kind of "spiritual" term, in the sense of being treated as the immaterial essence of humanity. So while dignitarian politics have been set against the material impact of politics, its seemingly immaterial nature has allowed it to be adapted to diverse situations. At the same time, because the material conditions of human life have precisely been at stake in dignitarian politics, dignity has always also been treated as an embodied reality. Dignity, after all, was born as a counterpolitics keyed to biopolitics. In this sense, embodied human life, in its most visceral aspects, has been a consistent concern.

If the unresolved tension between the spiritual and material aspects of dignity has proven productive in human rights and political theology, in bioethics it has proven a problem. To say that biology or biomedicine puts dignity at risk—as some bioethicists have done—invites a seemingly unanswerable question, What is it, precisely, about the relation between the human body as a material reality and dignity as a marker of inherent human worth that might be violated by science and technology? How are dignity and the body connected?

Talk of human dignity became a prominent part of bioethics in the United States and Europe in the mid-1990s and remained a matter of focused debate for the next fifteen years. After 2010, the controversy over the place of dignity in bioethics began to wane, although the debates have not gone away entirely. The United Nations and the European Union, for example, still periodically find themselves in disputes over dignity's meaning for, say, new reproductive technologies. But unlike in other domains, where the politics of human dignity have continued to thrive, talk of human dignity in bioethics has stultified.

In the United States, dignitarian bioethics reached its institutional apogee during the tenure of the President's Council on Bioethics (PCBE), the federal bioethics commission under the George W. Bush presidency. The PCBE was not the first to propose human dignity as a norm of bioethical reason in the United States. In the late 1960s, dignity had been advanced in response to developments in reproductive technology and end-of-life care, in particular by Roman Catholic theologians using language drawn from Vatican II. But human dignity had not became institutionally normative in bioethics. In the late 1980s and early 1990s things began to shift.[33] Bioethical funding and attention turned to the new genomic sciences, raising practical questions concerning privacy and safety, as well as conceptual questions concerning the "essence" of living beings. In the late 1990s, the specter of human cloning rose with Dolly the sheep, and, then, more consequentially still, scientists successfully derived stem cells from human embryos.[34] Talk of intrinsic worth, and its connection to the question of human nature and the ends of biotechnology, emerged as a defining concern, putting the ethics of human dignity front and center.[35]

In August 2001, George W. Bush gave his first live policy address, announcing his administration's decision to limit funding on human embryonic stem cell research. He surprised almost no one in saying he would "foster and encourage respect for life in America and throughout the world."[36] The statement reinforced familiar rhetorical connections between stem cells, in vitro fertilization (IVF), and abortion. More surprising, in explaining the reasons for his position, he did not appeal to the inviolability of the embryo, in the mode that the Catholic Church had pioneered. Bush proposed limited funding because stem cell research commodifies embryos and thereby "coarsens" Americans' collective moral sensibilities. Stem cell research, he said, using a dramatic phrase, subjected human life to "the threat of dehumanization." He went on to say that he was forming a bioethics council—the PCBE—to lead the way in resisting that threat. The council would be chaired by University of Chicago Professor Leon Kass.

The PCBE's inaugural meeting was to take place a month later. The events of September 11 intervened, driving stem cell research to the political sidelines and delaying the inaugural meeting until January 2002.[37] Kass opened that meeting with a provocation: he proposed that the events of 9/11, however devastating, were ultimately fortuitous for bioethics. They had awoken the American moral imagination to the fact of evil and its power to destroy a "way of life" taken to be "humanly good," even "truly human." The provocation was a rhetorical way forward in a situation blocked by talk of national security, as Kass acknowledged, "Everyone today is paying attention to terrorism. . . . the stakes of bioethics, which seemed so important only a few months ago, now appear to be less significant."[38] But Kass's framing was also substantively consequential because it allowed him to introduce the vision for bioethics that he had promoted for several decades, but that now seemed uniquely timely: a bioethics centered on the protection of human dignity.

Kass had long argued that the problem for bioethics is neither biology nor biotechnology per se. It is the relation between cultural appetites and technical capacity in late modernity. Kass argued that actions and choices made by individuals, taken in the name of personal and economic freedoms, can produce tragic outcomes over the long run. The outcomes are tragic because while acting in the name of seemingly fundamental goods (freedom of inquiry, medical advance, individual liberty), individuals can collectively generate worlds of indulgence, ennui, and injustice. Biotechnology, in Kass's view, had come to exemplify these tragic contradictions. Pursued in the name of seemingly good principles, it was unwittingly "taking us down the dehumanizing path toward a brave new world."[39]

In response, Kass proposed that bioethics get clearer about the meaning of the "bios," which conjoins "bio"science and "bio"ethics. Taking up a distinction that had become central to a critique of biopolitics in academic settings, Kass cautioned the members of the PCBE not to confuse bios with what the ancient Greeks called zōē, which designates "life as such, animate or animal life."[40] *Bios* designates a "course of life or a manner of living or a human life as lived." Other animals may have zōē, but humans also have bios: "life lived not merely physiologically but also mentally, socially, culturally, politically and spiritually." Debates over stem cell research, he argued, had reduced bioethics to a *logos* of zōē. Bioethics needs to produce truth about life humanly lived: a logos of bios.

Kass wanted the council to discern "the deep character of human individual and social 'bio,'" namely, human dignity. Human dignity might then be made a governing norm in relation to "the findings of biology and the technical powers they make possible."[41]

For its first year, the PCBE worked intensively on the question of what such a norm might look like and how it might be put to work. In their early publications, the members sought to provide what could be called an "ethical-empirical" account of human life "truly lived" and thereby establish the terms for an ethic of human dignity.[42] They did this by cataloguing examples of human experience that they took to exemplify, and thus verify, a truly human life—experiences of human finitude like the experience of disease; experiences of attachments like friendship, motherhood, or marriage; experiences of aspiration like athletic training or the cultivation of virtue. They then arrayed those examples in relation to pertinent areas of biotechnology and biomedicine, connecting the bios of bioethics and biology.

Working in this fashion, the council proposed a two-part answer to the question of a truly human life. First, such a life is one with naturally given limits, limits in our bodies, feelings, and relationships. Second, and at the same time, life is marked by a constant striving to overcome those limits. Because all aspects of human limitation and striving are natural and historical, they are also potential sites of biotechnical intervention. The tensions between limitation and striving, they concluded, constitute an anthropological universal against which developments in biotechnology can be judged.[43]

The council then offered two judgments.[44] First, the relation of limitation and striving is the site of things humanly worthwhile: longings, attachments, and virtue. This relation is normative in a strong sense. Second, the danger of biotechnology is that as its technical and economic power grows, it expands our sense of which aspects of human limitation should be dealt with technologically. Biotechnology inflames the desire to be free from all limitation. In this way it threatens to undo what makes us truly human.

At that time, the dominant model for how to confront the biopolitical with the archonic was human rights. But Kass and others on the council rejected rights talk as inescapably liberal and philosophically thin. Their assessment was half right. The figure of human dignity in human rights has been decidedly short on explicit philosophical substance. But where members of the PCBE got it wrong is that they failed to take stock of the considerable conceptual and institutional work that had to be done in order to assert human dignity as self-evident. In the end, Kass and the PCBE resolutely refused a presumption of self-evidence as sufficient to the task of connecting the bio of bioethics to the bio of biotechnology. Which is to say, their attempt to connect verified definitions of the truly human to science by way of a metric of dignity ultimately stalled.

In the wake of the PCBE's work, dignity briefly became a commonplace of bioethical concern and publication: the council's efforts to redefine the terms of bioethical practice had the effect of generating a conceptual and discursive ca-cophony around the term. This meant that dignity could no longer be mobilized as if self-justifying, and it certainly could not be treated as self-evident. In addi-tion, the PCBE had never made clear how human dignity could be turned into a regulative instrument of governance capable of regulating the relation of science and technology to embodied human life. But in attempting to do so they unwit-tingly transformed an archonic figure of human dignity into a political object that could no longer be taken for granted and that could thus no longer generate new practices beyond endless discursive binds.

Conclusion: Human Dignity as Ethical Practice

Human dignity in bioethics has suffered a kind of intellectual blackmail: one must either be for or against it. Those on one side urgently insist that more con-ceptual clarification of the term is needed. Those on the other argue the notion has never been a meaningful way to conceptualize human worth. Neither side has taken up human dignity as a historical event of social consequence, one in which the incessant redefinitions and denunciations themselves constitute im-portant social facts. I have tried to show that if one does take it up in that way, then the politics of human dignity begin to seem less the sort of thing one is for or against and more a dimension of our history as late moderns. We cannot "step outside" the politics of human dignity and its entanglement with biopolitics. Dignitarian politics are a part of our collective ethical imaginary.

Moreover, dignitarian politics are an integral part of our collective ethical im-aginary. The excesses and deficiencies of biopolitics are still with us, and we have few institutionally grounded ways of putting those excesses and deficiencies to the test. Dignitarian politics, in this light, are valuable because they serve as "eth-ical equipment" and not primarily because they offer a "grounding truth" for eth-ical theory. Talk of dignity equips us: it primes our attention to the excesses of biopower (those places where relativistic and unlimited impulses of biopolitics amplify existing discriminations) and to biopower's limitations (those places where the political mandate to make live is being institutionally neglected and where biopolitics effectively marginalizes other kinds of goods—goods that can't be squared with a logic of normalization).

Thus, to say that the legacy of dignitarian politics is part of who we are as late moderns is to say something more "normative" than it might sound. Recognizing how dignity has become part of our collective ethical imaginary is itself an important part of ethical practice. It brings into view the legacy of our collective ethical formation. Archonic human dignity may be a twentieth-century invention, but that "invention" is also an ethical achievement. As virtue ethics teaches, the transformation of moral habits and sensibilities requires tremendous labor. The "equipmental" dimension of the ethics of human dignity, in this sense, matters for reasons of not only philosophical anthropology (i.e., for thinking about the moral nature of being human), but also an anthropology of ethics (i.e., for thinking about how we go about the work of forming ourselves as moral beings).

All of this said, the critics of dignitarian politics are not altogether wrong. Human dignity is a term that has sometimes suffered a kind of philosophical "thinness," in the sense described by John Evans in Chapter 3 of this volume. It has thereby sometimes been victim to political opportunism: a moralism used to control the terms of the debate. Critics have thus derided the politics of human dignity as nothing more than what Robert Bellah once called a "life-style enclave," new, thin, and transient. The trouble with that criticism, however, is that it only holds if "old, thick, and permanent" are ethically preferable. Yet given the manner in which moderns have turned human dignity into a counterpolitics capable of confronting the power of sovereign states, global economies, and sometimes science and technology, such a preference is far from obvious. Indeed, the politics of human dignity invite us to take seriously the possibility that the most generative conceptual tools for engendering public deliberation about, and action in response to, biotechnology may not be those grounded in a definitive lexicon. The question of what concepts, norms, and vocabularies need nailing down as a precondition of deliberation versus what ambiguities are generative and what uncertainties might be tolerated or, indeed, engaged directly in order to foreground certain questions is one worth keeping open.

Admittedly, embracing dignitarian politics for pragmatic reasons introduces a tension. These politics have proven generative precisely because they resolutely lay claim to the idea that there is something intrinsically precious at stake in the exercise of power. To say that dignity is part of the historical fabric of who we are, and thus can be used as a tool of critique, is to beg the question of whether that precious aspect of human life is "real and true" or "merely" a technique of counterpolitics. This is only a tension, however, if we assume that something that comes into existence through specific circumstances or for pragmatic reasons cannot also be intrinsic or inviolable. In any event, it is a productive tension, worth tolerating.

In the face of new biotechnologies—to return to the theme of this volume—we must ask not only what we want to achieve in transforming ourselves through the manipulation of our bodies, but also what such transformations might violate. To ask whether there might be something inviolably precious about human life—or even about life more broadly—is to question the political economies that underwrite biotechnology. And to question the economies of biopower is to put into play the possibility that there might yet be things that matter to us that are not available through a politics of normalization.

Notes

1. Counterpolitics reject the idea that the dominant political or economic order, especially has it has been manifest in the modern capitalist and communist state, has moral resources or ethical practices sufficient to meeting the demands of the day.
2. Gaymon Bennett, *Technicians of Human Dignity: Bodies, Souls, and the Making of Intrinsic Worth* (Brooklyn, NY: Fordham University Press, 2016); Paul Rabinow, *Anthropos Today: Reflections on Modern Equipment* (Princeton, NJ: Princeton University Press, 2003).
3. Samuel Moyn, *The Last Utopia: Human Rights in History* (Cambridge, MA: Harvard University Press, 2012); Michael Rosen, *Dignity: Its History and Meaning* (Cambridge, MA: Harvard University Press, 2012).
4. Sheila Jasanoff, J. Benjamin Hurlbut, and Krishanu Saha, "CRISPR Democracy: Gene Editing and the Need for Inclusive Deliberation," *Issues in Science and Technology* 32 no.1 (Fall 2015): 25–32.
5. The most famous example of this is the United Nation's "Universal Declaration of Human Rights." The United Nations, *Universal Declaration of Human Rights*, 1948 http://www.un.org/en/universal-declaration-human-rights/.
6. For the classic treatment of "biopower," see Michel Foucault, *The History of Sexuality, Volume 1: An Introduction* (New York: Vintage, 2012). See also Paul Rabinow and Nikolas Rose, "Biopower Today," *BioSocieties* 1 no. 2 (2006): 195–217.
7. Andrew Lakoff, "Two Regimes of Global Health," *Humanity: An International Journal of Human Rights, Humanitarianism, and Development* 1, no. 1 (2010): 59–79; Didier Fassin, *Humanitarian Reason: A Moral History of the Present* (Berkeley: University of California Press, 2011).
8. Foucault, *History of Sexuality.*
9. Bennett, *Technicians.*
10. Ruth Macklin, "Dignity Is a Useless Concept," *BMJ* 327, no. 7429 (2003): 1419–1420; Clair Morrisey, "The Value of Dignity In and For Bioethics: Rethinking the Terms of the Debate," *Theoretical Medicine and Bioethics* 37, no. 3 (2016): 173–192.
11. Bennett, *Technicians*; Rabinow, *Anthropos Today*; Fassin, *Humanitarian Reason.*
12. Rosen, *Dignity.*
13. Moyn, *Utopia.*
14. Immanuel Kant, *Prolegomena to Any Future Metaphysics: That Will Be Able to Come Forward as Science: With Selections from the Critique of Pure Reason*, Cambridge Texts in the History of Philosophy, ed. Gary Hatfield (Cambridge: Cambridge University Press, 2004).

15. Bennett, *Technicians.*
16. Paul Rabinow, *French Modern: Norms and Forms of Social Environment* (Chicago: University of Chicago Press, 1995).
17. Georges Canguilhem, "The Normal and the Pathological," in *Knowledge of Life* (Brooklyn, NY: Fordham University Press, 2008): 121–133.
18. Michel Foucault, *Security, Territory, Population: Population: Lectures at the Collège de France 1977–1978*, ed. Michel Senellart and François Ewald (New York: Picador, 2009).
19. Klaus Dicke, "K. Dicke. Human Dignity in International Law," in *The Concept of Human Dignity in Human Rights Discourse*, ed. David Kretzmer and Eckart Klein (Leiden, the Netherlands: Brill, 2002); Rosa Freedman, *The United Nations Human Rights Council: A Critique and Early Assessment* (New York: Routledge, 2014); Roger Normand and Sarah Zaidi, *Human Rights at the UN: The Political History of Universal Justice* (Bloomington: Indiana University Press, 2008).
20. Normand and Zaidi, *Human Rights.*
21. Freedman, *Human Rights Council.*
22. The United Nations, *Universal Declaration of Human Rights*, 1948, http://www.un.org/en/universal-declaration-human-rights/
23. Dicke, *Human Dignity.*
24. Normand and Zaidi, *Human Rights.*
25. Freedman, *Human Rights Council.*
26. Foucault, *Security, Territory, Population.*
27. Rosen, *Dignity.*
28. See, for example, the papal encyclical *Rerum Novarum*, http://w2.vatican.va/content/leo-xiii/en/encyclicals/documents/hf_l-xiii_enc_15051891_rerum-novarum.html
29. Jaques Maritan, *Integral Humanism, Freedom in the Modern World, and a Letter on Independence* (Notre Dame, IN: University of Notre Dame Press, 1996).
30. Bennett, *Technicians.*
31. John Milbank, *Theology and Social Theory: Beyond Secular Reason*, 2nd ed. (New York: Wiley-Blackwell, 2006).
32. John W. O'Malley, *What Happened at Vatican II* (Cambridge, MA: Harvard University Press, 2010).
33. John Evans, *Playing God? Human Genetic Engineering and the Rationalization of Public Bioethical Debate* (Chicago: University of Chicago Press, 2002).
34. J. Benjamin Hurlbut, *Experiments in Democracy: Human Embryo Research and the Politics of Bioethics* (New York: Columbia University Press, 2017).
35. Bennett, *Technicians.*
36. The President's Council on Bioethics, *Beyond Therapy: Biotechnology and the Pursuit of Happiness* (New York: Harper, 2003).
37. See the President's Council's archive at https://bioethicsarchive.georgetown.edu/pcbe/.
38. PCBE archive at https://bioethicsarchive.georgetown.edu/pcbe/.
39. PCBE archive.

40. PCBE archive.
41. PCBE archive.
42. PCBE, *Beyond Therapy.*
43. PCBE, *Beyond Therapy.*
44. PCBE, *Beyond Therapy.*

17

Bioethics Contra Biopower

Ecological Humanism and Flourishing Life

Bruce Jennings

> The goal is to counter cultural orientations oscillating wildly between the stances of mastery, studied indifference, disappointment, and aggressive nihilism with an ethos of reflective attachment to a world that is rich in diverse meanings and purposes. . . . Today perhaps it is wise to try to transfigure the old humanisms . . . into multiple affirmations of entangled humanism in a fragile world.
>
> —William E. Connolly[1]

Will the significant advances in biotechnology made in the last few years by new techniques of genomic editing serve the human good and promote human flourishing? The twentieth century existed in the shadow of nuclear physics and nuclear weapons.[2] The twenty-first century does as well, but also faces the prospect of a rapidly advancing and ambitious medical-industrial complex of genetic engineering and synthetic biology, subsidized and reinforced by nation-states that have come in the past two centuries to play an ever-increasing role in the governance of life. The cardinal ethical challenge of the last century was to forbear in the face of a technology that would bring cosmic forces within the atmosphere of the planet, thereby destroying most life on Earth. The challenge of our time is not to forestall advancement but to prudently limit a biological technology that would transform much life on Earth into an artifact of human will. In question are nature and life, bodies and minds, agency and dignity—in a word, the questions associated with the ancient Greek concept of *bios*, which connotes not merely organic existence (*zōē*), but a form of life as it might be most fully realized and lived. Biopower and the fabrication of life is my subject, reflective attachment to a meaningful world, my theme.

As the concepts and styles of thought of the biotechnological revolution are absorbed into popular culture, biotechnology begins to shape the experience of all of us. This subtly alters both what we think is proper and what we desire.

It alters our relationship to the natural world and also to our own humanity. The viewpoint I propose in this chapter counsels caution here. We should look askance at anything that undermines the patience and humility fitting for a fallible being, that undermines a willingness (and intelligence) to set limits on our own behavior, or that lifts creativity and innovation out of a broader context of other values and embraces them for their own sakes. In the genomic engineering impulse is there something that will reinforce human arrogance just at a time of global ecological crisis when we need instead to cultivate its opposite: a stronger sense of limits and humility? Will we be mesmerized by our own biopower?[3]

Biopower and Humanism

An effective critique of biotechnology needs a searching conceptual vocabulary and a solid philosophical foothold to consider the broader psychological, social, and cultural effects, not only of particular uses of biotechnology, but also of the cultural embrace of the underlying philosophical ideas behind biotechnology and, beyond that, the institutionalization or routinization of those ideas.[4] In other words, the development of a biotechnical system integral to government and the economy raises the question of "biopower."

The concept of biopower denotes the realization that the modern state must be active in governing, manipulating, and intentionally using the vitality or life processes within its population and environment in order to achieve protection and security for the sake of productivity and prosperity. Biopower operates on both a collective or population level and an individual or subjective level. It also operates on two scales: a "molar" or macroscale of organic (including human) behavior and thought and a "molecular" or microscale of genomic, cellular, and biochemical processes within living organisms.[5] To some extent this has always been true in human history or even in prehistory for that matter. But, as Michel Foucault argues, since the eighteenth century the governance of biopower has become the modern foundation of sovereignty, and the scientific and technological advances of the past few decades have greatly facilitated and expanded the deliberate pursuit of biopower in human life.[6] It is pertinent then to pose questions such as, How are the nature of life and human knowledge understood by those who create and promote biotechnology? How does this technological self-understanding shape the meaning of humanness in contemporary society and shape our sense of self or personhood?[7]

It is at this level of analysis especially that a substantive philosophical theory of human flourishing and the human good are needed. Biotechnologies— understood, beyond mere apparatus or instrumentation, as cultural systems and as tokens of biopower—shape our imagination of self and world; they create a framework or worldview within which what it is to be human is defined and what is good about being human is characterized. Technology does not simply encounter a pregiven natural or social world; it engages in worldmaking.[8] The perceiving or understanding involved here is active, not passive; it does not simply reflect how individuals—even strategically positioned ones—think and feel beforehand but constitutes the very thoughts it is possible to think and the feelings it is possible for virtually everyone to experience.

In previous work on the social and ideological reception of synthetic biology, which aspires to genome authoring rather than merely editing, one might say, I identified three frameworks that react critically and skeptically to the extensions of biopower, now significantly advanced by CRISPR gene editing and gene drives. I called these the precautionary frame, or the argument from prudence; the liberal humanist frame, or the argument from dignity; and the ontological frame, or the argument from nature.[9] In this chapter I return to explore more fully the liberal humanist frame. I argue that humanism as a tradition has duty-based notions of respect and dignity historically ingrained and offers a critical framework that indicts biotechnology and genetic manipulation, in thought and deed, as intrinsically objectifying and reductionistic. Therefore, they are to be seen as culturally and ethically threatening to the notion of the inherent worth of human personhood and its capabilities for self-direction and agency. Liberal humanism offers an individualistic version of this critique; a more communitarian and social version of it would be a relational or ecological humanism—an "entangled humanism," in Connolly's suggestive phrase. I agree with the fundamental importance that the liberal humanist frame places on treating human beings as subjects to be respected and educated rather than as objects to be fabricated or reengineered. Thus far, however, the duty-based (deontological) arguments of liberal humanism have only been able to mount rearguard actions against the juggernaut of the molecular fabrication of life.

Ecological humanism would provide guidance about what to seek in a theory of human flourishing: pluralistic and developmental notions of good lives and a focus on constitutive practices—cultural patterns of meaning and institutional structures of power—rather than on either metaphysical essentialism or materialistic determinism.

The argument in this chapter is closely related to what Gaymon Bennett discusses in Chapter 16 of this volume under the rubric of "counterpolitics" and "dignitarian politics." He traces the recent intellectual history of the concept of human dignity, with special reference to the international human rights movement and developments in Roman Catholic social ethics, and shows how it has been the main challenger to the now-dominant biopolitical orientation in which biological processes and the activity of living things becomes one of the most important loci of control. Bennett analyzes a number of ways that an emphasis on dignity can confront the political economy of biotechnology. My thought is that in order to mount an effective bioethical response to biopower—something that, in Bennett's view, bioethics and its mainstream ethical discourse is ill-equipped to accomplish—what is needed is a relational, developmental, and practice-based theory of human flourishing that stresses (1) the importance of being recognized as a member with full moral standing of communities of equal dignity and parity of voice and agency and (2) the importance of being and becoming embedded within a lifeworld of mutuality and care.

If it can be rigorously developed, I believe that this perspective on the practices integral to the actualizing of human potential capabilities—the practices of membership recognition and mutual attentive care—offers a powerful critique of the mechanistic and reductionist ontology on which the ethical justifications of biotechnological engineering rests. The fact that the biological sciences themselves, in fields such as epigenetics, are discovering that mechanistic and reductionistic modes of interpreting nature and life are untenable does little to dampen the allure of biotechnology. Sobering assessments in this volume of the current state of bioethics by Bennett (Chapter 16) and John Evans (Chapter 3) reinforce my sense that the discourse needed here must engage with critical political and social theory.

Mechanistic Systems and Communicative Communities

The term *biotechnology* was coined in 1943 by the Royal Swedish Academy of Engineering Sciences to describe biological solutions to wartime food, energy, and pharmacological shortages. The academy's first director, Edy Velander, proposed the word *bioteknik* to describe "applications which arise while one is learning to influence biological processes scientifically and exploit them technologically in an industrially organized activity."[10] In the domain of bioteknik, nature, or the natural, is not a set point from which deviations can be measured and condemned. But in this regard biotechnology is caught in a contradiction. It rejects the notion of natural form (such as the notion of homeostasis in medicine) that would provide a standard for assessing appropriate and inappropriate states of being. Therefore, it must seek control without such a standard and without nature's cooperation. Biotechnology must seek control in the face of a dynamic ontology that belies predictability and control. Nature—organic nature, at any rate—comprises emergent properties, sudden tipping points, and developmental capabilities. Human-caused alterations coexist with other change factors in dynamic natural systems.[11]

Consequently, the line between the evolved operational limits of biological systems and technologically mediated human intervention pressing against those limits is becoming harder to locate, and it is being crossed with increasing frequency. Without nature as a reference, we more readily—but not necessarily— enter a discourse reflecting biopower, which significantly expands the scope of what human beings can and should fabricate. As noted, biopower promotes the efficient exploitation and normalized functioning of biological life, including human bodies and minds. In the age of biopower, respect for evolved forms or natural wholes in life has no moral foothold; everything is seen as decomposable and fungible bits of DNA.

Nikolas Rose provided a striking description of this new style of seeing what nature and human beings are:

> The biomedical knowledges and techniques that are currently taking shape have many differences, but they do have one thing in common. It is now at the molecular level that human life is understood, at the molecular level that its processes can be anatomized, and at the molecular level that life can now be engineered. At this level, it seems, there is nothing mystical or incomprehensible about our vitality—anything and everything appears, in principle, to be intelligible, and hence to be open to calculated interventions in the service of our desires about the kinds of people we want ourselves and our children to be. . . . Molecularization strips tissues, proteins, molecules, and drugs of their specific affinities—to a disease, to an organ, to an individual, to a species—and enables them to be regarded, in many respects, as manipulatable and transferable elements or units, which can be delocalized—moved from place to place, from organism to organism, from disease to disease, from person to person. . . . "Molecular biopolitics" now concerns all the ways in which such molecular elements of life may be mobilized, controlled, and accorded properties and combine into processes that previously did not exist.[12]

Homo sapiens have been probing the secrets of life through the domestication of plants and animals for many thousands of years without any understanding of the underlying molecular and genetic processes invisibly at work. However, during the past century, science has entered the molecular domain, and technologies have been devised to manipulate life processes at that level. This I believe is a genuine and significant discontinuity. Human beings are doing something new: fabricating living entities that neither natural evolution nor human husbandry has ever produced.

What are the terms of the conflict between the molecular gaze of biopower and biotechnology and the understanding of human beings offered by liberalism and more broadly by the Western humanistic tradition? The humanistic gaze sees the molecular gaze as objectifying and reductionistic and therefore as threatening to the notion of the inherent worth and value of human personhood and free, intentional agency. What is the nature of this disagreement and of the humanistic concern for the loss of something integral or constitutive of our humanity?

There are two broad outlooks or worldviews that stand behind the confrontation of molecular biopower and an ecological humanism in bioethics. [13] The first is a worldview of "mechanistic systems." It is based on explanatory reductionism and an analytic method of breaking complex wholes and networks down into component parts and generalizing their properties and behavior in a decontextualized (abstract) way. It grew out of the explosion of intellectual and practical reform movements in Europe during the seventeenth and eighteenth centuries commonly known as the Enlightenment. The second is a worldview of "communicative communities."[14] It is based on the interpretive understanding of holistic complexity and of purposive, relational agency. The communicative communities orientation grew out of an intellectual reaction against the Enlightenment in transcendental philosophy and romanticism in the late eighteenth and early nineteenth centuries.[15]

The mechanistic worldview orients human aspiration and agency toward reshaping and reengineering nature and the conditions of life—a stance of improvement and enhancement. The holistic or communicative communities worldview inclines human aspiration and agency toward accommodating and working within evolved forms and natural limits. It is not primarily a stance of fabrication and control, but one of cocreation with other human agents, nonhuman living beings, and material things. It is a stance of respect for the givenness of the world and its constraints and limits, as well as gratitude for what the world affords us.

The mechanistic worldview is material, empirical, reductionistic, and objectifying. It breaks things down into component parts and reassembles or rearranges them. In ontological terms—in terms of how we understand being—it views human beings as objects comprised of matter (bodies and brains) that can be understood and manipulated in the same way as the matter comprising the nonhuman world. In ethical terms (in terms of what we should do), it views human beings as users of nonhuman nature, constrained only by their own species needs and interests. In epistemological terms (in terms of what we can know), it is oriented toward the discovery of observable regularities in nature that can be set forth (albeit provisionally and rebuttably) as causal laws. The fundamental endeavor is to explain why something exists now so that the conditions of its existence can be predicted and therefore better controlled in the future.

Unlike the mechanistic worldview, humanism tries to hold on to the idea that there is a distinctive kind of materiality in human life that is real and objective, but is not objectifying or reductive—a materiality in which both function and form are constitutive. Such a materiality endows humankind with a complex mental life, self-consciousness, and vast symbolic and linguistic communicative capabilities. The goal of understanding here is less prediction and control than mutual recognition and meaning.

In the seventeenth century, followers of Descartes and Locke rejected the unity contained in the Aristotelian tradition in which life is a self-organizing and self-maintaining form that operates through its material embodiment. Aristotelian ontology—and in particular Aristotelian biology—is materialistic, but not in the modern mechanistic sense. Matter is not only content, but also is a unity of form and content, and matter maintains continuity of form over time and thereby expresses or exhibits a purposiveness, agency, and intelligence. The early modern scientific revolution and the Enlightenment moved from construing purposiveness as an integral property of the organismal or bodily world to construing it as a separate property of the mind. Philosopher Charles Taylor summarizes the shift: "Dualism . . . attributes all these functions of intelligence to a mind which is heterogeneous from body, so that matter is left as something which is to be understood purely mechanistically. In this way, Cartesian-empiricist dualism has an important link to mechanism."[16]

By contrast, the holistic worldview revitalizes an idea of unity, reminiscent of Aristotelian thought, particularly in the realm of life, and especially in the domain of human being and becoming:

> A living thing is a functioning unity and not just a concatenation of parts. . . . The living thing is . . . not just a functioning unity, but also something in the nature of an agent; and this places it in a line of development which reaches its apex in the human subject. . . . [This development] restored the sense of continuity of living things which was damaged by Cartesianism. But there is not just continuity between ourselves and animals; there is also continuity within ourselves between vital and mental functions, life and consciousness. On [a holistic] view these cannot be separated out and attributed to two parts, or faculties, in man. . . . We can never understand man as an animal with rationality added; on the contrary, he is a quite different kind of totality, in which the fact of reflective consciousness leaves nothing else unaltered.[17]

A world of communicative communities requires *explication* and interpretation, not *explanation* and prediction. It does not present objects to be explained by cause and effect regularities, but systems and structures of meaning to be interpreted and engaged dialogically. Interpretive dialogue results eventually in increased insight and self-understanding by the knowing subject rather than increased control over the object known. Human knowledge is embedded in the reality it seeks to understand. It seeks relationships of interdependence and seeks to comprehend them in their context and particularity; it does not seek to abstract from them into more general theoretical constructs and covering laws.

From an ethical perspective, the holistic worldview offers norms of right relationship among people and between humans and nonhuman nature. It is within these webs of living nature and social meaning that human experience of the world has developed; in it we have come to comprehend, not only the natural environment, but also ourselves. The holistic worldview is an entangled, ecological humanism in which the purpose of knowledge and the intention of action are not simply controlling and refabricating but also conserving and celebrating the social mutuality and natural symbiosis that is the groundwork for human flourishing.

Because the holistic worldview does not prescind from embedded or lived experiences of the material world in its quest for knowledge, it embraces its own embeddedness. An important implication of this for our purposes was underscored by Hubert Dreyfus and Charles Taylor:

> If we return to our most basic, primordial way of being in the world, when we are led to respond to the things in it as affordances, we understand ourselves as at grips with a world that aids us and at the same time sets limits on what we can do. We have to adopt the right stance to it; else we will suffer frustration or worse. The things that are showing up for us as obstacles, supports, facilitators, in short as affordances, have as it were an ontic solidity and depth. They set boundary conditions on our activities. They have what philosophy has come to call their "nature," which we have to respect and adjust ourselves to.[18]

By contrast, the mechanistic worldview maintains that life, as the molecular gaze comprehends it, has no inherent solidity or depth: what biochemistry affords to human beings is not an inherent property of molecules—DNA, RNA, proteins, and the rest—but an artifact for our manipulation. Dreyfus and Taylor suggested that our views of what *is*—in other words, our understanding of being—are linked to our understanding of ethical limits. Natural things with inherent solidity set limits on what human beings can and should do. They call for respect and accommodation or adjustment, not re-creation and reengineering. Discussions of biotechnology and human flourishing need to refresh the vocabulary of inherent or intrinsic value and to revisit our understanding of the right relationship between humans and nature.[19]

Properly interpreted, the idea of human flourishing need not entail a separation of human beings from the rest of nature and the material world, and it does not need to embrace a theory of value that puts humans at the center. For these reasons, flourishing can be appropriately used as a moral touchstone for justice and an ethical justification for science and technology. Taylor's discussion points that out clearly: an ecological humanism that attempts to restore unity between human freedom (agency) and full self-realization (flourishing) rejects a human-centered ethics as one more expression of dualism. To emphasize the distinctiveness of human beings among fellow living creatures, as the communicative communities worldview does, is surely not to deny that moral consideration is due to nonhuman beings and ecological webs that support all life.

Moral considerability is not ontologically rooted but it is conceptually constituted, and one fundamental aspect of that is the difference between relational standing as a subject among subjects or as an object among objects. To see a being (whether it be another human being, a nonhuman being, or an interdependent ecosystem) as an object, or as a set of component biochemical processes, is to acknowledge only the use value of that being. To see a being as a subject is to acknowledge the inherent value of being and becoming as such. Recognition of subjects comes from an impartial and inclusive—that is to say, a welcoming—point of view. The capability theory of human flourishing has its application in nonhuman species being as well.

If we are not mindful of these points, it is tempting for bioethics to take the program of biopower at face value and to sign on to its promise for promoting and enhancing human flourishing. But for bioethics to do this is to miss a profound irony and predicament. Biopower and the molecular gaze strip matter and nonhuman forms of life of their purposiveness and agency and thereby objectify them in ways that undermine their moral status. Biopower cannot resist doing this to human beings as well, collectively or individually, when the molecular gaze is turned on them and insofar as they are regarded as living objects rather than subjects of a life. We should bear in mind that discourses of domination and defining gazes that dehumanize human beings, by turning them from subjects into objects, do not promote human flourishing, but undermine it for each and all. This predicament—the dialectic of enlightenment—has been noticed before.

The Flourishing of Subjects

I said that properly interpreted the idea of human flourishing need not imply human separation from the material world or mandate human control of the natural. But what is a proper interpretation of human flourishing? How is our understanding of human beings as subjects (persons and agents) affected by the emergence of biopower as a fundamental aspect of our social and cultural imagination? Of course, the answer to this question will depend on what substantive account we give of human flourishing. Biopower and biotechnology privilege control over the material conditions of life and, within our overall self-understanding, privilege the fabricating aspect of our humanity—the self as *Homo faber*.

What aspects of flourishing are served by this view, and what aspects are distorted or eclipsed? I believe the answer is revealed in the account of human flourishing centered on the recognition of just membership in a moral community and on just relations of mutual care and regard among members of such a community. In several ways, my argument concerning biotechnology as a whole runs parallel to Maartje Schermer's analysis in Chapter 15 in this volume of the effects of reproductive biotechnology on the public good, both in terms of social justice or equitable access to the new technologies and in terms of social values such as freedom, solidarity, and diversity, which reproductive biotechnology can possibly fulfill or undermine but will definitely redefine.

Moreover, biopower on the whole is an objectifying and totalizing vision, demanding normalization and standardization—the logic of one correct measurement, one correct appraisal. As Schermer notes in Chapter 15 of this volume, "a collection of clones . . . could never make up a flourishing society." Aldous Huxley already in the 1930s was quite prescient about this aspect of the biopolitical state in *Brave New World*, which depicted a society of dubious flourishing whose population was largely comprised large contingents of clones of varying levels of ability. A fabricated caste system of manufactured diversity covered over by a mass of identical faces: e pluribus unum, genetically fabricated and semantically edited. Dystopian thought experiments aside, the ways in which biopower and biotechnology are being institutionalized in the global political economy make it all the more important that we assess the molecular gaze for its potential to become *the one true way* we see ourselves and the rest of our world.

Cultural embeddedness and natural embodiment are not silent backdrops in our lives; at least, they are not only that. They are made self-aware and self-reflective through ideas and language, concepts, and discourse. It is within the interplay of these discourses and social imaginaries that concrete social interactions become purposive and reflective activities and, thereby, ground human flourishing. The plurality of ways of being human is essential here. Some older philosophies of the good life called for the imposition of one set of substantively constraining master values, as in Plato's *Republic* or More's *Utopia*, for example. Contemporary notions of flourishing have something quite different in mind. They call for the creation of an associational environment of rights, equality, dignity, and respect in which each person has the social supports and opportunities necessary to develop many capabilities and to realize many pathways of self-development and meaningful self-identity.

Indeed, there is no single, uniquely right way to flourish as a human being.[20] Accounts of the human good must be multifaceted; flourishing inheres the interplay of virtues lived, dispositions carried out, capabilities operationalized. We should not treat aspects of flourishing—like being happy; feeling a sense of accomplishment; being treated with dignity and civility; having the joy of listening to birdsong, gardening, or crafting something with your hands—as if they were abstract mental or emotional events cut off from patterns of relational activity.[21] Human flourishing is located at specific times and in specific places—culturally embedded in practices of human agency and naturally embodied in symbiotic selves.

In other words, flourishing is not a lading list of things doable or done; it is a pattern of life that is social and relational, both internally (the inner dialogue of thought) and externally (in social dialogue with other persons and interaction with the material world). Further in the chapter I point to the so-called capability theory of social justice and human flourishing developed by Martha C. Nussbaum and others as the most promising starting point for reflecting on the human good in connection with biotechnology. But, in my view, its formulation tends to be too oriented around discrete functions, as though the person who flourishes is putting his or her life together from a menu of component parts.[22] I realize that this is a strategy that some thinkers have used to make their account of the human good more compatible with the individualism of the liberal tradition. Nonetheless, I think that the holistic character of living well requires more emphasis, and I argue that such an emphasis is compatible with the tradition of humanistic social and ethical thought. By consistently interpreting capabilities (or "functionings") as the exercise of agency within relational contexts, we can push the tradition of liberal humanism forward to a new ecological humanism.

As I see it, the philosophy behind the current molecular sciences and technologies and the biopolitical governance of life impedes the ecological turn and relational agency–centered perspective due to its impulse toward objectification, simplification, and reductionism. Biotechnology rejects ontological unity in favor of an abstract and universal view of separate and interchangeable units (isolated sequences of DNA as "legos," "biobricks," and the like). It seeks the refabrication of life functions by breaking down complex living networks into component parts or fragments and then reassembling them to perform new molecular functions and to support new observable traits. This mechanistic worldview is able to articulate the value of flourishing only in instrumental terms. And its instrumental values are essentially hedonistic because it whittles the notion of inherent goodness down to felt benefit. By contrast, capabilities and agencies within patterns of just recognition of membership and just relations of care offer a basis for the intrinsic value of flourishing. This has ethical consequences that are rights and duty based and that countenance a notion of living well as a dynamic narrative of self-development rather than as a calculus of felt benefit and satisfaction.

Subjects are persons to be respected and allowed to flourish via lives lived in their own way and enabled by communal support. Subjects alone enjoy moral considerability, moral standing, or moral recognition. (But moral standing as subjects need not be restricted exclusively to human beings.) Objects are things to be understood as lacking in interiority; they respond exclusively to external forces of causal determinism or probability. The mode of being of objects invites extrinsic manipulation and control: The mode of being of subjects permits self-rule and self-control, and their mode of becoming (self-development) requires the space for this.

The subject is an active being, one whose well-being comprises not only external material conditions or circumstances, but also an inner capacity for freedom, self-direction, and self-actualization. Agency is both *intentional* (directed toward some object or goal) and *evaluative* (motivated and restrained by senses of right, wrong, virtue, and appropriateness). The intentional face of agency seeks to alter the world to meet some need, fulfill some desire, or produce something useful. The evaluative face of agency expresses the person or character of the agent: it presents the self in light of values that are shared with others. In human life, being a subject and an agent has distinctive expression. By dint of the human capacity for highly complex symbolic language, and consequently also for historical memory and imagination, human agency not only conforms to social values, but also can interpret them afresh and reenact them anew.

Thus, the exercise of evaluative agency can only be undertaken in conditions of freedom, autonomy, and reflective awareness. Then the agent can be meaningfully said to be the author of the act, rather than merely being the medium of the causal forces at work bringing the act about. Factors that prevent such freedom negate agency. Intentional agency—acts that aim to bring about consequences—need not be conceptualized outside a causal nexus linking the agent's mind with the world. But evaluative agency—acts that express a judgment about the worth of an action and the character of the agent—calls for explication in terms of reasons and values rather than explanation in terms of causes. We have difficulty grasping the evaluative face of human agency when we think of actions as causing external things to happen in the material world, and when we think of actions, in turn, as being caused by the prior thoughts or feelings in the mind, or neurochemical activity in the brain, of the agent. However, for humans doing or not doing something is more than simply triggering a causal chain; it is sending a signal to others and embracing a meaning in one's own eyes. That is to say, it is dialogic and relational.[23]

Again, to be a full-fledged person in the worldview of communicative communities is to be a moral subject and to have a broad scope of voluntary activity and choice. It is to be free from domination by other individuals, from institutionalized forms of social power, and from cultural structures of stigma,

disgust, or transgression. Autonomous agency, properly understood as the absence of domination and the presence of support, is not a possible achievement
for an individual isolated from culture and society. It both depends on and is
actualized by a surrounding ecology of relational respect and recognition, membership, and supportive institutional and cultural structures.[24]

Philosophies of the human good are legion. In contemporary scholarship
they have been criticized roundly as metaphysically essentialist, ideologically
totalizing, and historically prone to reinforce cultural and ethnic hegemony and
domination. However, there is an approach to the analysis of varieties of living
well and flourishing that I believe avoids these pitfalls. One of the most promising accounts of human flourishing is the so-called capability theory of freedom
and justice.[25] In this theory, flourishing refers to what individuals or societies
experience when both institutional structures and cultural frameworks of
meaning permit the actualization of a wide range of those constructive and just
capabilities potentially inherent in all human beings. Flourishing occurs when
capabilities for self-direction, creativity, intelligence, understanding, emotional
development, and other positive human potentialities take shape in the lives of
individuals and societies.[26]

The idea of flourishing is not perfectionist, but it is holistic and relational. It
need not deny evil or sanction unjust relationships or activity. Flourishing is
not essentialist; but it is developmental. It is not defined as coming into alignment with a timeless pattern of being that we have either lost or not yet attained.
Flourishing is a normative, value-laden notion of developmental human self-
realization, and it is pluralistic in its affirmation of the realization of human
possibility in its multiple varieties and forms. It recognizes that physical and
mental health facilitate the actualization of many potential capabilities in actual
lives of freedom and well-being, but it does not valorize the "normal" or species-
typical functioning as such, it need not hold that all potential capabilities must be
actualized for a specific person to live well, and thus, while not recommending
physical or cognitive impairment, it does not stigmatize it, either. A philosophy
of human flourishing can and should hold that self-realization and development
are possible within broad parameters of biological function and a wide range
of accomplishment. This renders problematic any notion of human enhancement that seeks to facilitate convergence on a homogeneous pattern of capability
or value.

Finally, on the capability view, flourishing is not individualistically achievable,
let alone genetically determined. Flourishing is a dialectic between nature and
culture, the molecular and the molar. It represents the connection between the
realization of generic human capabilities and agency, on the one hand, and background social structures that provide (or close off) opportunities for agency, on
the other hand. The constitutive condition of human flourishing is a symbiosis

between individual and society so that potential capabilities of individual persons are actualized as socially enacted performances or functionings.

Relationality per se cannot be left as a placeholder or a value-neutral element in a theory of human flourishing. The substantive normative content of relationality is crucial. Right or just relationality has many components, but as noted earlier, I regard the notions of "membership recognition" and "attentive mutuality" as particularly important. Recognition, membership, attentiveness, and mutuality are just when they are institutionalized as practices of free and equal self-realization; equal moral considerability; parity of voice, power, and wealth; civic respect; and dignity. Such practices convey ethical standing, belonging, and concern. I do not intend these categories to refer to the dispositions or virtues of individual agents. Nor do these categories simply describe discrete acts. I understand recognition and mutuality to provide criteria for assessing the legitimacy of background structures of opportunity and institutionalized power.

The Relational Interpretation of Flourishing: Membership and Mutuality

Just recognition of membership involves the acknowledgment of interdependence among all human and nonhuman beings when it comes to the flourishing of each form of life relative to its repertoire of capabilities, development, and behavior. It also involves the affirmation of the moral standing of others who contribute to and are active, symbiotic citizens of a commonwealth of shared life.

Again, a bit more fully, one can say that membership is a status that confers access to certain modes of relationality: namely, equal dignity, concern, and respect. It carries with it correlative obligations of reciprocity and consideration. The recognition of membership reflects and echoes across each person in the community. Membership status requires that one be granted equity, parity of participation, engagement, and the exercise of free agency within the web of institutionalized relational rules and roles that make up the basic structure of a society. The denial of parity in relational participation—disenfranchisement, exclusion, marginalization—is at one and the same time an exclusion from membership and an imposition of domination on a person.

For its part, just mutuality involves actually lived and enacted practices of attentive care and concern. These norms reinforce the capability theory of human flourishing and give it more concrete ethical shape, while still reinforcing its pluralism and the strong value it places on individual personhood, self-direction, and agency. Indeed, the mutuality of attentive care and concern are keystones of human flourishing and living a life fully realized and deeply experienced.

Membership and mutuality are closely linked, and their common ethical ground is the valuing of others by the self (respect) and the valuing of the self by others (social esteem). To be in a condition of membership and mutuality is to be interdependently self-aware. Membership is conferred but it is also lived, earned, constructed, and reconstructed by actions and transactions over time. Mutuality involves the realization of an imaginative capability to see the linkages between the condition of others and the condition of the self and to act on the basis of those linkages.

Membership confers standing; mutuality enables standing together. The site within human flourishing where both membership in a moral community and mutuality of concern and respect converge is solidarity.[27] Solidarity has a developmental trajectory of membership recognition and mutuality of care and concern. It involves the reflective encounter of personal horizons, the imaginative meeting of minds, the ability to discover others' humanity in the mirror of one's own self-understanding and to perceive one's humanity in the self-understanding of others. Although never fully achieved in practice, the perspective of ecological humanism is committed to the notion that moral awareness and sensibility are potential capabilities of most human beings, and their achievement as realized functions or agencies is a linchpin of human flourishing.

Conclusion

Will the legitimation of biopower, and the use of biotechnology to alter the human body, erode the concepts of personhood and agency? These concepts were forged in the development of humanist traditions, both religious and secular, and in the democratic and human rights revolutions that grew out of them. These concepts, and the understanding of human flourishing built around them, warn us against totalizing and objectifying ideas of any kind, including those, such as biopower, that travel under the banners of technological progress and liberation from a host of maladies.

Global biopower, biopolitics, and bioeconomics may carry on the modern historical narrative of human betterment through scientific and technological progress—better living through chemistry, as one might say. But biotechnological progress should not march alone; it should be placed in the context of other values and facets of the human good.

If nature as a standard by which to guide human agency and the use of technology won't hold still, as Gregory Kaebnick keenly observes in Chapter 6 of this volume, while nature as a standard of duty, restraint, and appropriate agency is fading from view, what can bring biopower under prudent and humble precautionary governance and responsible use? Can biopower be constrained by bioethics? If so, where will we find the vocabulary with which to argue the case for a bioethics of technological humility and restraint? Can such a bioethics emerge from the intellectual traditions, frameworks of moral imagination, and forms of practical activity of an ecological humanism? I think it can.

Notes

1. William E. Connolly, *Facing the Planetary: Entangled Humanism and the Politics of Swarming* (Durham, NC: Duke University Press, 2017), 119, 168.
2. William J. Perry, *My Journey at the Nuclear Brink* (Stanford, CA: Stanford University Press, 2015).
3. Ben Minteer, "Is It Right to Reverse Extinction?" *Nature*, 509 (May 15, 2014): 261.
4. On these points, see Langdon Winner, *Autonomous Technology* (Cambridge, MA: MIT Press, 1977).
5. Paul Rabinow and Nikolas Rose, "Biopower Today," *BioSocieties* 1, no. 2 (2006): 195–217.
6. Michel Foucault, *Society Must Be Defended: Lectures at the Collège de France, 1975–76* (New York: Picador, 2003).
7. This mode of inquiry remains relatively neglected and underdeveloped in bioethics. A pioneering exception to which I am indebted is Erik Parens, *Shaping Ourselves: On Technology, Flourishing, and a Habit of Thinking* (New York: Oxford University Press, 2015).
8. See Craig Calhoun, "Imagining Solidarity: Cosmopolitanism, Constitutional Patriotism, and the Public Sphere," *Public Culture* 14, no. 1 (2002): 152:

   > World-making is a way of approaching culture that emphasizes agency and history in the constitution of the languages and understandings by which populaces give shape to social life. To speak of the social imaginary is to assert that there are no fixed categories of external observation adequate to all history; that ways of thinking and structures of feeling make possible certain social forms, and that such forms are thus products of action and historically variable.

9. Bruce Jennings, "Biotechnology as Cultural Meaning: Reflections on the Moral Reception of Synthetic Biology," in *Synthetic Biology and Morality: Artificial Life and the Bounds of Nature*, ed. Gregory Kaebnick and Thomas H. Murray (Cambridge, MA: MIT Press, 2013), 149–176.
10. Quoted in Sopia Roosth, "Screaming Yeast: Sonocytology, Cytoplasmic Milieus, and Cellular Subjectivities," *Critical Inquiry* 35, no. 2 (2009): 332n2.
11. See Connolly, *Facing the Planetary*; Paisley Livingston, *Literary Knowledge: Humanistic Inquiry and the Philosophy of Science* (Ithaca, NY: Cornell University Press, 1988); Karen Barad, *Meeting the Universe Halfway: Quantum Physics and the Entanglement of Matter and Meaning* (Durham, NC: Duke University Press, 2007); and Sandra D. Mitchell, *Unsimple Truths: Science, Complexity, and Policy* (Chicago: University of Chicago Press, 2009). Mitchell's discussion is particularly pertinent for

our discussion. She argues that the mechanistic worldview has been unduly influential in the philosophy of science because philosophers have focused on theoretical physics rather than biology. Indeed, if one takes the biological sciences seriously one is led toward a more interpretive form of knowledge than a reductionistic and mechanistic one:

> The old Newtonian aspirations of reduction to the simple, most basic properties and most basic motions has been replaced by a world of multilevel causal interactions and emergence. A world of only necessary truths cannot engage productively with the degrees of contingent causation that characterize historically evolved natural systems. The universal has given way to the contextual and local, and a search for the one, singular, absolute truth must be replaced by humble respect for the plurality of truths that partially and pragmatically represent the world. . . . To begin to understand our complex world, I have argued that we need to expand our conceptual frameworks to accommodate emergence, contingency, dynamic robustness, and deep uncertainty. Our conception of the nature of nature must shift away from the expectation of always finding regularities and causal powers that are universal, deterministic, and predictable. The truths that attach to our world are rarely simple, global, and necessary. Rather, nature organizes itself in a plurality of ways, and what we validate as "knowledge" should reflect that diversity. (*Unsimple Truths*, 118, 105–106)

12. Nikolas Rose, *The Politics of Life Itself: Biomedicine, Power, and Subjectivity in the Twenty-first Century* (Princeton, NJ: Princeton University Press, 2006), 4, 15.

13. See the discussion of the "root metaphors" of mechanism, contextualism, and organicism in Stephen C. Pepper, *World Hypotheses: A Study in Evidence* (Berkeley: University of California Press, 1942), 186–314.

14. See Charles Taylor, *Hegel and Modern Society* (Cambridge: Cambridge University Press, 1979) and Richard J. Bernstein, *Beyond Objectivism and Relativism: Science, Hermeneutics, and Praxis* (Philadelphia: University of Pennsylvania Press, 1983). Taylor referred to this as "expressivism," while Bernstein discussed it as "relativism." For our purposes here the nuances of these constructs are less important than the way they deploy the fundamental distinction between subjectification and agency or objectification and determinism.

The gist of these contrasting perspectives has been succinctly characterized in the following ways: Bernstein contrasted "objectivism" with "relativism" as follows:

> By "objectivism" I mean the basic conviction that there is or must be some permanent, ahistorical matrix or framework to which we can ultimately appeal in determining the nature of rationality, knowledge, truth, reality, goodness, or rightness. . . . Relativism is the basic conviction that . . . all such concepts must be understood as relative to a specific conceptual scheme, theoretical framework, paradigm, form of life, society, or culture. (*Beyond Objectivism and Relativism*, 8)

Taylor compared the mechanistic view of the Enlightenment with a holistic view he called "expressivism":

The mainstream Enlightenment . . . was a philosophy which was utilitarian in its ethical outlook, atomistic in its social philosophy, analytic in its science of man, and which looked to a scientific social engineering to reorganize man and society and bring men happiness through perfect mutual adjustment.

In the perspective of expressivism, however,

Human life was seen as having a unity . . . where every part or aspect only found its proper meaning in relation to all the others. . . . To see a human being as in some compounded of different elements: faculties of reason and sensibility, or soul and body, or reason and feeling was to lose sight of the living, expressive unity. (Taylor, *Hegel and Modern Society*, 1–2)

15. See Allen W. Wood, *The Free Development of Each: Studies on Freedom, Right, and Ethics in Classical German Philosophy* (New York: Oxford University Press, 2014).

16. Taylor, *Hegel and Modern Society*, 17.

17. Taylor, *Hegel and Modern Society*, 19.

18. Hubert Dreyfus and Charles Taylor, *Retrieving Realism* (Cambridge, MA: Harvard University Press, 2015), 138. Erik Parens expressed a similar point when he said, "Learning to let some things be may be one of the hardest problems to which we need to apply our ability to think creatively. . . . If we in the United States suffer from a status quo bias, it may be a bias toward the notion that the more we creatively transform ourselves and the world the better. For all that is marvelous in our ability to do just that, we have to get better at grappling with the ways in which such transformation cannot alone make us happier" (*Shaping Ourselves*, 173–174).

19. The Aristotelian tradition has persisted in humanistic thought, and neo-Aristotelian themes are also a part of contemporary work on the philosophy of technology and environmental ethics. Consider, for instance, the following formulation of intrinsic value by the philosopher of technology Keekok Lee:

Human beings are intrinsically valuable "in themselves" in virtue of the unique type of consciousness they possess. Biotic beings are intrinsically valuable "for themselves" in virtue of the fact that they strive to maintain their own function integrity. But biotic and abiotic beings and the natural processes underpinning them are valuable "by themselves" in virtue of the fact that they have come into existence and will continue to exist independent of humankind. They had existed and will exist in a world without humankind. [Keekok Lee, *The Natural and the Artefactual: The Implications of Deep Science and Deep Technology for Environmental Philosophy* (Lanham, MD: Lexington Books, 1999), 9]

20. In her explication of the capability approach to human flourishing, Nussbaum expressed the point this way: "The Capabilities Approach departs from a tradition in economics that measures the real value of a set of options by the best use that can be made of them. Options are freedoms, and freedom has intrinsic value. Some political views deny this: they hold that the right thing for government to do is to make people lead healthy lives, do worthwhile activities, exercise religion, and so on. We deny this: we say that capabilities, not functionings, are the appropriate political goals because room is thereby left for the exercise of human freedom" (Martha C. Nussbaum,

Creating Capabilities: The Human Development Approach (Cambridge, MA: Harvard University Press, 2011), 25–26).

21. For a wonderful account of a human experience of materiality, see George Sturt, *The Wheelwright's Shop*, passages selected and edited by A. F. Collins (1930; repr. Redditch, England: Read Books, 2013).

22. Nussbaum's list of basic human capabilities comprises the following domains: life and awareness; bodily health and integrity; imagination and intellect; emotional attachments; critical reflection on one's own life-plan; forming relationships, having social supports for self-esteem and respect; being concerned for the non-human (animals and nature); being able to play; having some measure of control over one's political and material environment. See Martha C. Nussbaum, *Creating Capabilities*, 33–34.

23. Moreover, an important element in the tradition of liberal humanism is the view that the individual human being has inherent, although not exclusive, ethical value and worth. As noted previously, inherent or intrinsic value means value as such, in and of itself, not simply the instrumental value that comes from the benefit or worth the individual may have to others. Such inherent value calls forth care and concern for the individual's health, happiness, and well-being. It also calls forth respect and recognition of the individual's equal status as a member of the moral community—be they concurrent local communities of concrete mutuality or imagined aspirational communities of a more flourishing mutuality that may prevail in the future. Two clarifications are important here. First, in addition to the belief in the moral worth or value of the human being, humanism has often held a separate belief in the ontological moral superiority of humankind. I am not avowing that doctrine here. Second, the assertion of the moral value of the individual human being need not deny the significant ways in which each individual is born into, develops within, and interacts within a set of social relationships. The moral worth of the individual does not depend on the social isolation of the individual. The value of autonomy does not entail the value of isolation or even the possibility of a nonrelational condition of life. When autonomy is understood as negative liberty—noninterference—it may seem to be linked to this kind of ontological individualism, but when autonomy is understood as a condition of nondomination, it can readily be understood as a condition of relationality, a social and cultural condition—an unfortunately rare and historically unusual social and cultural condition, to be sure, but a social and cultural condition nonetheless.

24. In the liberal humanist tradition there have often been exaggerated and unrealistic conceptions of independence, self-sufficiency, and isolation. However, this negative individualism is not a necessary logical corollary of the notion of autonomous agency, which is more adequately understood in social and relational terms. See Bruce Jennings, "Reconceptualizing Autonomy: The Relational Turn in Bioethics," *Hastings Center Report* 46, no. 3 (May/June 2016): 11–16.

25. In addition to Nussbaum, *Creating Capabilities*, see Martha C. Nussbaum and Amartya Sen, eds., *The Quality of Life* (Oxford: Oxford University Press, 1993). See also Jennifer Prah Ruger, *Health and Social Justice* (New York: Oxford University

Press, 2010) and Sridhar Venkatapuram, *Health Justice: An Argument from the Capabilities Approach* (Cambridge, England: Polity Press, 2011).

26. In Nussbaum's work the relationship between capabilities and functionings is theoretically complex. Characterizing capabilities as inherent potential that may or may not be actualized can be misunderstood. This formulation is not genetically reductionistic or deterministic, as she makes clear: "We now know that the development of basic capabilities is not hard-wired in the DNA: maternal nutrition and prenatal experience play a role in their unfolding and shaping. In that sense, even after a child is born, we are always dealing with very early internal capabilities, already environmentally conditions, not with a pure potential. Nonetheless, the category is a useful one, so long as we do not misunderstand it. Basic capabilities are the innate faculties of the person that make later development and training possible" (*Creating Capabilities*, 23–24).

27. See Bruce Jennings and Angus Dawson, "Solidarity in the Moral Imagination of Bioethics," *Hastings Center Report* 45, no. 5 (September–October 2015): 31–38; and Bruce Jennings, "Solidarity and Care as Relational Practices," *Bioethics* 32 (2018): 553–561.

Index